D1168495

Kidney and Urinary Tract
DISEASES AND DISORDERS
SOURCEBOOK

Health Reference Series

Volume Twenty-one

Kidney and Urinary Tract

DISEASES AND DISORDERS

SOURCEBOOK

RC
900
. K53
1997

Basic Information about Kidney Stones, Urinary Incontinence, Bladder Disease, End Stage Renal Disease, Dialysis, and More, Along with Statistical and Demographic Data and Reports on Current Research Initiatives

Edited by
Linda M. Ross

Omnigraphics, Inc.

Penobscot Building / Detroit, MI 48226

BIBLIOGRAPHIC NOTE

This volume contains documents from the following government agencies: the Agency for Health Care Policy and Research (AHCPR), Department of Health and Human Services (DHHS), the National Cancer Institute (NCI), the National Institute on Aging (NIA), National Institutes of Health (NIH), and the National Kidney and Urologic Disease Information Clearinghouse (NKUDIC). In addition, information from the NCI's CancerNet online service and articles *FDA Consumer*, *NIH Record*, and *NIH Consensus Statements* are included.

This volume also contains copyrighted information from the following sources: the American Kidney Fund, the American Society of Nephrology, *Cancer*, Dowden Publishing Company, the *Journal of Obstetrics, Gynecology and Neonatal Nursing*, the National Kidney Cancer Association, the National Kidney Foundation, the Polycystic Kidney Research Foundation, Medical Economics (*Contemporary Urology* and *Patient Care*), Springhouse Corporation, VHL Family Alliance, and William Morrow Company. Information from OncoLink, the University of Pennsylvania's online cancer information service is also contained in this volume. Full citation information is located on the first page of each article. Copyrighted material is used with permission. Every effort has been made to secure all necessary rights to reprint the copyrighted material. If any omissions have been made, contact Omnigraphics to make corrections for future editions.

Edited by
Linda M. Ross

Peter D. Dresser, Managing Editor, *Health Reference Series*
Karen Bellenir, Series Editor, *Health Reference Series*

Omnigraphics, Inc.
Matthew P. Barbour, Production Manager
Laurie Lanzen Harris, Vice President, Editorial
Peter E. Ruffner, Vice President, Administration
James A. Sellgren, Vice President, Operations and Finance
Jane Steele, Marketing Consultant

Frederick G. Ruffner, Jr., Publisher
Copyright ©1997, Omnigraphics, Inc.

Library of Congress Cataloging-in-Publication Data

Kidney and urinary tract diseases and disorders sourcebook: basic information about kidney stones, urinary incontinence, bladder disease, end stage renal disease, dialysis, and more, along with statistical and demographic data and reports on current research initiatives/edited by Linda M. Ross.
    p.   cm. — (Health reference series; v.21)
    Includes bibliographical references and index.
    ISBN 0-7808-0079-6 (lib.bdg.: alk.paper)
    1. Urinary organs — Diseases.   2. Kidneys —Diseases.
    I. Ross, Linda M. (Linda Michelle) II. Series.
RC900.K53 1997
616.6 — dc21
                                        97-16533
                                        CIP

∞

This book is printed on acid-free paper meeting the ANSI Z39.48 Standard. The infinity symbol that appears above indicates that the paper in this book meets that standard.

Printed in the United States.

CAK4131

Contents

Part III—Kidney Disorders in Children

Part IV—Understanding Adult Kidney Disorders

Part V—Cancer of the Kidney

Part VI—End-Stage Renal Disease, Dialysis, and Amyloidosis

Part VII—General Information on Urinary Tract Disorders

Part VIII—Children and Urinary Tract Disorders

Part IX—Understanding Adult Urinary Tract Disorders

Part X—Cancer of the Urinary Tract

Preface

About This Book

According to the National Kidney Foundation, kidney and urinary tract diseases and disorders affect more than 20 million Americans. This volume provides essential information for those who suffer from these problems and for concerned friends and family members. It contains numerous publications from government and private agencies including the National Institutes of Health (NIH), the National Kidney and Urologic Diseases Information Clearinghouse (NKUDIC), the National Cancer Institute (NCI), the Department of Health and Human Services (DHHS), the National Kidney Cancer Association, the National Kidney Cancer Foundation, *Professional Guide to Diseases*, *Physician's Guide to Rare Diseases*, *Contemporary Urology*, *Patient Care*, the Polycystic Kidney Research Foundation, Dowden Publishing, *Journal of Obstetrics and Neonatal Nursing* (JOGGN), the American Kidney Fund, VHL Family Alliance, and online services including OncoLink from the University of Pennsylvania and CancerNet from the National Cancer Institute.

How to Use This Book

This book is divided into 10 parts to provide easy access to specific kidney and urinary tract problems.

Part I: *General Information on Kidney Disease Resources* provides general information on and contacts for organizations that support patients with kidney disease. In addition, the Glossary of Terms gives clear, concise definitions of terms associated with kidney disease.

Part II: *Introduction to the Kidneys* explains normal kidney function and the complications that result from a nonfunctioning organ. Also included in this section is information about kidney disease among African Americans, a population in which the incidence of various kidney diseases is disproportionately high.

Part III: *Kidney Disorders in Children* discusses the diagnosis, treatment, and follow up care for those with Wilms' Tumor (a form of kidney cancer that most often appears in children) and Childhood Nephrotic Syndrome.

Part IV: *Understanding Adult Kidney Disorders* describes the symptoms, diagnosis and treatment options available to those with common and rare kidney problems. This section also contains numerous citations of additional information sources for the patient and concerned support people.

Part V: *Cancer of the Kidney* contains the most recent information about the diagnosis and treatment of kidney cancer. Since the field of cancer research is ongoing and dynamic, the online service for kidney cancer patients will be especially helpful in obtaining up-to-the-minute material of concern to these individuals and their families.

Part VI: *End-Stage Renal Disease, Dialysis, and Amyloidosis* presents invaluable material on the differences between the various treatments of End-Stage Renal Disease (ESRD), the nutritional needs of ESRD patients, and related health concerns such as the risk of AIDS and amyloidosis in dialysis patients.

Part VII: *General Information on Urinary Tract Disorders* gives basic facts about urologic diseases and disorders, including when to be concerned about blood in the urine, and explains what information can be obtained from a urinalysis.

Part VIII: *Children and Urinary Tract Disorders* addresses such common but perplexing problems as bedwetting, frequent urination, and urinary reflux in children. Strategies for aiding children with these disorders and additional resources for help and support are also included.

Part IX: *Understanding Adult Urinary Tract Disorders* supplies indepth information about incontinence, interstitial cystitis, and urinary tract infections. Though these problems are common, they are often difficult to discuss with family members and medical professionals. The resources in this section allow the patient and concerned loved ones to gain basic information about the causes and treatment of these problems and can provide a basis of discussion with a health professional. Additional resources for further information and support are offered as well.

Part X: *Cancer of the Urinary Tract* delineates diagnosis, treatment, and coping strategies for those faced with cancer of the bladder and urethra.

Acknowledgements

The editor wishes to thank everyone at Omnigraphics for their flexibility and professional support, Margaret Mary Missar for the unflagging research efforts that made this volume possible, Sarah Schneider for looking after lots of the details and surfing the 'Net for the most up-to-date information, Karen Edwards for her delicate balance of creativity and practicality, Karen Bellenir for direction and practical insight, Bruce Bellenir for scanning scores of pamphlets, and Peter Dresser for his leadership and patience.

Note from the Editor

This book is part of the Omnigraphics' *Health Reference Series*. The series provides basic information about a broad range of medical concerns. It is not intended to serve as a tool for diagnosing illness, in prescribing treatments, or as a substitute for the physician/patient relationship. All persons concerned about medical symptoms or the possibility of disease are encouraged to seek professional care from an appropriate health care provider.

Part One

General Information on Kidney and Urologic Disease Resources

Chapter 1

Facts from the National Kidney and Urologic Disease Information Clearinghouse

What Are Kidney and Urologic Diseases?

The kidneys and urinary tract form the organ system primarily responsible for cleaning and filtering excess fluid and waste material from the blood. The kidneys also function as glands that produce hormones necessary for building red blood cells and regulating blood pressure.

Kidney and urologic diseases affect more than 13 million people, or about 5 percent of the United States population, and claim about 260,000 lives annually. The number of people affected by these diseases is expected to grow as the populations of older adults and racial and ethnic minorities, groups disproportionately affected by the diseases, increase. Kidney and urologic diseases impose a large social and economic burden on the population costing the Nation an estimated $50 billion annually.

The most serious and debilitating of these diseases include end-stage renal disease (ESRD), urinary stone disease, urinary incontinence, benign prostatic hyperplasia (BPH), interstitial cystitis, urinary tract infection, and polycystic kidney disease. In addition, other seemingly unrelated diseases have a tremendous impact on the disability and death associated with kidney and urologic diseases. For instance, diabetes can, over time, damage many parts of the body including the kidneys. Additionally, 30 percent of ESRD cases are

Unnumbered pamphlet from the National Kidney and Urologic Disease Information Clearinghouse (NKUDIC), a division of the NIH.

attributed to hypertension. Among black Americans, these percentages double. Experts estimate that 60 percent of black Americans on dialysis have ESRD because of hypertension, a potentially avoidable outcome.

What is the National Kidney and Urologic Diseases Information Clearinghouse?

The National Kidney and Urologic Diseases Information Clearinghouse (NKUDIC) is an information and referral service of the National Institute of Diabetes and Digestive and Kidney Diseases (NIDDK), National Institutes of Health. The clearinghouse, authorized by Congress in 1987, is designed to increase the knowledge and understanding about kidney and urologic diseases and health among patients and their families, health care professionals, and the general public. To accomplish this mission, NKUDIC works closely with professional, patient, and voluntary associations; Government agencies; and other kidney and urologic diseases organizations forming a unique network that identifies and responds to information needs about these diseases.

How Can the Clearinghouse Help You?

The NKUDIC provides the following products and services:

- Information about kidney and urologic diseases—from patient and professional educational materials to reprints of selected journal articles.

- Publications developed by NKUDIC and NIDDK about specific kidney and urologic diseases.

- Literature searches about kidney and urologic diseases from the Combined Health Information Database (CHID). The CHID is a database of references to thousands of materials produced for patients and health care professionals. CHID searches identify fact sheets, brochures, books, articles, audiovisual materials, and other educational materials and include information about how to obtain the item.

- *KU Notes*, the NKUDIC newsletter that features news about kidney and urologic diseases research, special events, professional and patient organizations, and publications available from NKUDIC and other organizations.

How Can You Help Us?

The NKUDIC's key sources of information are the individuals and organizations involved in providing informational and educational services related to kidney and urologic diseases. By informing the clearinghouse of your materials and programs, you expand the information base of products and services available through NKUDIC. Please inform the clearinghouse about your resources and needs and add us to your mailing list.

National Kidney and Urologic Diseases
Information Clearinghouse
Box NKUDIC
9000 Rockville Pike
Bethesda, MD 20892
(301) 654-4415

Chapter 2

Directory of Kidney and Urologic Diseases Organizations

This directory lists voluntary, governmental, and private organizations involved in kidney and urologic disease related activities. Some of the organizations offer educational materials and other services to patients and the public; others primarily serve health care professionals.

Alport Syndrome Study

410 Chipeta Way
Room 156
University of Utah Health Sciences Center
Salt Lake City, Utah 84108-1297
(801) 581-5479

Mission: To support research in the genetic basis of various forms of hereditary nephritis (Alport Syndrome) and the ongoing collection of clinical family histories and laboratory samples, which are maintained in a confidential genetic database.

American Association of Clinical Urologists

955 D North Plum Grove Road
Schaumburg, Illinois 60173
(708) 517-1050
FAX (708) 517-7229

Unnumbered document from the U.S. Department of Health and Human Services, July 1994.

Mission: To stimulate interest in the science and practice of urology and to promote understanding of socioeconomic and political affairs affecting medical practice among clinical urologists who are members of the American Urological Association and the American Medical Association.

Publications: AACU News (bimonthly) and AACU FAX (monthly legislative update FACSIMILE).

American Association of Genitourinary Surgeons

University of Virginia Hospital
Box 422
Charlottesville, Virginia 22908
(804) 924-2224

Mission: Professional society of urologists elected into membership due to their outstanding contributions to urology.

American Association of Kidney Patients

100 South Ashley Drive, Suite 280
Tampa, Florida 33602
(800) 749-2257 or (813) 223-7099
FAX (813) 223-0001

Mission: To serve the needs and interests of kidney patients and their families. Founded by kidney patients to help others with kidney failure cope with its physical and emotional impact on their lives.

Publications: Renalife (semi-annual journal) and The AAKP Bulletin (quarterly newsletter).

American Board of Urology

31700 Telegraph Road, Suite 150
Bingham Farms, Michigan 48025
(810) 646-9720

Mission: To identify for the public's knowledge those physicians who have satisfied the Board's criteria for certification and recertification in the speciality of urology.

American Foundation for Urologic Disease, Inc.

300 West Pratt Street, Suite 401
Baltimore, Maryland 21201
(800) 242-2383 or (410) 727-2908

Mission: To provide research grants, patient and public education, government relations, and patient support group activities.

Publications: Informational brochure about AFUD, Foundation Focus (quarterly newsletter), and patient education brochures.

Councils: Prostate Health Council, Bladder Health Council, Pediatric Council.

American Kidney Fund

6110 Executive Boulevard, Suite 1010
Rockville, Maryland 20852
(800) 638-8299 or (301) 881-3052

Mission: To provide direct financial assistance, comprehensive educational programs, research grants, and community service projects for the benefit of kidney patients.

Publications: AKF Nephrology Letter, AKF Torchbearer, AKF Newsletter for Health Professionals, and patient and public education brochures.

American Lithotripsy Society

13 Elm Street
Manchester, Massachusetts 01944
(508) 526-8330

Mission: Professional membership society dedicated to addressing all aspects of lithotripsy as a medical treatment for both renal stones and biliary disease.

Publication: ALS Quarterly News.

American Nephrology Nurses' Association

East Holly Avenue
Box 56
Pitman, New Jersey 08071-0056
(609) 256-2320
FAX (609) 589-7463

Mission: To protect the future of quality renal care through continuing education, research, standards of clinical practice, quality assurance activities, certification, and interdisciplinary communication and cooperation.

Publications: ANNA Journal, ANNA Update (bi-monthly newsletter), Core Curriculum for Nephrology Nursing, position statements, and clinical monographs.

American Prostate Association

P.O. Box 4206
Silver Spring, Maryland 20914
(301) 384-9405

Mission: To offer patient support, education, and research information about prostate disorders, including non-cancerous prostate enlargement, prostatitis, and prostate cancer.

American Prostate Society

1340 Charwood Road
Hanover, Maryland 21076
(410) 859-3735

Mission: To increase awareness about prostate diseases and establish centers for diagnosis and treatment.

Publications: What You Don't Know About Your Prostate Can Kill You (brochure), Medication Versus Surgery (brochure), and quarterly newsletter.

American Society for Artificial Internal Organs, Inc.

National Office
P.O. Box C
Boca Raton, Florida 33429-0468
(407) 391-8589

Mission: To promote the increase of knowledge about artificial internal organs and their utilization.

Publications: ASAIO Journal (quarterly peer-reviewed journal), ASAIO Abstracts (for annual meeting).

American Society of Histocompatibility and Immununogenetics

P.O. Box 15804
Lenexa, Kansas 66285-5804
(913) 541-0009

Mission: To provide investigators in the field with a mechanism for education and communication and to influence regulatory efforts, provide a forum for the exchange of research and clinical data, and offer technical workshops at an annual education meeting.

Publications: Topics in Clinical Histocompatibility Testing, Volumes 1-3; Cellular Immunology, 1983; Paternity Testing, Data Analysis and Management in the Immunogenetics Lab; Third American Histocompatibility Workshop Report of HLA-A,B,C; Serology (Phases I and II) and B-Cell Serology (Phase II); Clinical Histocompatibility Testing; Laboratory Procedures Manual; Human Immunology Journal; membership directory.

American Society of Nephrology

1101 Connecticut Avenue, NW
Suite 700
Washington, DC 20036
(202) 857-1190

Mission: To contribute to the education of member nephrologists and to improve the quality of patient care.

Publications: Journal of the American Society of Nephrology (JASN), Training Program Directory, and Highlights (member newsletter).

American Society of Pediatric Nephrology

Department of Pediatrics
Children's Hospital of Buffalo
219 Bryant Street
Buffalo, New York 14222
(716) 878-7300

Mission: To promote public and professional educational programs in pediatric nephrology.

American Society of Transplant Surgeons

c/o Wright Organization, Inc.
716 Lee Street
Des Plaines, Illinois 60016
(708) 824-5700
FAX (708) 824-0394

Mission: To promote and encourage education and research with respect to transplantation surgery through applying funds, gifts, bequests, and endowments. Offers accreditation of training programs for transplant surgeons.

American Uro-Gynecologic Society

401 N. Michigan Avenue
Chicago, Illinois 60611-4267
(312) 644-6610
FAX (312) 527-6640
Deene Alongi, Executive Director

Mission: To promote research and education in uro-gynecology and to improve care for women with lower urinary tract disorders.

Publication: Quarterly newsletter.

American Urological Association

1120 North Charles Street
Baltimore, Maryland 21201
(410) 727-1100

Mission: To encourage research, experiments, investigations, and analysis of conditions of the genitourinary tract and their treatments and corrections; to develop scientific methods for the diagnosis, prevention, and treatment of disorders of the genitourinary tract; to benefit the general public by encouraging the study of and maintaining the highest possible standards for urological education, practice, and research; and to promote the publication of and encourage contributions to medical and scientific literature pertaining to urology.

Publication: American Journal of Urology.

American Urological Association Allied, Inc.

11512 Allecingie Parkway
Richmond, Virginia 23235
(804) 379-5513

Mission: To unite urologic allied health professionals and promote the highest quality of urologic education and professional standards for the better and safer care of the urologic patient/client.

Publication: Program Newsletter, Urologic Nursing (official journal of AUAA), and Standards of Urologic Nursing Practice.

Continence Restored, Inc.

407 Strawberry Hill Avenue
Stanford, Connecticut 06902
(914) 285-1470 (daytime) or
(203) 348-0601 (evening)

Mission: To disseminate information about bladder control problems to all interested parties, to establish a network of continence support groups throughout the United States, to provide a resource for the public and professionals, and to work with manufacturers who produce incontinence products.

Endourology Society

c/o Department of Urology
Long Island Jewish Medical Center
270–05 76th Avenue
New Hyde Park, New York 11042
(718) 470-7221

Mission: To educate urologists about research and treatment in the management of endourological problems.

Publication: Journal of Endourology.

The Geddings Osbon, Sr., Foundation

P.O. Box 1593
Augusta, Georgia 30903
(800) 433-4215

Mission: To improve the quality of life for those suffering from sensitive medical disorders. Through the nonprofit organization's seminars and educational materials, patients and their partners learn about the treatment of impotence so they can make an informed choice.

Publication: Educational booklets and slide/video programs for consumers and medical professionals.

Help for Incontinent People, Inc.

Member Address:
P.O. Box 544
Union, South Carolina 29349
Business Address:
P.O. Box 8306
Spartanburg, South Carolina 29305
(800) BLADDER or (803) 579-7900
FAX (803) 579-7902

Mission: To improve the quality of life for people with incontinence. HIP is a leading source of education, advocacy, and support to the public and to the health profession about the causes, prevention, diagnosis, treatment, and management alternatives for incontinence.

Publication: The HIP Report.

Hereditary Nephritis Foundation

P.O. Box 57294
Murray, Utah 84107
(801) 581-7790

Mission: To promote research into the causes of and cures for hereditary nephritis and to provide up-to-date general information about Alport Syndrome and related conditions to patients, families, and physicians.

Publication: HNF Newsletter (semi-annual).

IgA Nephropathy Support Network

234 Summit Avenue
Jenkintown, Pennsylvania 19046
(215) 884-9038

Mission: To assist patients with IgA Nephropathy and their families. To serve as a clearinghouse for dissemination of information about IgA Nephropathy and to promote research for a possible cure.

Publications: Newsletter and pamphlets.

Impotence Institute of America

8201 Corporate Drive, Suite 320
Landover, Maryland 20785
(800) 669-1603 or (301) 577-0650

Mission: To inform and educate the public about impotence and its causes and treatments, and to maintain a referral list of urologists who will treat and diagnose impotence.

Publications: It's Not All In Your Head (book), Impotence Worldwide (newsletter), Impotence: Help and Hope (videotape).

International Pediatric Nephrology Association

Albert Einstein College of Medicine
1825 Eastchester Road
Bronx, New York 10461
(212) 904-2857

Mission: To promote public and professional education and symposia.

Publication: Pediatric Nephrology.

International Society of Nephrology

Department of Nephrology
University of Florida
P.O. Box 100224
Gainesville, Florida 32610-0231
(904) 392-4008

Mission: To educate nephrologists about research and patient care.

Publication: Kidney International.

International Society for Peritoneal Dialysis

c/o James F. Winchester, M.D.
Georgetown University School of Medicine
F–6003–PHC
3800 Reservoir Road, NW
Washington, DC 20007
(202) 784-3662

Mission: To advance knowledge of peritoneal dialysis.

Publication: Peritoneal Dialysis International.

International Transplant Nurses Society

Foster Plaza 5, Suite 300
651 Holiday Drive
Pittsburgh, Pennsylvania 15220
(513) 223-9765

Mission: Professional membership organization of transplant nurses dedicated to improving patient care through dissemination of information and symposia.

Publication: ITNS Newsletter.

Intersociety Council for Research for the Kidney and Urinary Tract

2020 Zonal Avenue
IDR-220
Los Angeles, California 90033
(213) 226-7591

Mission: To develop testimony about kidney and urologic diseases for Congress.

Interstitial Cystitis Association

P.O. Box 1553
Madison Square Station
New York, New York 10159
(800) ICA-1626 or (212) 979-6057
FAX (212) 979-6058

Mission: To assist patients with interstitial cystitis (IC), to educate the medical community about IC, to promote IC research.

Publications: ICA (brochure), ICA Update (quarterly newsletter), transcripts of annual meetings, and patient and professional education materials.

National Association of Nephrology

Technologists and Technicians
60 Revere Drive, Suite 500
Northbrook, Illinois 60062
(708) 480-7675

Mission: To emphasize and promote interaction between practitioners and industry, and to provide training and certification.

Publications: Bi-monthly newsletter, educational and technical manuals.

National Kidney Cancer Association

1234 Sherman Avenue, Suite 200
Evanston, Illinois 60202
(708) 332-1051
FAX (708) 328-4425

Mission: To provide information to patients and physicians; to sponsor research on kidney cancer; to act as an advocate on behalf of patients with the Federal government, insurance companies, and employers.

Publications: We Have Kidney Cancer (56-page booklet for patients), Kidney Cancer News (quarterly newsletter), and public policy papers. Chapters: New York, Los Angeles, Chicago.

Annual Convention: In July for both patients and physicians.

Other Services: Free information on kidney cancer and clinical trial information by E-mail: 708-332-1052.

National Kidney Foundation, Inc. (NKF)

30 East 33rd Street
New York, New York 10016
(800) 622-9010 or (212) 889-2210

Mission: To seek the total answer to diseases of the kidney and urinary tract through prevention, treatment, and cure; and to conduct programs in research, professional education, patient and community services, public education, and organ donation.

Publications: The Kidney, American Journal of Kidney Diseases, CNSW Perspectives, CRN Quarterly, CNNT Action Update, Family Focus (newsletter), and patient and public education materials.

Other Services: Council of Nephrology Nurses and Technicians (CNNT), Council of Nephrology Social Workers (CNSW), Council on Renal Nutrition (CRN), Council on Clinical Nephrology (CCN), Council on Dialysis and Transplantation (CDT), and Council on Urology.

National Kidney Patients Association

804 Second Street Pike
Southhampton, Pennsylvania 18966
(215) 953-8883

Mission: To help kidney patients obtain quality treatments, to increase patient awareness and rights, to obliterate the current practice of reusing medical disposables, and to urge strict government enforcement of manufacturers' labels.

National Organization for Rare Disorders (NORD)

P.O. Box 8923
New Fairfield, Connecticut 06812-1783
(800) 999-6673 or (203) 746-6518

Mission: To act as a clearinghouse for information about rare disorders and provide a network for mutual support to match families with similar disorders; to foster communication among rare disease voluntary agencies, government bodies, industry, scientific researchers, academic institutions, and concerned individuals; and to encourage and promote research and education about rare disorders and orphan drugs.

Publications: Fact sheets and reprints on rare disorders and Orphan Drug Update (newsletter).

North American Society for Dialysis and Transplantation

c/o Wadi N. Suki, M.D.
6550 Fannin, Suite 1273
Houston, Texas 77030

Mission: To disseminate current information about dialysis and transplantation, to provide an update for the status of the management of renal transplantation and its complications, and to provide an update on the mechanisms involved in the progression of renal disease.

North American Transplant Coordinators

P.O. Box 15384
Lenexa, Kansas 66285-5384
(913) 492-3600

Mission: To enhance the role of the transplant coordinator, and to provide training courses for professionals.

Publications: In Touch/Journal of Transplant Coordinator and patient care brochures.

Organ Transplant Fund

1027 South Yates Road
Memphis, Tennessee 38119
(800) 489-3863 or (901) 684-1697

Mission: To provide financial and support assistance to transplant patients and their families.

Oxalosis and Hyperoxaluria Foundation

P.O. Box 1632
Kent, Washington 98035
(800) 484-9698 ext. 5100 or (206) 631-0386

Mission: To inform the public, especially patients, parents, families, physicians, and medical professionals about hyperoxaluria and the related conditions, i.e., oxalosis and calcium-oxalate kidney stones; to provide a support network for those affected by hyperoxaluria, and to support and encourage research to find a cure for hyperoxaluria.

Polycystic Kidney Research Foundation

922 Walnut Street, Suite 411
Kansas City, Missouri 64106
(800) PKD-CURE or (816) 421-1869
FAX (816) 421-7208

Mission: To promote research in the cause and cure of polycystic kidney disease.

Publications: Polycystic Kidney Disease (patient manual); PKR Progress (quarterly newsletter); Fifth International Workshop Book; Autosomal Recessive PKD, Questions and Answers.

Psychonephrology Foundation

c/o New York Medical College
Psychiatric Institute
Valhalla, New York 10595
(914) 285-8424

Mission: To conduct conferences devoted to psychological issues surrounding patients with kidney failure.

Publications: Psychonephrology I: Psychological Factors in Hemodialysis and Transplantation, and Psychonephrology II: Psychological Problems in Kidney Failure and Their Treatment.

Renal Physicians Association

2011 Pennsylvania Avenue, NW, Suite 800
Washington, DC 20006-1808
(202) 835-0436
(202) 835-0436

Mission: To ensure optimal care under the highest standards of medical practice for patients with renal disease and related disorders, to act as a national representative for physicians engaged in the study and management of patients with renal disease and related disorders, and to serve as a major resource for the development of national health policy concerning renal disease.

Publication: RPA News, bi-monthly, available at no cost to members.

The Simon Foundation for Continence

P.O. Box 815
Wilmette, Illinois 60091
(800) 23-SIMON

Mission: To remove the stigma from incontinence and provide help to sufferers, their families, and the professional care giver.

Publications: Informer (quarterly newsletter), Managing Incontinence: A Guide to Living With the Loss of Bladder Control, and other educational materials.

Society of Government Service Urologists

P.O. Box 6810587
San Antonio, Texas 78280
(512) 681-0587

Mission: Professional membership organization of government service urologists.

Society for Pediatric Urology

c/o Dr. Richard M. Ehrlich
100 UCLA Medical Plaza
Los Angeles, California 90024
(310) 825-6865

Mission: To advance the knowledge of pediatric urology. Members have demonstrated interest and significant experience in pediatric urology.

Society of Urologic Oncology

Urology Department
Brigham and Women's Hospital
75 Francis Street
Boston, Massachusetts 02115
(617) 732-6325

Mission: Professional society for those with primary interest in the field of urologic oncology.

The Transplant Foundation

8002 Discovery Drive, Suite 310
Richmond, Virginia 23229
(804) 285-5115
FAX (804) 288-2408

Mission: To provide information and direct grants nationally to post-transplant recipients to offset the costs of immunosuppressive medications.

Transplant Society

c/o Felix Rapaport, M.D.
University Hospital
Department of Surgery, Health Science Center
T-19, Room 040
Stony Brook, New York 11794-8192

Mission: To further knowledge in transplantation biology and medicine.

Publication: Transplantation and Transplantation Proceedings.

United Network for Organ Sharing (UNOS)

1100 Boulders Parkway
Suite 500
P.O. Box 13770
Richmond, Virginia 23225
(800) 24-DONOR or (804) 330-8500

Mission: To administer the national organ procurement and transplantation network and the national organ transplantation scientific registry under contracts with the Health Resources and Services Administration, a division of the U.S. Department of Health and Human Services. UNOS' purpose is to promote, facilitate, and scientifically advance organ procurement and transplantation and to administer an equitable organ allocation for all the Nation. The UNOS Scientific Registry is a comprehensive organ transplantation data system enabling scientists and other interested individuals to access information for all liver, heart, heart-lung, pancreas, kidney, and small bowel donors and recipients in the United States since October 87.

Publications: UNOS Update, UNOS Communique, and educational materials.

United Ostomy Association

36 Executive Park, Suite 120
Irvine, California 92714
(800) 826-0826 or (714) 660-8624

Mission: To offer practical assistance and emotional support to ostomy patients through trained UOA members, and to produce and distribute materials about ostomy care and management.

Publications: Ostomy Quarterly, (magazine); and patient education materials.

Urodynamics Society

6431 Fannin
Suite 6018
Houston, Texas 77030
(713) 792-5640

Mission: To act for charitable, scientific, and educational purposes, particularly in the advancement and dissemination of scientific knowledge in the fields of urology and dynamics and bioengineering of the genitourinary system and the application of such knowledge in the diagnosis and treatment of urologic diseases.

Publications: Urology and Urodynamics.

National Kidney and Urologic Diseases Information Clearinghouse

Box NKUDIC
9000 Rockville Pike
Bethesda, Maryland 20892
(301) 654-4415

Mission: The National Kidney and Urologic Diseases Information Clearinghouse is a service of the National Institute of Diabetes and Digestive and Kidney Diseases, part of the National Institutes of Health, under the U.S. Public Health Service. The clearinghouse was authorized by Congress to focus a national effort on providing information about kidney and urologic diseases to the public, patients and their families, and doctors and other health care professionals. The clearinghouse works with organizations to educate people about kidney and urologic diseases; answers inquiries; develops, reviews, and distributes publications; and coordinates informational resources.

Chapter 3

Information about the National Kidney Foundation

Mission Statement

The ultimate goal and mission of the National Kidney Foundation is the eradication of all diseases of the kidney and urinary tract. Our lay volunteers, working in tandem with health professionals, are seeking the means to the prevention of kidney disease, while at the same time, ensuring that those now suffering from these diseases receive the finest possible care.

The ultimate goal can be met only if the National Kidney Foundation (NKF) achieves a series of smaller goals. These are:

- Gaining adequate support for research and research training;
- Fostering the continuing education of health care professionals;
- Expanding and developing patient services and community resources;
- Increasing the public's knowledge about kidney disease;
- Monitoring health policy development;
- Increasing fund raising to allow for the continuation of present programs and the development of new ones.

Unnumbered publication from the National Kidney Foundation. Used by permission.

The Problem of Kidney Disease

Kidney and urinary tract diseases continue to be one of the major causes of work-loss among men and women. Approximately 27 million American outpatients' visits result from kidney and urinary tract problems.

The statistics are dramatic, but not nearly as moving as watching someone being dialyzed on an artificial kidney machine or knowing someone who has literally been given the "Gift of Life" by receiving a transplant.

Since diseases of the kidney and urinary tract remain a major cause of illness and death in the United States, a concerted effort by the government, the private sector and lay and medical volunteers is needed to ease their toll on society. The National Kidney Foundation, and its 52 Affiliates with over 200 chapters nationwide, comprise the major voluntary health organization in the U.S. whose purpose and efforts are directed solely to this end.

- More than 20 million Americans suffer from diseases of the kidney and urinary tract. More than 90,000 die each year because of these diseases.

- About 200,000 Americans suffer from chronic kidney failure and need an artificial kidney machine to stay alive.

- Diabetes is the leading cause of chronic kidney failure; diabetes accounts for approximately one third of new cases of chronic kidney failure in the United States each year.

- Uncontrolled or poorly controlled high blood pressure is the second leading cause of chronic kidney failure in the United States; it accounts for about 30 percent of all cases.

- More than 27,000 patients are waiting for kidney transplants, but only about 11,000 will receive transplants this year because of a shortage of suitable organ donors.

- Benign prostatic hyperplasia (prostate problems) affect 60 percent of men by age 50 and more than 80 percent of men by age 80.

- Currently, some 1 million Americans are treated each year for kidney stones.

The Foundation's History and Leadership

Since its inception in 1950, the Foundation has sought to improve the care and treatment of those afflicted with diseases of the kidney and urinary tract through advances in detection, diagnosis and treatment. The ultimate goal is eradication of these diseases.

The affairs of the Foundation are governed by Delegate Trustees who are elected by the members of each local Affiliate, and by Trustees-at-Large elected by the other voting Trustees. These Trustees elect the Foundation's Volunteer Officers and a Board of Directors that meets regularly to attend to the ongoing affairs of the Foundation. All are unpaid volunteers.

Public Education

Educating the public on the causes and effects of kidney and urologic diseases has always been a top priority for the National Kidney Foundation. These public education efforts concentrate on eight major goal areas:

- general information on the role of the kidneys in maintaining good health
- diseases of the kidney and urinary tract
- treatment
- nutrition and kidney disease
- rehabilitation of kidney patients
- early intervention and prevention
- organ donation
- information regarding National Kidney Foundation programs and services

More than 62 brochures cover a wide variety of topics within these areas, and the National Kidney Foundation is continuously expanding its educational resources to reach out to new audiences.

The Organ Donor Program

Through its nationwide Organ Donor Program, the National Kidney Foundation is working to increase the number of organs available for transplantation. By distributing the Uniform Donor Card and developing and disseminating public and professional education materials, and developing comprehensive public and professional education programs, more people have been made aware of transplantation and will be offered the option of organ donation.

Research

The support, encouragement and promotion of research and other activities relating to the prevention, diagnosis, cause and treatment of diseases of the kidney and urinary tract have always been a major concern of the National Kidney Foundation. The outlook for patients suffering from kidney and urinary tract diseases has changed greatly in the past 44 years. Although improvements in the current therapies allow patients to live longer and more comfortably, the capability of finding the causes and cures that will eventually lead to the prevention of these diseases is still lacking.

Through its Research and Fellowship Grants Program, the National Kidney Foundation and its Affiliates award more than $2 million annually to support post-doctoral research fellows conducting basic research in kidney and urinary tract disorders.

The problems of hypertension, kidney failure, and polycystic kidney disease are also being investigated by many of the researchers the Foundation supports in laboratories throughout the United States. Through its Young Investigator Grant Program, The National Kidney Foundation provides grants to young physician-scientists who have completed their training and are junior faculty members.

Another NKF research support category is the Clinical Scientist Award. This program provides salary support of $50,000 per year for three years to experienced scientists throughout the United States.

Encouraging young people to pursue careers in biomedical research, the NKF conducts a Science Scholars Program which offers select students the opportunity to receive a stipend to work in nephrology labs during the summer. Each year, the winner of the Science Scholars Award receives a four year college scholarship for use towards a degree in medicine.

In addition to supporting scientific research, the NKF awards grants through its allied health professional councils—Council of Nephrology Social Workers, Council of Nephrology Nurses and Technicians and the Council on Renal Nutrition—to encourage research on a variety of topics in the different disciplines.

Patient and Community Services

The National Kidney Foundation and its Affiliates sponsor a wide variety of programs in treatment, service, education and prevention designed to aid the patient in the community. Examples of programs carried out by some Affiliates include information and referral for patients and their families, drug banks, summer camps for children on dialysis, counseling, screening, transportation services and four national patient and family publications: NKF Family Focus, Transplant Chronicles, Straight Talk and Parent Connection.

Professional Education

The National Kidney Foundation and its Affiliates sponsor symposia, conferences and meetings to encourage dialogue about diseases of the kidney and urinary tract among members of the medical, professional and allied health sciences. Leadership in professional education is provided by the following Scientific Councils of the Foundation:

- Council on Diabetic Kidney Disease;
- Council on Dialysis;
- Council on Glomerulonephritis;
- Council on Hypertension;
- Council of Nephrology Nurses and Technicians (CNNT);
- Council of Nephrology Social Workers (CNSW);
- Council on Pediatric Nephrology and Urology;
- Council on Polycystic Kidney Disease;
- Council on Renal Nutrition (CRN);
- Council on Transplantation;
- Council on Urology.

NKF professional publications include:

- Advancements in Renal Replacement Therapy;
- American Journal of Kidney Diseases;
- CNSW Newsletter;
- CNNT Newsletter;
- The Journal of Renal Nutrition;
- Nutrition and Blood Pressure Reviews;
- Perspectives.

The National Kidney Foundation Dollar

In fiscal year 1994, the National Kidney Foundation and its Affiliates spent 81% of their total expenditures on the programs noted, while 19% of the funds spent went to management and general and fund raising costs. A detailed annual report with a full explanation of income and expenditures is available upon written request. The National Kidney Foundation is a 501C3 organization.

The National Kidney Foundation is a participating member of the following agencies:

- Combined Health Appeal of America;
- Foundation for Biomedical Research;
- International Society on Hypertension in Blacks;
- Intersociety Council for the Research of the Kidney and Urinary Tract;
- National Health Agencies for the Combined Federal Campaign;
- National High Blood Pressure Education Program;
- National Organization of State Kidney Programs; and
- United Network for Organ Sharing.

The Future

The National Kidney Foundation faces the challenge of its growing responsibility with determination and confidence. With the financial support of philanthropic individuals, corporations, foundation and civic organizations, the search for the causes and cures of kidney disease can continue. Without that support, the National Kidney Foundation cannot survive. The voluntary health movement, regardless of the problem being fought, is a signpost of what makes our country great. The National Kidney Foundation and its Affiliates deserve your support.

Chapter 4

Glossary of Terms

Alport Syndrome. Alport syndrome is a form of genetic kidney disease characterized by persistent blood in the urine and deafness, especially to high frequency sounds.

Benign Prostatic Hyperplasia. Benign prostatic hyperplasia is the noncancerous enlargement of the prostate gland that occurs in almost all men as they age. In many men, the tissue growth inside the prostate eventually obstructs the bladder outlet, causing difficulties with urination. The enlargement may lead to destruction of the normal storing and emptying functions of the bladder resulting in difficulty urinating, increased day and night urinary frequency, urgency and incontinence. Ultimately, it may result in severe infection of the urinary tract and kidney failure.

Bladder Cancer. Malignant bladder tumors can develop on the lining of the bladder wall or extend into the bladder wall and spread rapidly to the underlying muscle. They may metastasize (spread) to distant sites through the venous or lymphatic systems. Blood in the urine is the most common sign of bladder cancer. Other symptoms may include pain during urination and a feeling of urgency or a need to urinate frequently.

Unnumbered pamphlet from the American Society of Nephrology. Used with permission.

Bladder Dysfunction. The term bladder dysfunction encompasses a wide range of bladder disorders and includes any disorder related to urine storage or emptying including urinary incontinence, interstitial cystitis and neurogenic voiding dysfunction.

Congenital Disorders. Congenital disorders are those that are present at birth. Some are genetic, or inherited; others arise from disturbances of development in utero. One example of the latter is the transmission of the human immunodeficiency virus from mother to fetus which can lead to the development of AIDS and associated kidney disease.

Cystitis. Cystitis refers to infection or inflammation of the lower urinary tract. Symptoms can include a frequent urge to urinate, a painful, burning sensation when urinating, blood in the urine, pain in the area of the bladder and in some cases a fever.

End-stage Renal Disease. End-stage renal disease is the irreversible loss of kidney function. It is most commonly due to diabetes, hypertension, or glomerulonephritis but may also result from kidney damage due to other diseases, primarily progressive chronic renal disease and occasionally acute renal injury. The result is severe systemic intoxication that may eventually lead to coma due to retained waste products and imbalances in salt and water composition and acid/base balance. Unless the condition is treated with dialysis or transplantation the patient will die.

Genetic Disorders. Genetic disorders are inherited and may be congenital, that is, apparent at birth or may appear years later. Examples of genetic kidney diseases are polycystic kidney disease and Alport syndrome.

Genital Herpes and Genital Warts. Genital herpes and genital warts are viral infections contracted by both sexes through sexual contact. Herpes is characterized by small blisters on the genitals that usually recur. Genital warts are usually small growths on the genitals or anal region, but with time they may become quite large. They may also occur inside the male urethra.

Glomerulonephritis. Primary diseases of the glomerulus, the filtering mechanism of the kidney, are usually classified as glomerulonephritis.

Hypertensive Renal Disease. Hypertension, or high blood pressure, has been implicated as a cause of progressive renal disease called nephrosclerosis and as a contributor to the rate of progression of established renal disease. However, the precise nature of the linkage between renal disease and hypertension remains incompletely understood.

Impotence. Impotence is the inability of a man to achieve or maintain a satisfactory erection. It can be the result of physical causes such as drugs, blood flow abnormalities, injuries, nerve impulse abnormalities, or hormonal imbalances; psychological causes, including depression, stress, or performance anxiety; or a combination of both.

Infertility (male). Infertility may be suspected when a couple has been trying to conceive for at least 1 year without success. About 50 percent of infertility is due to a male factor. Among the factors that can cause male infertility are semen disorders, systemic disease, obstruction of the ductal system, genital infection, genetic defects, and drugs.

Interstitial Cystitis. Interstitial cystitis is a bladder disorder that primarily affects women. It causes painful and frequent urination and often, bladder and/or pelvic pain. The cause is unknown.

Kidney Cancer (Wilms' Tumor). Adult kidney cancer has no known cause and may be discovered incidentally through examination for other conditions. It is often widespread when initially found. Major symptoms include blood in the urine, a lump or mass in the abdomen, and pain in the side. Childhood kidney cancer, known as Wilms' tumor, occurs primarily in children younger than 7 years of age. A swelling on one side of the upper abdomen is the most common symptom of the disease. At least 30 percent of Wilms' tumor cases are caused by genetic factors.

Kidney Disease of Diabetes Mellitus. Kidney disease of diabetes mellitus is a renal disease unique to diabetic patients that consists principally of a specific progressive scarring of the glomerulus (the filtering mechanism of the kidneys), leading ultimately to end-stage renal disease. Among the early signs of kidney disease in persons with diabetes are swelling of the legs and high blood pressure.

Neurogenic Voiding Dysfunction. Neurogenic voiding dysfunction refers to all types of lower urinary tract dysfunction caused by interruption of the innervation (nerve supply) of the bladder and bladder outlet. This condition can be caused by brain or spinal cord disorders and injuries, peripheral nerve damage, metabolic disturbances, some acute infectious diseases, and vascular diseases.

Obstructive Uropathy. Obstructive uropathy results in the progressive destruction of renal function due to the failure of the urinary tract to empty. This is most commonly due to structural obstruction but may also occur because the bladder fails to properly contract and empty. Obstructive uropathy is a common congenital disorder that also occurs in adults.

Orchitis and Epididymitis. Orchitis and epididymitis are inflammations of the testis and/or surrounding structures characterized by pain, redness, and swelling of the scrotum. The condition may affect one or both testes. Orchitis is usually caused by infection that reaches the testes through the blood, lymph vessels, or vas deferens and epididymitis.

Polycystic Kidney Disease. Polycystic kidney disease is a genetic disease characterized by multiple clusters of fluid-filled cysts within the kidney. The cysts enlarge the kidney, compressing and eventually replacing the organ's functioning tissue, causing kidney failure.

Primary Renal Diseases. Primary, or intrinsic, renal diseases are disorders in which the kidney appears to be the predominant or only organ affected. Many forms involve the glomeruli (the tiny filtering structures where urine formation begins), but the tubules into which the glomerular filtrate passes to continue urine formation as well as the intervening tissue may also be affected.

Prostate Cancer. Prostate cancer is the most commonly diagnosed cancer and the second leading cause of cancer deaths in American males. When symptoms occur they are most often due to metastatic spread of the cancer to the bones, resulting in chronic back pain. Other symptoms such as weak or interrupted flow of urine, inability to urinate, blood in the urine, or need to urinate frequently are similar to those of benign prostatic hyperplasia.

Prostatitis. Prostatitis is an acute or chronic inflammation of the prostate. Symptoms of acute prostatitis include fever, chills, low back pain, and frequent painful urination. Symptoms of chronic prostatitis are similar but much less severe than those of the acute form, although in many cases the chronic form is asymptomatic.

Pyelonephritis. Pyelonephritis is the inflammation of the kidney due to bacterial infection. In acute pyelonephritis, the infection is characterized by fever, chills, and pain in the sides and back. In chronic pyelonephritis, the infection often leads to kidney failure because the kidneys may become small and scarred.

Renal failure. Renal failure can be acute or chronic. Acute renal failure is the sudden interruption of kidney function—most frequently by shock, trauma, embolism, blood loss, sudden obstruction, or reactions to drugs—causing the retention of toxic wastes and fluids. The result is a severe and frequently lethal intoxication affecting every organ system in the body. Chronic renal failure results from gradual reduction in functional kidney mass and leads to permanent kidney failure, known as end-stage renal disease. Acute renal failure is potentially reversible; chronic renal failure is not.

Secondary Renal Disease. Secondary renal disease is produced by a variety of system diseases that affect other organs or tissues in addition to the kidney. The major causes of secondary renal diseases are diabetes, systemic lupus erythematosus, systemic vasculitis, and Wegener's granulomatosis.

Testicular Cancer. Testicular cancer is the most common solid tumor occurring in males between the ages of 13 and 34 years. Symptoms include a lump in the testicle, swelling or a change in consistency of the testicle, and a dull ache in the lower abdomen, groin, or scrotum.

Urethritis and Gonococcal Infections. Urethritis is the inflammation of the urethra caused by gonorrhea or by a nonspecific or other venereal infection such as chlamydia. Symptoms include frequent and painful urination and often a urethral discharge.

Urinary Incontinence. Incontinence is the loss of urinary control, ranging from occasional slight losses of urine to severe, frequent wetting.

Urinary Stone Disease. In the United States, urinary stones most commonly occur in the kidneys and ureters, the tubes that connect the bladder to the kidneys. Stones develop when mineral crystals form a hard mass in the urinary tract. The first symptom of a stone is usually severe pain in the back, side, or lower abdomen.

Urinary Tract Infection. A urinary tract infection is an inflammation of tissue caused by bacteria found anywhere in the urinary tract—from the tip of the urethra (the tube through which urine is expelled from the body) to the kidney.

Vesicoureteral Reflux. Vesicoureteral reflux is usually a childhood condition that causes urine in the bladder to back up (reflux) into the ureters and kidneys. Patients with vesicoureteral reflux often develop urinary tract infections, which are among the major results of the disorder. Vesicoureteral reflux can lead to injury to or scarring of the kidneys, called reflux nephropathy—the most common cause of end-stage renal disease in children, as well as hypertension in adolescents and young adults.

Part Two

Introduction to the Kidneys

Chapter 5

Your Kidneys: Master Chemists of the Body

"Bones can break, muscles can atrophy, glands can loaf, even the brain can go to sleep without immediate danger to survival. But should the kidneys fail, neither bones, muscles, gland nor brain could carry on."

—Dr. Homer W. Smith

Kidneys perform crucial functions which affect all parts of the body. As Dr. Smith says in the quote above, many other organs in our body depend upon the kidneys to function normally. The kidneys perform complex operations which keep the rest of the body in balance. But when the kidneys become damaged by disease, the other organs are affected as well.

Kidney problems can range from a minor urinary tract infection to progressive kidney failure. Scientific advances over the past three decades have improved our ability to diagnose and treat those who suffer from kidney disorders. Even when the kidneys no longer function, treatments such as dialysis and transplantation have brought hope and literally new life to hundreds of thousands of people.

Medical scientists continue to learn more about the function and structure of the kidneys and the diseases that affect them. There is still much to learn and a need for continued support of research.

National Kidney Foundation © 1989, revised 1995. Used by permission.

Why Are the Kidneys So Important?

Most people know that a major function of the kidneys is to remove waste products and excess fluid from the body. These waste products and excess fluid are removed through the urine. The production of urine involves highly complex steps of excretion and reabsorption. This process is necessary to maintain a stable balance of body chemicals.

The critical regulation of the body's salt, potassium and acid content is performed by the kidneys. The kidneys also produce hormones and vitamins which affect the function of other organs. For example, a hormone produced by the kidneys stimulates red blood cell production. In addition, other hormones produced by the kidneys help regulate blood pressure and others help control calcium metabolism.

The kidneys are powerful chemical factories that perform the following functions:

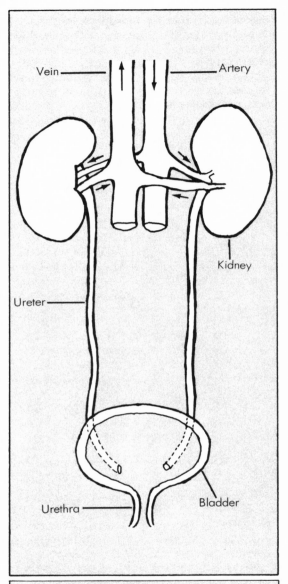

The kidneys are located behind your other abdominal organs. The vessels that connect them with the circulatory system are shown above. The large vessel at the right is the aorta; that at the left, the vena cava. Descending from the kidneys are the ureters, which empty into the bladder (at bottom of drawing).

Figure 5.1.

42

- remove waste products from the body
- balance the body's fluids
- release hormones which regulate blood pressure
- synthesize the vitamins which control growth
- control the production of red blood cells

Where Are the Kidneys and How Do They Function?

There are two kidneys, each about the size of one's fist, located on either side of the spine at the lowest level of the rib cage. Each kidney contains about one million functioning units called nephrons. A nephron consists of a filtering unit of tiny blood vessels called a glomerulus attached to a tubule. When blood enters the glomerulus, it is filtered and the remaining fluid then passes along the tubule. In the tubule, chemicals and water are either added to or removed from this filtered fluid according to the body's needs, the final product being the urine we excrete.

The kidneys perform their life-sustaining job of filtering and returning to the bloodstream about 200 quarts of fluid every 24 hours. Approximately two quarts are eliminated from the body in the form

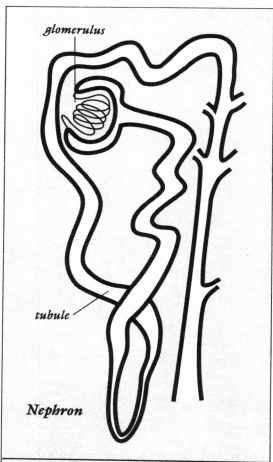

Each kidney is made up of about 1 million working units, called nephrons. Each nephron consists of a filtering unit of tiny blood vessels, called a glomerulus, attached to a tubule. When blood enters the glomerulus, it is filtered and the remaining fluid passes along the tubule, where chemicals and water are either added to or removed from the filtered fluid according to what the body needs.

Figure 5.2.

43

of urine, and about 198 quarts are retained in the body. The urine we excrete has been stored in the bladder for approximately 1-8 hours.

What Are Some of the Types and Causes of Kidney Disease?

Kidney disease usually affects both kidneys. If the kidneys' ability to remove and regulate water and chemicals is seriously damaged by disease, waste products and excess fluid build up, causing severe swelling and symptoms of uremia (kidney failure).

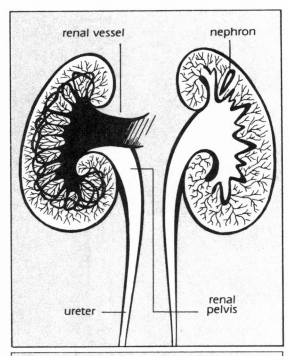

A cross section of the kidney shows two aspects of its internal structure. Shown at the left is the circulation of the kidney. At the right the blood vessels have been eliminated to show the renal pelvis and the ureter, into which the urine empties. At the upper right in the right hand drawing is the outline of the individual unit of kidney function, the nephron. Each kidney of man contains about a million nephrons.

Figure 5.3.

There are many different types and causes of kidney disease, and these can be characterized as either hereditary, congenital, or acquired.

Hereditary disorders. Hereditary disorders can be transmitted to both males and females and generally produce clinical symptoms from teenage years to adulthood. The most prevalent hereditary kidney condition is polycystic kidney disease. Other hereditary conditions include Alport's Syndrome, hereditary nephritis, primary hyperoxaluria, and cystinuria.

Congential disease. Congenital disease usually involves some malformation of the genitourinary tract, usually leading to some type of obstruction which subsequently produces infection and /or destruction of kidney tissue. Eventually the destruction can progress to chronic kidney failure.

Acquired kidney diseases. Acquired kidney diseases are very numerous, the general term being nephritis (meaning inflammation of the kidney). The most common type of nephritis is glomerulonephritis, and again this has many causes. Your doctor can explain what is known and not known about the various forms of acquired kidney diseases.

Kidney stones are very common, and when they pass the pain can be extremely severe in your side and back. Stone formation can be an inherited disorder, secondary to a malformation and/or infection in the kidney, or can occur without any prior problem. The pain can appear suddenly, occur in waves, and disappear just as rapidly when the stone is passed. Evaluation by your doctor can reveal a cause for the kidney stone formation in about 1/3 of patients who have their first stone. When kidney stones get stuck in the kidney and ureter (and cannot pass), a new form of shock wave treatment has been used to destroy the stone. This treatment is called extracorporeal shock wave lithotripsy.

Nephrotic syndrome refers to a large protein loss in the urine, frequently in association with low blood protein (albumin) levels, an elevated blood cholesterol and severe retention of body fluid causing swelling (edema). This disease can be a primary disorder of the kidney or secondary to an illness affecting many parts of the body (for example, diabetes mellitus). Your doctor can explain the best approach to this serious problem which can attack people of any age.

45

Long-standing high blood pressure (hypertension) can cause kidney disease itself or be a result of a kidney disorder. Uncontrolled high blood pressure can accelerate the natural course of any underlying kidney disease.

Drugs and toxins. Years of heavy use of headache compounds can slowly produce kidney failure. Certain other medications, toxins, pesticides, and "street" drugs (i.e., heroin) can also produce kidney damage. Your doctor can explain the problems associated with long-standing use or abuse of these different agents.

Can Kidney Disease Be Successfully Treated?

Unfortunately, many kidney diseases are still of unknown cause. Some of the kidney diseases noted above can be successfully treated and others progress to advanced kidney failure, requiring dialysis and/or transplantation. For example, kidney infections and kidney stones can often be successfully treated. Chronic inflammation of the glomerulus (called glomerulonephritis) is the most common kidney disease which slowly progresses to kidney failure (see the National Kidney Foundation's brochure Glomerulonephritis).

How Do We Treat Advanced Kidney Failure?

Research is now being considered on the effect of special diets in slowing or halting progressive kidney failure, especially if the problem is approached early. Treatments to slow the progress of kidney failure hold promise for the future. When these therapies are no longer successful, there are now several ways by which chronic, irreversible kidney failure can be treated. These methods are listed below and often more than one type of treatment is suitable for any one person.

Treatment with hemodialysis (the artificial kidney) may be performed at a dialysis unit or at home. Hemodialysis treatments are usually performed in three separate sessions per week. Peritoneal dialysis is generally done daily at home. Continuous Cycling Peritoneal Dialysis requires the use of a machine while Continuous Ambulatory Peritoneal Dialysis does not. A kidney specialist can explain the different approaches and suggest what may be best for the individual patient.

Finally, there has been increasing success with kidney transplantation. In some cases, the kidney may come from a relative who donates one of his or her own kidneys to the patient. Kidney transplantation from cadaveric donors, however, is more common in the United States. Under these circumstances, individuals who have died have donated their kidneys for potential transplantation. More information about hemodialysis, peritoneal dialysis, kidney transplantation and organ donation is available from your local National Kidney Foundation.

1. Hemodialysis (artificial kidney machine)
   * Hospital or center hemodialysis
   * Home hemodialysis

2. Peritoneal dialysis
   * Continuous ambulatory (CAPD)
   * Continuous cycling peritoneal dialysis (CCPD)

3. Kidney transplantation
   * Living-related donor
   * Cadaveric donor

What Are the Warning Signs of Kidney Disease?

Although, many forms of kidney disease do not produce symptoms until late in the course of the disease, there are six warning signs of kidney diseases:

* burning or difficulty during urination;
* an increase in the frequency of urination;
* passage of bloody urine;
* puffiness around eyes, swelling of hands and feet;
* pain in small of back just below ribs;
* high blood pressure.

How Common Is Kidney Disease in the USA?

It is estimated that at least 20 million Americans suffer from kidney or urinary tract related diseases. Of these, over 100,000 per year will need dialysis or transplantation in order to survive.

Ultimately, the National Kidney Foundation hopes through research to eradicate these diseases altogether. Until that time comes, the National Kidney Foundation stands ready to provide continuing, education and support to kidney patients and their families. Many thousands of people have returned to active, productive lives with the help of dialysis and transplantation. But we still need a cure. When research renders the kidney machine obsolete, one mission of the National Kidney Foundation will have been realized.

More than 20 million Americans have some form of kidney or urologic disease. Millions more are at risk. The National Kidney Foundation, Inc., a major voluntary health organization, is working to find the answers through prevention, treatment and cure. Through its 52 Affiliates nationwide, the Foundation conducts programs in research, professional education, patient and community services, public education and organ donation. The work of the National Kidney Foundation is funded entirely by public donations.

Chapter 6

Statistical and Demographic Information about Kidney Disease

Chapter Contents

Section 6.1

African Americans Struck by High Rate of Kidney Disease

The NIH Record, Vol. XLII, No. 24, November 27, 1990.

Four hours a day, three days a week, and probably for the rest of his life, 39-year-old Joe Henderson Jr. goes to his "job" at Walter Reed Army Medical Center's dialysis clinic. There he is joined to a machine that removes his blood a pint at a time, cleans it, and returns it to his body.

Joe Henderson's kidneys don't work. His job is dialysis, and it keeps him alive. Maybe long enough to receive a donated kidney. Maybe not.

"Kidney failure is no longer fatal, thanks to maintenance dialysis and kidney transplantation," said Dr. Lawrence Agodoa, who directs NIDDK's research program in chronic kidney failure and treats patients with kidney disease at Walter Reed Army Medical Center. "But even with these effective treatments, most people with chronic kidney failure have a vastly shortened lifespan, with survival rates comparable to those for prostate, colon and lung cancers."

The main reason for this shortened survival is heart disease. Heart-related problems were the immediate cause of death in 65 percent of kidney failure patients who died in 1988. "Some of the deaths were due to an accelerated buildup of cholesterol in the arteries," said Agodoa. But cholesterol is not the heart's only enemy. Because dialysis is not a perfect replacement for the kidneys, patients with kidney failure must control the amount of potassium-rich foods they eat. Too much or too little potassium can disrupt the heart's rhythm, causing sudden heart failure.

Under normal conditions, the kidneys, nestled on each side of the body under the rib cage, remove waste and regulate blood pressure. They also balance body fluids and salts and release erythropoietin, a hormone that tells the bone marrow to produce red blood cells.

The filtering units of the kidney, called glomeruli, are made up of clusters of microscopic blood vessels. When these units are damaged by a disease such as diabetes or high blood pressure, the remaining healthy units work harder to compensate for the loss. As the disease progresses, more units are destroyed until the kidneys are working at only 5 or 10 percent of capacity. At this point, a person is diagnosed with end-stage kidney disease, or kidney failure, and must have dialysis or a kidney transplant to survive.

During 1988, 172,506 people in the United States were treated for kidney failure. More than 36,000 were newly diagnosed cases—nearly a nine percent increase over 1987. Whites accounted for 67 percent of those treated for kidney failure, and African-Americans accounted for 29 percent—more than double their representation in the U.S. population, which is only 12 percent. Most patients with kidney failure have access to treatment—dialysis and transplantation—through the Medicare program administered by the Health Care Financing Administration (HCFA). According to a report from the U.S. Renal Data System, an NIDDK-supported program, treatment for chronic kidney failure cost more than $5.4 billion in 1988.

The four main causes of kidney failure are diabetes, hypertension, glomerulonephritis and polycystic kidney disease. African-Americans are at higher risk than whites for all causes except polycystic kidney disease, but researchers are finding that African-Americans are hit especially hard by high blood pressure, which they tend to get at a younger age than whites. Between ages 25 to 44, African-Americans have nearly 20 times the rate of kidney failure from high blood pressure as whites, and between ages 45 to 64, their risk is about 11 times higher.

"High blood pressure is basically what did my kidneys in," said Joe Henderson. "My feet and legs started swelling, so I went to the doctor." By the time Henderson found out he had high blood pressure, his kidneys had already been severely damaged. Fifteen years later he had kidney failure.

As treatment for high blood pressure has improved, death rates for stroke and heart disease have declined. In contrast, kidney failure due to high blood pressure is on the rise, particularly in African-Americans. As one researcher pointed out, doctors know how to protect the heart and brain from hypertension but not the kidneys.

An NIDDK research initiative on kidney disease in African-Americans is aimed at filling this gap of information. "We need to find out why African-Americans seem more vulnerable to renal injury from high blood pressure, if some drugs are better than others in preventing blood pressure related renal injury in African-Americans, and if the target blood pressure should be lower for African-Americans than whites," said Dr. Gary Striker, director of NIDDK's Division of Kidney, Urologic, and Hematologic Diseases.

People with kidney failure must decide, with the help of their doctors and families, which treatment—dialysis or transplantation—is best for them. Factors such as age, other illnesses, emotional support of family and friends, religious beliefs and trust in the medical profession influence a patient's decision.

Dialysis is a life-saving procedure and the treatment choice of most chronic kidney failure patients. Hemodialysis, done three times a week, uses a machine connected to a special filter to remove, clean and return the patient's blood minus wastes. Various forms of peritoneal dialysis, done three times a week to four times a day, depending on the form, use the patient's abdominal wall to filter wastes from the bloodstream into a solution in the abdomen. The waste-filled fluid is periodically replaced with a clean solution. Surgery is required to insert a permanent device that allows easy access to the bloodstream for hemodialysis or the abdominal cavity for peritoneal dialysis. All dialysis patients must cut down on calories, fluids, protein and salts.

Side effects of dialysis include blood clots and infections of the access site and the abdominal wall in peritoneal dialysis. New hemodialysis patients can also experience headache, nausea, muscle cramps, anorexia, dizziness and seizures.

African-Americans most often opt to remain on dialysis, possibly because they tend to do well on it. Among African-Americans with kidney failure at the end of 1988, 86 percent were on dialysis compared to 69 percent of their white counterparts. African-Americans on dialysis have fewer complications that require hospitalization, and they live longer than whites on dialysis. According to Henderson, "It's not a physically active life, but I don't have any noticeable problems. If I didn't tell you that I was on dialysis, you wouldn't know. I feel well and I have adjusted well to the diet and regular visits to the dialysis center."

Kidney transplantation has important advantages over dialysis that, for many people, outweigh the risk of organ rejection, infection, osteoporosis and kidney damage. Although transplant patients must take immunosuppressive drugs to prevent rejection, they are freed from dialysis and tend to have an improved quality of life, close to that experienced before the onset of kidney disease.

In 1989, 8,882 people got their wish for a new kidney. Unfortunately, another 14,669 were still waiting. Kidney donations have not kept pace with need, so most patients wait a year or more for a kidney transplant, according to the U.S. Renal Data System.

Henderson does not want a kidney transplant. "Maybe if I was to get worse I would think about it," he said. But even if he wanted a transplant, he would not accept a kidney from a family member. "It would be too much to put on them. What if they got sick and died, and I was still alive? I couldn't live with that."

But for patients who receive a transplant, the success rate is encouraging. African-Americans and whites who received a transplant in 1987 had about the same 2-year survival. Up to 96 percent of patients who received a kidney from a living relative and up to 93 percent of those who received a kidney from a deceased, unrelated donor lived at least 2 years.

Graft survival, or survival of the new kidney, is lower in African-Americans than whites regardless of whether the kidney came from a living relative or deceased, unrelated donor. Researchers do not know why some patients keep a transplant when others who seem as well matched reject the transplant. Why graft survival is lower in African-Americans compared to whites is not well understood, but researchers are beginning to find genetic clues.

A donor kidney is matched with a recipient on the basis of six antigens, or tissue types, found on the HLA gene of each person. These antigens are part of the immune system and have been linked to kidney rejection. According to Agodoa, "Graft survival is best when all six antigens match. The next best is when five of six match. Beyond that, graft survival is similar for four or fewer matching antigens."

Researchers have found that African-Americans have a more diverse genetic makeup and a wider range of HLA antigens than whites. This diversity decreases the chances of finding a donor kidney with matching antigens.

Finding Answers

In recommendations to NIDDK, a panel of researchers in epidemiology, genetics, immunogenetics, hypertension and nephrology has called for more studies, including a clinical trial to help answer questions about kidney disease in hypertensive African-Americans. The NIDDK is now planning a pilot clinical trial that will test the feasibility of a full-scale study of kidney disease in hypertensive African-Americans.

The NIDDK is also supporting U.S. Renal Data System, the source of most of the data presented in this chapter. The data system began collecting and analyzing data in 1988 with the help of the HCFA and is now the largest database on kidney disease in the U.S. Current studies are comparing patient and graft survival considering severity of illness at the onset of treatment; prognosis based on renal biopsy results; and quality of life of patients treated with erythropoietin, which relieves the anemia of kidney failure.

These and other NIDDK-supported studies will improve the understanding of kidney disease and, one day, will lead to the treatment and prevention of kidney failure.

— by Mary Harris

Section 6.2

Additional Resources on Kidney Disease and Black Americans

Searches on File, NKUDIC.

Legend

TI   Title
AU Author
CN Corporate Author
SO Source
PD Product
AV Producer/Availability

TI   **African Americans and Organ Donors.**
AU George, A.R.
SO *Journal of the National Medical Association*. 83(12): 1057–1060. December 1991.
AV Available from SLACK Incorporated, 6900 Grove Road, Thorofare, NJ 08086. (609) 848-1000.

TI   **Association of HLA Phenotypes with Hypertension in African Americans and Caucasoid Americans with Type II Diabetes, a Population at Risk for Renal Disease.**

AU   Acton, R.T., et al.

SO   *Transplantation Proceedings*. 25(4):2400–2403. August 1993.

AV   Available from Appleton & Lange, Paramount Publishing, 25 Van Zant Street, E. Norwalk, CT 06885. (203) 838-4400, extension 550.

TI   **Black Americans and the ESRD Program.**

AU   De Palma, J.R.

SO   *Contemporary Dialysis and Nephrology*. 10(4): 33-37. April 1989.

AV   Available from Contemporary Dialysis, Inc. 6300 Variel Avenue, Suite I, Woodland Hills, CA 91367. (818) 704-5555.

TI   **Black Americans: Diabetes and Obesity.**

SO   *Diabetes Forecast*. 43(2): 74-75. February 1990.

AV   Available from American Diabetes Association, Inc. 1660 Duke Street, Alexandreia, VA 22314. (800) 232-3472.

TI   **Educating the African-American Community on Organ Donation.**

AU   Thompson, V.L.S.

SO   *Journal of the American Medical Association*. 85(1): 17-19. January 1993.

TI   **Effect of Race on Access and Outcome in Transplantation.**

AU   Kasiske, B.L., et al.

SO   *New England Journal of Medicine*. 324(5): 302-307. January 31, 1991.

TI   **End-Stage Renal Disease and Race: An Overview and Perspective.**

AU   Ferguson, R.

SO   *Journal of the National Medical Association*. 83(9): 794-798. September 1991.

AV   Available from SLACK Incorporated, 6900 Grove Road, Thorofare, NJ 08086. (609) 848-1000.

TI   **End-Stage Renal Disease in US Minority Groups.**
AU Feldman, H.I., et al.
SO *American Journal of Kidney Diseases.* 19(5): 397-410. May 1992.
AV Available from National Kidney Foundation. 30 East 33rd Street, New York, NY 10016; (212) 889-2210 or (800) 622-9010.

TI   **End-Stage Renal Disease in Minorities (editorial).**
AU Cruz, I.A.; Hosten, A.O.
SO *Journal of the National Medical Association.* 83(4): 309-312. April 1991.
AV Available from SLACK Incorporated, 6900 Grove Road. Thorofare. NJ 08086.(609) 848-1000.

TI   **Factors Affecting the Waiting Time of Cadaveric Kidney Transplant Candidates in the United States.**
AU Sanfilippo, F.P., et al.
SO *Journal of the American Medical Association (JAMA).* 267(2): 247-252. January 8, 1992.

TI   *Generate a Life/Genere Una Vida: Sign an Organ Donor Card/Firma una Tarjeta de Donante de Organos.*
SO Houston, TX: LifeGift Organ Donation Center. 1993. 7 p.
AV Available from LifeGift Organ Donation Center. 7505 South Main, Suite 500, Houston, TX 77030. (713) 799-9115 or (800) 633-6562. Single copy free.

TI   *High Blood Pressure and Your Kidneys.*
SO New York: National Kidney Foundation. 1990. 4 p.
CN National Kidney Foundation, Inc.
AV Available from National Kidney Foundation, Inc. 30 East 33rd Street. New York. NY 10016. (800) 622-9010. Free.

TI   *Hypertension and Chronic Renal Failure: National High Blood Pressure Education Program (NHBPEP) Working Group Report.*
SO Bethesda, MD: National Institutes of Health. August 1990. 28 p.
CN National Institutes of Health
AV Available from Information Center for the National Heart, Lung and Blood Institute, 7200 Wisconsin Avenue, Box 329, Bethesda, MD 20814. (301) 951-3260. Single copy free. Order Number 90-3032.

TI **Hypertension in the Black Population: Revisited.**
AU Baskin, S.
SO *Nephrology News and Issues.* 4(11): 24-27. November 1990.
AV Available from Nephrology News and Issues. 13901 N. 73rd Street, Suite 214, Scottsdale, AZ 85260-9804. (602) 443-4635.

TI **Hypertension: Racial Differences.**
AU Eisner, G.M.
SO *American Journal of Kidney Diseases.* 16(4 Supplement 1): 35-40. October 1990.
AV Available from National Kidney Foundation. 30 East 33rd Street, New York, NY 10016. (212) 889-2210 or (800) 622-9010.

TI **Hypertensive Renal Disease in Blacks.**
AU Retta, T.M.; Afre, G.M.; Randall, O.S.
SO *Transplantation Proceedings.* 25(4): 2421-2422. August 1993.
AV Available from Appleton & Lange, Paramount Publishing, 25 Van Zant Street, E. Norwalk, CT 06885. (203) 838-4400, extension 550.

TI **IG's Report Uncovers Racial Disparities in Organ Distribution.**
AU Oday, L.A.
SO *Contemporary Dialysis and Nephrology.* 11(11): 38, 54. November 1990.
AV Available from Contemporary Dialysis, Inc. 6300 Variel Avenue, Suite I, Woodland Hills, CA 91367. (818) 704-5555.

TI **Incidence of Treatment for End-Stage Renal Disease Attributed to Diabetes Mellitus, by Race/Ethnicity-Colorado, 1982-1989.**
AU Hamman, R.F., et al.
SO *Morbidity and Mortality Weekly Report (MMWR).* 41(44): 845-848. November 6, 1992.
AV Available from Superintendent of Documents, U.S. Government Printing Office, Washington, DC 20402-9325. (202) 783-3238.

TI **Increasing Organ Donation in the Black Community.**
AU Plawecki, H.M.; Freiberg, G.; Plawecki, J.A.
SO *American Nephrology Nurses Association Journal (ANNA Journal).* 16(5): 321-324. August 1989.

AV   Available from American Nephrology Nurses' Association. Box 56, North Woodbury Road, Pitman, NJ 08071. (609) 589-2187.

TI   Increasing Organ Donation in the Black Community.
AU   Plawecki, H.M.; Freiberg, G.; Plawecki, J.A.
SO   *Perspectives (Journal of the Council of Nephrology Social Workers)*. Volume 12:39-47. 1991.

TI   Organ Donation and Approaching the African-American Family: A Case for Understanding Over Expectation.
AU   Lynch, J.
SO   *Contemporary Dialysis and Nephrology*. 11(12): 21–22. December 1990.
AV   Available from Contemporary Dialysis, Inc. 6300 Variel Avenue, Suite I, Woodland Hills, CA 91367. (818) 704-5555.

TI   Organ Donation and Blacks: A Critical Frontier.
AU   Callender, C.O., et al.
SO   *New England Journal of Medicine*. 325(6): 442–444. August 8, 1991.

TI   *Organ Donation: A Dilemma for Black Americans.*
SO   Chapel Hill, NC: Health Sciences Consortium. 1992. (videocassette).
PD   ½ in VHS videocassette (13 min), col.
AV   Available from Health Sciences Consortium (HSC). 201 Silver Cedar Court, Chapel Hill, NC 27514-1517. (919) 942-8731. Price: $195.00, HSC members $136.50. Order Number N911-VI-061.

TI   *Organ Donation: The Gift of Life.*
AU   Owens, A.
SO   Washington, DC: National Kidney Foundation-National Capital Area. 1989. (videocassette).
CN   National Kidney Foundation, National Capital Area.
PD   ½ in. VHS videocassette (approximately 18 min), col.
AV   Available from National Kidney Foundation-National Capital Area, Inc. 5335 Wisconsin Avenue, N.W., Suite 830, Washington, DC 20015. (202) 244-7900. Price: Free loan program, includes shipping and handling. Videocassette may be duplicated.

TI **Problem of Diabetic Renal Failure in the United States: An Overview.**
AU Teutsch, S.; Newman, J.; Eggers, P.
SO *American Journal of Kidney Diseases.* 13(1): 11–13. 1989.
AV Available from National Kidney Foundation. 30 East 33rd Street, New York, NY 10016. (212) 889-2210 or (800) 622-9010.

TI **Racial Discrepancies in U.S. Organ Allocation.**
SO *Contemporary Dialysis and Nephrology.* 11(11): 14–15. November 1990.
AV Available from Contemporary Dialysis, Inc. 6300 Variel Avenue, Suite I, Woodland Hills, CA 91367. (818) 704-5555.

TI **Racial Equity in Renal Transplantation: The Disparate Impact of HLA-Based Allocation.**
AU Gaston, S.L., et al.
SO *Journal of the American Medical Association (JAMA).* 270(11): 1352–1356. September 15, 1993.

TI ***Reducing Transplant Rejection in Blacks: News Briefings for Science Writers on Transplantation, Dialysis and Kidney Research*** (memorandum).
AU Hurley, C.K.
SO New York, NY: National Kidney Foundation, Inc. March 26–27, 1990. 6 p.
AV Available from National Kidney Foundation, Inc. 30 East 33rd Street, New York, NY 10016. (800) 622-9010 or (212) 889-2210.

TI **Renal Disease in Hypertensive Adults: Effect of Race and Type II Diabetes Mellitus.**
AU Tierney, W.M.; McDonald, C.J.; Luft, F.C.
SO *American Journal of Kidney Diseases.* 13(6): 485–493. 1989.
AV Available from National Kidney Foundation. 30 East 33rd Street, New York, NY 10016. (212) 889-2210 or (800) 622-9010.

TI **Renal Function in Black Americans With Type II Diabetes.**
AU Palmisano, J.J.; Lebovitz, H.E.
SO *Journal of Diabetic Complications.* 3(1): 40–44. January-March 1989.

AV   Available from J.B. Lippincott Company, at Downsville Pike, Route 3, Box 20-B, Hagerstown, MD 21740. (800) 638-3030.

TI   **Risk Factors for End-Stage Renal Disease Among Minorities.**
AU   Ferguson, R.; Morrissey, E.
SO   *Transplantation Proceedings*. 25(4): 2415–2420. August 1993.
AV   Available from Appleton & Lange, Paramount Publishing, 25 Van Zant Street, E. Norwalk, CT 06885. (203) 838-4400, extension 550.

TI   *Second Chance.*
SO   Washington, DC: National Kidney Foundation-National Capital Area. 1990. (videocassette).
CN   National Kidney Foundation, National Capital Area.
PD   ½ in. VHS videocassette (approximately 12 min), col.
AV   Available from National Kidney Foundation-National Capital Area, Inc. 5335 Wisconsin Avenue, N.W., Suite 830, Washington, DC 20015. (202) 244-7900. Price: Free loan program, includes shipping and handling. Videocassette may be duplicated.

TI   **Understanding and Increasing Black Kidney Donation.**
AU   Rosen, S.L.
SO   *American Nephrology Nurses Association Journal (ANNA Journal)*. 18(2): 195–198. April 1991.
AV   Available from American Nephrology Nurses' Association. Box 56, North Woodbury Road, Pitman, NJ 08071. (609) 589-2187.

TI   **US Minority Groups and End-Stage Renal Disease: A Disproportionate Share (editorial).**
AU   Rostand, S.G.
SO   *American Journal of Kidney Diseases*. 19(5): 411–413. May 1992.

Part Three

Kidney Disorders in Children

Chapter 7

Wilms' Tumor

Chapter Contents

Section 7.1

PDQ on Wilms' Tumor

National Cancer Institute, CancerNet online information service.

What is Wilms' Tumor?

Wilms' tumor is a disease in which cancer (malignant) cells are found in certain parts of the kidney. The kidneys are a "matched" pair of organs found on either side of the backbone. The kidneys are shaped like a kidney bean. Inside each kidney are tiny tubes that filter and clean the blood, taking out unneeded products, and making urine. The urine made by the kidneys passes through a tube called a ureter into the bladder where it is held until it is passed from the body.

Wilms' tumor occurs most commonly in children under the age of 15 and is curable in the majority of affected children. Like most cancers, Wilms' tumor is best treated when it is found (diagnosed) early.

If your child has symptoms, your child's doctor will usually feel your child's abdomen for lumps and run blood and urine tests. Your doctor may order a special x-ray called an intravenous pyelogram (IVP). During this test, a dye containing iodine is injected into your child's bloodstream. This allows your child's doctor to see the kidney more clearly on the x-ray. Your child's doctor may also do an ultrasound, which uses sound waves to make a picture, or a special x-ray called a CT scan to look for lumps in the kidney. A special scan called magnetic resonance imaging (MRI), which uses magnetic waves to make a picture, may also be done. Chest and bone x-rays may also be taken.

If tissue that is not normal is found, your child's doctor will need to cut out a small piece and look at it under the microscope to see if there are any cancer cells. This is called a biopsy.

Your child's chance of recovery (prognosis) and choice of treatment depend on the stage of your child's cancer (whether it is just in the kidney or has spread to other places in the body), how the cancer cells look under a microscope (histology), and your child's age and general health.

Stages of Wilms' Tumor

Once Wilms' tumor has been found, more tests will be done to find out if cancer cells have spread from the kidney to other parts of the body. This is called staging. Your child's doctor needs to know the stage of the disease to plan treatment. The following stages are used for Wilms' tumor:

Stage I. Cancer is found only in the kidney and can be completely removed by surgery.

Stage II. Cancer has spread to the areas near the kidney, such as to fat or soft tissue, lymph nodes (small, bean-shaped structures found throughout the body that produce and store infection-fighting cells), or blood vessels. The cancer can be completely removed by surgery.

Stage III. Cancer has spread to areas near the kidney, but cannot be completely removed by surgery. The cancer may have spread to important blood vessels or organs near the kidney or the cancer may have spread throughout the abdomen, so that the doctor cannot remove all the cancer during surgery.

Stage IV. Cancer has spread to organs further away from the kidney, such as the lungs, liver, bone, and brain.

Stage V. Cancer cells are found in both kidneys.

Recurrent. Recurrent disease means that the cancer has come back (recurred) after it has been treated. It may come back where it started or in another part of the body.

In Wilms' tumor, how the cancer cells look under a microscope (histology) is also very important. The cancer cells can be of favorable histology or unfavorable histology (which includes diffuse anaplastic and clear cell sarcoma of the kidney).

How Wilms' Tumor is Treated

There are treatments for all patients with Wilms' tumor. Three kinds of treatment are used: surgery (taking out the cancer in an operation), chemotherapy (using drugs to kill cancer cells) and radiation therapy (using high-dose x-rays or other high-energy x-rays to kill cancer cells).

- Surgery is a common treatment for Wilms' tumor. Your doctor may take out the cancer using one of the following:

  1. Partial nephrectomy removes the cancer and part of the kidney around the cancer. This operation is usually used only in special cases, such as when the other kidney is damaged or has already been removed.

  2. Simple nephrectomy removes the whole kidney. The kidney on the other side of the body can take over filtering blood.

  3. Radical nephrectomy removes the whole kidney with the tissues around it. Some lymph nodes in the area may also be removed.

- Chemotherapy uses drugs to kill cancer cells. Chemotherapy may be taken by pill, or it may be put into the body by a needle in a vein or muscle. Chemotherapy is called a systemic treatment because the drugs enter the bloodstream, travel through the body, and can kill cancer cells throughout the body. Chemotherapy given after surgery or radiation therapy has removed all cancer cells that can be seen is called adjuvant chemotherapy. When very high doses of chemotherapy are used to kill cancer cells, these high doses can destroy the blood-forming tissue in the bones (the bone marrow). If very high doses of chemotherapy are needed to treat the cancer, bone marrow may be taken from the bones before therapy and frozen until it is needed. Following chemotherapy, the bone marrow is then given back through a needle in a vein. This is called autologous bone marrow reinfusion.

- Radiation therapy uses x-rays or other high-energy rays to kill cancer cells and shrink tumors. Radiation for Wilms' tumor usually comes from a machine outside the body (external radiation therapy). Radiation may be used before or after surgery and/or chemotherapy.

Treatment of Wilms' Tumor by Stage

Treatments for Wilms' tumor depend on the stage of your child's disease, the cell type (histology), and your child's age and general health.

Your child may receive treatment that is considered standard based on its effectiveness in a number of patients in past studies, or you may choose to have your child take part in a clinical trial. Not all patients are cured with standard therapy and some standard treatments may have more side effects than are desired. For these reasons, clinical trials are designed to test new treatments and to find better ways to treat cancer patients. Clinical trials are going on in most parts of the country for most stages of Wilms' tumor. If you want more information, call the Cancer Information Service at 1-800-4-CANCER (1-800-422-6237).

Stage I Wilms' Tumor

Your child's treatment depends on the histology of your child's cancer.

If your child has favorable histology or diffuse anaplastic Wilms' tumor, your child's treatment will probably be surgery to remove the cancer followed by chemotherapy. A clinical trial (the National Wilms' Tumor Study) is comparing different schedules of chemotherapy.

If your child has clear cell sarcoma of the kidney, your child's treatment will probably be surgery to remove the cancer followed by chemotherapy plus radiation therapy. A clinical trial (the National Wilms' Tumor Study) is testing whether different schedules of chemotherapy may be used.

Stage II Wilms' Tumor

Your child's treatment depends on the histology of the cancer.

If your child has favorable histology cancer, your child's treatment will probably be surgery to remove the cancer followed by chemotherapy. A clinical trial (the National Wilms' Tumor Study) is comparing different schedules of chemotherapy to see whether a shorter schedule of chemotherapy may be used.

If your child has unfavorable histology cancer (diffuse anaplastic or clear cell sarcoma of the kidney), your child's treatment will probably be surgery to remove the cancer followed by chemotherapy plus radiation therapy. A clinical trial (the National Wilms' Tumor Study) is testing whether different schedules of chemotherapy may be used.

Stage III Wilms' Tumor

Your child's treatment will probably be surgery to remove the cancer followed by chemotherapy and radiation therapy. The dose of radiation therapy may be lower if your child has a favorable histology cancer. A clinical trial (the National Wilms' Tumor Study) is testing whether different schedules and types of chemotherapy may be used in some patients.

Sometimes the cancer cannot be removed during surgery because it is too close to important organs or blood vessels or because it too big to remove. In this case, the doctor may only perform a biopsy, and then give chemotherapy with or without radiation therapy. Once the cancer has become smaller, surgery can be performed, followed by additional chemotherapy and radiation therapy.

Stage IV Wilms' Tumor

Your child's treatment will probably be surgery to remove the cancer followed by chemotherapy, with or without radiation therapy to the abdomen. If the cancer has spread to the liver, radiation therapy may be given to the liver when the cancer can't be removed surgically. If the cancer has spread to the lungs, radiation therapy is given to the lungs. A clinical trial (the National Wilms' Tumor Study) is testing whether different schedules and types of chemotherapy may be used in some patients.

Stage V Wilms' Tumor

Because both kidneys contain cancer, it is not usually possible to remove both kidneys. Your child's doctor will probably take out a piece of the cancer in both kidneys and remove some of the lymph nodes around the kidney to see whether they contain cancer. Following surgery, chemotherapy is given to shrink the cancer. A second operation is then performed to remove as much of the cancer as possible, while leaving as much of the kidneys as possible. Surgery may be followed by more chemotherapy and/or radiation therapy.

Recurrent Wilms' Tumor

If your child's cancer comes back (recurs), treatment depends on the treatment he or she received before, how much time has passed since the first cancer was treated, the histology of the cancer, and where the cancer came back.

Depending on the above factors, your child's treatment may be surgery to remove the cancer, plus radiation therapy and chemotherapy.

Clinical trials are evaluating new treatments, such as new chemotherapy drugs and combinations, and very high doses of chemotherapy followed by bone marrow reinfusion.

To Learn More

To learn more about Wilms' tumor, call the National Cancer Institute's Cancer Information Service at 1-800-4-CANCER (1-800-422-6237). By dialing this toll-free number, you can speak with someone who can answer your questions.

The Cancer Information Service can also send you free booklets. The following booklet about kidney cancers may be helpful to you:

— Research Report: Adult Kidney Cancer and Wilms' Tumor

The following booklets on childhood cancer may be helpful to you:

— Young People with Cancer: A Handbook for Parents
— Talking with Your Child About Cancer
— When Someone in Your Family Has Cancer
— Managing Your Child's Eating Problems During Cancer Treatment

The following general booklets on questions related to cancer may also be helpful:

— Taking Time: Support for People with Cancer and the People Who Care About Them
— What Are Clinical Trials All About?
— Chemotherapy and You: A Guide to Self-Help During Treatment
— Radiation Therapy and You: A Guide to Self-Help During Treatment
— What You Need to Know About Cancer

There are many other places you can get material about cancer treatment and services to help you. You can check the social service office at your hospital for local and national agencies that help with your finances, getting to and from treatment, care at home, and dealing with your problems. The American Cancer Society, for example, has many free services. Candlelighters Childhood Cancer Foundation (1-800-366-2223) has free services and publications including newsletters, bibliographies, and information for parents and brothers and sisters of children with cancer. It can also refer you to a local parent peer support group in the United States or abroad. Local offices for these organizations are listed in the white pages of the telephone book.

You can also write to the National Cancer Institute at this address:

National Cancer Institute
Building 31, Room 10A24
9000 Rockville Pike
Bethesda, MD 20892

What is PDQ?

PDQ is a computer system that gives up-to-date information on cancer treatment. It is a service of the National Cancer Institute (NCI) for people with cancer and their families, and for doctors, nurses, and other health care professionals.

PDQ tells about the current treatments for most cancers. The information in PDQ is reviewed each month by cancer experts. It is updated when there is new information.

PDQ also lists information about research on new treatments (clinical trials), doctors who treat cancer, and hospitals with cancer programs. The treatment information in this summary is based on information in the PDQ treatment summary for health professionals on this cancer.

How to use PDQ

Cancer in children is not common, with about 7,000 new cases diagnosed each year in the United States. The majority of children with cancer are treated at cancer centers with special facilities to treat children with cancer. There are organized groups of doctors and other health care professionals who work together to improve treatments for children with cancer by doing clinical trials.

A clinical trial is a study that tries to improve current treatment or find new treatments to care for patients. Each trial is based on past studies and what has been learned in the laboratory. Each trial answers certain scientific questions in order to find new and better ways to help cancer patients. During clinical trials, more and more information is collected about new treatments, their risks, and how well they do or do not work.

If clinical trials show that the new treatment is better than the one currently being used, the new treatment may become the "standard" treatment. Children who are treated on clinical trials have the advantage of getting the best available therapy. In the United States, about two thirds of children with cancer are treated on a clinical trial at some point in their illness. Listings of clinical trials are a part of PDQ. In the United States, there are two major groups (called cooperative groups) that organize clinical trials for childhood cancers: the Childrens Cancer Group (CCG) and the Pediatric Oncology Group (POG). Doctors who belong to these groups or who take part in other clinical trials are listed in PDQ.

You can use PDQ to learn more about current treatments for your child's kind of cancer. Bring this material from PDQ with you when you see your child's doctor. You can talk with the doctor, who knows your child and has the facts about your child's disease, about which treatment would be best.

If you want to know more about cancer and how it is treated, or if you wish to learn about clinical trials for your child's kind of cancer, you can call the National Cancer Institute's Cancer Information Service. The number is 1-800-4-CANCER (1-800-422-6237). The call is free and a trained information specialist will talk with you and answer your questions. PDQ may change when there is new information. Check with the Cancer Information Service to be sure that you have the most up-to-date information.

Section 7.2

Additional Resources on Wilms' Tumor

NCI / PDQ CancerLit Search: Wilms' Tumor,
Citations and Abstracts from the NCI's CancerLit Database
from the National Cancer Institute,
CancerNet online information service, January 1996.

Legend

TI Title
AU Author
SO Source
AD Address

Citations and Abstractions

TI ***Expression of Resistance-Related Proteins in Nephroblastoma after Chemotherapy***
AU Volm M; Mattern J; Stammler G; Royer-Pokora B; Schneider S; Weirich A; Ludwig R
SO Int J Cancer 1995;63(2):193–7
AD German Cancer Research Center, Heidelberg, Germany.

TI ***Relationship Between Dose Schedule and Charges for Treatment on National Wilms' Tumor Study-4. A Report from the National Wilms' Tumor Study Group.***
AU Green DM; Breslow NE; Evans I; Moksness J; Finklestein JZ; Evans AE; D'Angio GJ
SO Monogr Natl Cancer Inst 1995;(19):21–5
AD Department of Pediatrics, Roswell Park Cancer Institute, Buffalo, NY 14263, USA.

TI *National Wilms' Tumor Study: Economic Perspective*
AU Buxton MJ
SO Monogr Natl Cancer Inst 1995;(19):27–9
AD Health Economics Research Group, Brunel University, Uxbridge, Middx, U.K.

TI *Regulation of the Proto-oncogenes Bcl-2 and C-myc by the Wilms' Tumor Suppressor Gene Wt1*
AU Hewitt SM; Hamada S; McDonnell TJ; Rauscher FJ 3rd; Saunders GF
SO Cancer Res 1995;55(22):5386–9
AD Department of Biochemistry and Molecular Biology, University of Texas M.D. Anderson Cancer Center, Houston 77030, USA.

TI *Constitutional and Somatic Mutations in the Wt1 Gene in Wilms' Tumor Patients*
AU Nordenskjold A; Friedman E; Sandstedt B; Soderhall S; Anvret M
SO Int J Cancer 1995;63(4):516–22
AD Department of Molecular Medicine, Karolinska Hospital, Stockholm, Sweden.

Chapter 8

Childhood Nephrotic Syndrome

This chapter has been written to tell you some facts about a kidney disease called the nephrotic syndrome. This illness also is called nephrosis or minimal change disease. The chapter will give you and your family information about your child's illness. It will tell you what will happen with this illness. You also should talk to your doctor. The more you know, the more you can help your child.

What Do the Kidneys Do?

The kidneys are two fist-sized organs found in the lower back. When they are working well, they clean the blood and get rid of waste products and excess salt and water. When diseased, the kidneys may get rid of things that the body needs to keep, such as blood cells and protein.

What Is the Nephrotic Syndrome?

This is an illness where the kidney loses protein in the urine. This causes protein in the blood to drop, and water moves into body tissues, causing swelling (edema). You will see the swelling around the child's eyes, in the belly, or in the legs. Your child will not go to the bathroom as often as usual and will gain weight with the swelling.

Kidney and Urology Facts on Childhood Nephrotic Syndrome, National Kidney Foundation. Used by permission.

Do Other Kidney Diseases Cause Edema and Protein in the Urine?

Yes. Edema and protein in the urine are common in other types of kidney disease, especially a disease called glomerulonephritis.

What Causes the Nephrotic Syndrome?

In the majority of cases, the cause is not known. The National Kidney Foundation has active research programs into causes and treatments of the nephrotic syndrome.

Who Gets It?

Usually, young children between the ages of 1½ and 5. It happens twice as often in boys as girls. However, children of all ages and adults also can get it.

How Can You Tell If Your Child Has It?

You may see that your child has swelling around the eyes in the morning. You may think that your child has an allergy. Later, the swelling may last all day, and you may see swelling in your child's ankles, feet and belly. Also, your child may be:

- more tired
- more irritable
- eating less
- pale looking

The child may have trouble putting on shoes or buttoning clothes because of swelling.

How Is the Nephrotic Syndrome Treated?

The treatment will try to stop the loss of protein in the urine, and increase the amount of urine. Usually, the doctor will start your child on a drug called prednisone. Most children get better with this drug.

What Does Prednisone Do?

Prednisone is used to stop the loss of protein from the blood into the urine. After one to four weeks of treatment, your child should begin going to the bathroom more often. As your child makes more urine, the swelling will go away.

When there is no protein in the urine, the doctor will begin to reduce the amount of prednisone over several weeks. The doctor will tell you exactly how much prednisone to give your child each day. Never stop prednisone, unless the doctor tells you to do so. If you stop this drug or give your child too much or too little, he or she may get very ill.

Sometimes, your child will stay healthy after treatment. Your child may relapse (get sick again) at any time, even after a long time with good health. Getting sick may happen after a viral infection, such as a cold or the flu.

What Problems Can Occur with Prednisone?

Prednisone can be a very good drug, but it has a number of side effects. Some of these side effects are:

- being hungry
- gaining weight
- acne (pimples)
- mood changes (very happy, then very sad)
- being overactive
- slowing of growth rate
- more chance of infection

Side effects are more common with larger doses and if it is used for a long time. Once prednisone is stopped, most of these side effects go away.

What If Prednisone Does Not Work?

If prednisone does not work for your child or if your child has serious side effects, the doctor may order another kind of medicine, called an immunosuppressive drug. These drugs decrease the activity of the body's immune system. They are effective in most, but not all, children.

Your doctor will discuss in detail with you the good and bad things about the drug. The side effects of these drugs include: increased susceptibility to infections, hair loss and decreased blood cell production.

Parents also should be aware that children taking immunosuppressive drugs may become ill if they develop chicken pox. Therefore, you should notify your doctor any time that your child is exposed to chicken pox while on these medications.

Your child also may be given diuretics (water pills). These drugs help the kidney get rid of salt and water. The most common water pill used in children is called furosemide. If your child starts to have a problem with vomiting or diarrhea, you should call your doctor as the child can lose too much fluid and become even sicker. Once protein disappears from the urine, diuretics should be stopped.

What Other Problems Happen with the Nephrotic Syndrome?

Most children will have problems only with swelling. However, a child with nephrotic syndrome can develop a serious infection in the belly. If your child has a fever or starts complaining of severe pain in the belly, you should call your doctor at once.

Sometimes, children with nephrotic syndrome get blood clots in their legs. If this happens, your child will complain of:

- severe pain in arm or leg
- swelling of arm or leg
- changes in color or temperature of arm or leg

If any of these things happens, you should call your doctor right away.

What Can Parents Do?

Much of your child's care will be given by you. Pay attention to your child's health, but do not overprotect the child. If your child is ill or taking prednisone, the doctor will recommend a low salt diet. This type of diet will make your child more comfortable by keeping the swelling down. Try to give your child foods that he or she likes but that are low in salt. Ask the dietitian for suggestions.

Usually, the child will be allowed to drink as much as he or she wants. A child's natural thirst is the best guide as to how much to drink. You should also weigh your child and keep a record of weight to spot a change in the disease.

The first sign that your child is getting sick again is the return of protein in the urine. Because of this, many doctors ask you to check your child's urine regularly. To do this, a special plastic strip with a small piece of paper on the end is dipped into the urine. The paper will change color when protein is in the urine. This test can be done easily at home and it can detect a relapse before any swelling is seen. Check with your doctor to learn how to do the test and how often to do it.

When there is swelling, check that your child's clothing is not too tight because the clothing can rub the child's skin over the swollen areas. This can make the skin raw, and it may get infected.

Your child will probably have this disease several years. It is very important to treat your child as normally as possible. Your child needs to continue his or her usual activities, such as going to school and seeing friends. Your child should be treated just like other children in the family in terms of discipline. Occasionally, your child may not go to school for a time. Your doctor will let you know if this is necessary. Keeping your child out of school or not letting him or her see friends will not change the illness.

Does the Disease Ever Go Away?

Sometimes. Even though the nephrotic syndrome does not have a specific cure, the majority of children "outgrow" this disease in their late teens or early adulthood. Some children will have only one attack of the nephrotic syndrome. If your child does not have another attack for three years after the first one, the chances are quite good that he or she will not get sick again.

Still, most children will have two or more attacks. The attacks are more frequent in the first one to two years after the nephrotic syndrome begins. After ten years, less than one child in five is still having attacks. Even if a child has a number of attacks, most will not develop permanent kidney damage. The major problem is to control their accumulation of fluid using prednisone and diuretics. Children with this disease have an excellent long-term outlook.

What Else Should I Know?

1. Most children with the nephrotic syndrome respond to treatment.
2. Most children with the nephrotic syndrome have an excellent long-term outcome.
3. You should feel free to ask your child's doctor any questions.

What If I Have More Questions?

If you have more questions, you should speak to your doctor. You also can get additional information by contacting your local National Kidney Foundation Affiliate.

What Is the National Kidney Foundation and How Does it Help?

Twenty million Americans have some form of kidney or urologic disease. Millions more are at risk. The National Kidney Foundation, Inc., a major voluntary health organization, is working to find the answers through prevention, treatment and cure. Through its 50 Affiliates nationwide, the Foundation conducts programs in research, professional education, patient and community services, public education and organ donation. The work of The National Kidney Foundation is funded entirely by public donations.

Part Four

Understanding Adult Kidney Disorders

Chapter 9

Kidney Stones in Adults

Overview

Kidney stones are one of the most painful disorders to afflict humans. This ancient health problem has tormented people throughout history. Scientists have even found evidence of kidney stones in an Egyptian mummy estimated to be more than 7,000 years old.

Kidney stones are one of the most common disorders of the urinary tract. More than 1 million cases of kidney stones were diagnosed in 1985. It is estimated that 10 percent of all people in the United States will have a kidney stone at some point in time. Men tend to be affected more frequently than women.

Most kidney stones pass out of the body without any intervention by a physician. Cases that cause lasting symptoms or other complications may be treated by various techniques, most of which do not involve major surgery. Research advances also have led to a better understanding of the many factors that promote stone formation.

An Introduction to the Urinary Tract

The urinary tract, or system, consists of the kidneys, ureters, bladder, and urethra. The kidneys are two bean-shaped organs located below the ribs toward the middle of the back. The kidneys remove extra water and wastes from the blood, converting it to urine. They

NIH Publication No. 94–2495, April 1994.

also keep a stable balance of salts and other substances in the blood. The kidneys produce hormones that help build strong bones and help form red blood cells.

Narrow tubes called ureters carry urine from the kidneys to the bladder, a triangle-shaped chamber in the lower abdomen. Like a balloon, the bladder's elastic walls stretch and expand to store urine. They flatten together when urine is emptied through the urethra to outside the body.

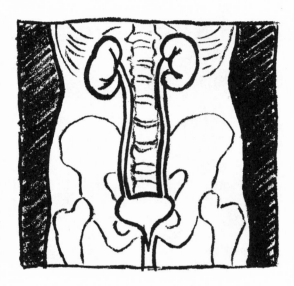

Figure 9.1. *The urinary tract.*

What Is a Kidney Stone?

A kidney stone develops from crystals that separate from urine and build up on the inner surfaces of the kidney. Normally, urine contains chemicals that prevent or inhibit the crystals from forming. These inhibitors do not seem to work for everyone, however, and some people form stones. If the crystals remain tiny enough, they will travel through the urinary tract and pass out of the body in the urine without even without even being noticed.

Kidney stones may contain various combinations of chemicals. The most common type of stone contains calcium in combination with either oxalate or phosphate. These chemicals are part of a person's normal diet and make up important parts of the body, such as bones and muscles.

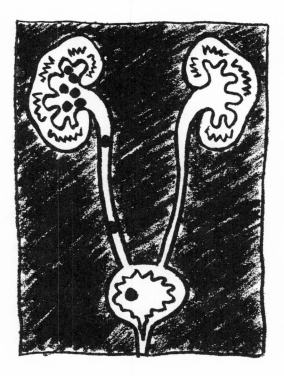

Figure 9.2. Kidney stones in kidney, ureter and bladder.

A less common type of stone is caused by infection in the urinary tract. This type of stone is called a struvite or infection stone. Much less common are the uric acid stone and the rare cystine stone.

Urolithiasis is the medical term used to describe stones occurring in the urinary tract. Other frequently used terms are urinary tract stone disease and nephrolithiasis. Doctors also use terms that describe the location of the stone in the urinary tract. For example, a ureteral stone (or ureterolithiasis) is a kidney stone found in the ureter. To keep things simple, the term "kidney stones" is used throughout this text document.

Gallstones and kidney stones are not related. They form in different areas of the body. If a person has a gallstone, he or she is not necessarily more likely to develop kidney stones.

Who Gets Kidney Stones?

For some unknown reason, the number of persons in the United States with kidney stones has been increasing over the past 20 years. White people are more prone to kidney stones than are black people. Although stones occur more frequently in men, the number of women who get kidney stones has been increasing over the past 10 years, causing the ratio to change. Kidney stones strike most people between the ages of 20 and 40. Once a person gets more than one stone, he or she is more likely to develop others.

What Causes Kidney Stones?

Doctors do not always know what causes a stone to form. While certain foods may promote stone formation in people who are susceptible, scientists do not believe that eating any specific food causes stones to form in people who are not susceptible.

A person with a family history of kidney stones may be more likely to develop stones. Urinary tract infections, kidney disorders such as cystic kidney diseases, and metabolic disorders such as hyperparathyroidism are also linked to stone formation.

In addition, more than 70 percent of patients with adequate hereditary disease called renal tubular acidosis develop kidney stones.

Cystinuria and hyperoxaluria are two other rare inherited metabolic disorders that often cause kidney stones. In cystinuria, the kidneys produce too much of the amino acid cystine. Cystine does not dissolve in urine and can build up to form stones. With hyperoxaluria, the body produces too much of the salt oxalate. When there is more oxalate than can be dissolved in the urine, the crystals settle out and form stones.

Absorptive hypercalciuria occurs when the body absorbs too much calcium from food and empties the extra calcium into the urine. This high level of calcium in the urine causes crystals of calcium oxalate or calcium phosphate to form in the kidneys or urinary tract.

Other causes of kidney stones are hyperuricosuria (a disorder of uric acid metabolism), gout, excess intake of vitamin D, and blockage of the urinary tract. Certain diuretics (water pills) or calcium-based antacids may increase the risk of forming kidney stones by increasing the amount of calcium in the urine.

Calcium oxalate stones may also form in people who have a chronic inflammation of the bowel or who have had an intestinal bypass operation, or ostomy surgery. As mentioned above, struvite stones can form in people who have had a urinary tract infection.

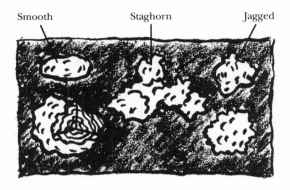

Figure 9.3. *Sizes and shapes of various stones.*

What Are the Symptoms?

Usually, the first symptom of a kidney stone is extreme pain. The pain often begins suddenly when a stone moves in the urinary tract, causing irritation or blockage. Typically, a person feels a sharp, cramping pain the back and side in the area of the kidney or in the lower abdomen. Sometimes nausea and vomiting occur with this pain. Later, the pain may spread to the groin.

If the stone is too large to pass easily, the pain continues as the muscles in the wall of the tiny ureter try to squeeze the stone along into the bladder. As a stone grows or moves, blood may be found in the urine. As the stone moves down the ureter closer to the bladder, a person may feel the need to urinate more often or feel a burning sensation during urination.

If fever and chills accompany any of these symptoms, an infection may be present. In this case, a doctor should be contacted immediately.

How Are Kidney Stones Diagnosed?

Sometimes "silent" stones—those that do not cause symptoms—are found on x-rays taken during a general health exam. These stones would likely pass unnoticed.

More often, kidney stones are found on an x-ray or sonogram taken on someone who complains of blood in the urine or sudden pain. These diagnostic images give the doctor valuable information about the stone's size and location. Blood and urine tests help detect any abnormal substance that might promote stone formation.

The doctor may decide to scan the urinary system using a special x-ray test called an IVP (intravenous pyelogram). Together, the results from these tests help determine the proper treatment.

How Are Kidney Stones Treated?

Fortunately, most stones can be treated without surgery. Most kidney stones can pass through the urinary system with plenty of water (2 to 3 quarts a day) to help move the stone along. In most cases, a person can stay home during this process, taking pain medicine as needed. The doctor usually asks the patient to save the passed stone(s) for testing.

The First Step: Prevention

People who have had more than one kidney stone are likely to form another. Therefore, prevention is very important. To prevent stones from forming, their cause must be determined. The urologist will order laboratory tests, including urine and blood tests. He or she will also ask about the patient's medical history, occupation and dietary habits. If a stone has been removed, or if the patient has passed a stone and saved it, the lab can analyze the stone to determine its composition.

A patient may be asked to collect his or her urine for 24 hours after a stone has passed or been removed. The sample is used to measure urine volume and levels of acidity, calcium, sodium, uric acid, oxalate, citrate, and creatinine (a byproduct of protein metabolism). The doctor will use this information to determine the cause of the stone. A second 24-hour urine collection may be needed to determine if the prescribed treatment is working.

Lifestyle Changes. A simple and most important lifestyle change to prevent stones is to drink more liquids—water is best. A recurrent stone former should try to drink enough liquids throughout the day to produce at least 2 quarts of urine in every 24-hour period.

Patients with too much calcium or oxalate in the urine may need to eat fewer foods containing calcium and oxalate.

Not everyone will benefit from a low-calcium diet, however. Some patients who have high levels of oxalate in their urine may benefit from extra calcium in their diet. Patients may be told to avoid food with added vitamin D and certain types of antacids that have a calcium base.

Patients who have a very acid urine may need to eat less meat, fish, and poultry. These foods increase the amount of acid in the urine.

To prevent cystine stones, patients should drink enough water each day to reduce the amount of cystine that escapes into the urine. This is difficult because more than a gallon of water may be needed every 24 hours, a third of which must be drunk during the night.

Medical Therapy. The doctor may prescribe certain medications to prevent calcium and uric acid stones. These drugs control the amount of acid or alkali in the urine, key factors in crystal formation. The drug allopurinol may also be useful in some cases of hypercalciuria and hyperuricosuria.

Another way a doctor may try to control hypercalciuria, and thus prevent calcium stones, is by prescribing certain diuretics, such as hydrochlorothiazide. These drugs decrease the amount of calcium released by the kidneys into the urine.

Some patients with absorptive hypercalciuria may be given the drug sodium cellulose phosphate. This drug binds calcium in the intestine and prevents it from leaking into the urine.

If cystine stones cannot be controlled by drinking more fluids, the doctor may prescribe the drug Thiola. This medication helps reduce the amount of cystine in the urine.

For struvite stones that have been totally removed, the first line of prevention is to keep the urine free of bacteria that can cause infection. The patient's urine will be tested on a regular basis to be sure that bacteria are not present.

If struvite stones cannot be removed the doctor may prescribe a new drug called acetohydroxamic acid (AHA). AHA is used along with long-term antibiotic drugs to prevent the infection that leads to stone growth.

To prevent calcium stones that form in hyperparathyroid patients, a surgeon may remove all of the parathyroid glands (located in the neck). This is usually the treatment for hyperparathyroidism as well. In most cases, only one of the glands is enlarged. Removing the gland ends the patient's problem with kidney stones.

Surgical Treatment

Some type of surgery may be needed to remove a kidney stone if the stone:

- does not pass after a reasonable period of time and causes constant pain,
- is too large to pass on its own,
- blocks the urine flow,
- causes ongoing urinary tract infection,
- damages the kidney tissue or causes constant bleeding, or
- has grown larger (as seen on follow up x-ray studies).

Until recently, surgery to remove a stone was very painful and required a lengthy recovery time (4 to 6 weeks). Today, treatment for these stones is greatly improved. Many options exist that do not require major surgery.

Extracorporeal Shockwave Lithotripsy. Extracorporeal shockwave lithotripsy (ESWL) is the most frequently used surgical procedure for the treatment of kidney stones. ESWL uses shockwaves that are created outside of the body to travel through the skin and body tissues until the waves hit the dense stones. The stones become sand-like and are easily passed through the urinary tract in the urine.

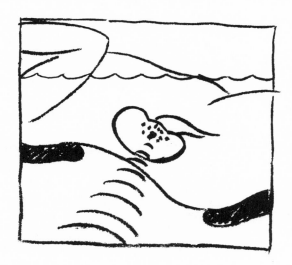

Figure 9.4. ESWL.

There are several types of ESWL devices. One device positions the patient in the water bath while the shock waves are transmitted. Other devices have a soft cushion or membrane on which the patient lies. Most devices use either x-rays or ultrasound to help the surgeon pinpoint the stone during treatment. For most types of ESWL procedures, some type of anesthesia is needed.

In some cases, ESWL may be done on an outpatient basis. Recovery time is short, and most people can resume normal activities in a few days.

Complications may occur with ESWL. Most patients have blood in the urine for a few days after treatment. Bruising and minor discomfort on the back or abdomen due to the shockwaves are also common. To reduce the chances of complications, doctors usually tell patients to avoid taking aspirin and other drugs that affect blood clotting for several weeks before treatment.

In addition, the shattered stone fragments may cause discomfort as they pass through the urinary tract in the urine. In some cases, the doctor will insert a small tube called a stent through the bladder into the ureter to help the fragments pass. Sometimes the stone is not completely shattered with one treatment and additional treatments may be required.

Percutaneous Nephrolithotomy. Sometimes a procedure called percutaneous nephrolithotomy is recommended to remove a stone.

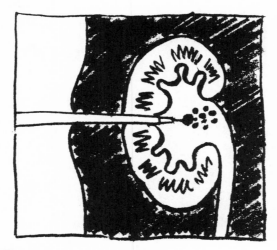

Figure 9.5. *Percutaneous nephrolithotomy.*

This treatment is often used when the stone is quite large or in a location that does not allow effective use of EWSL.

In this procedure, the surgeon makes a tiny incision in the back and creates a tunnel directly into the kidney. Using an instrument called a nephroscope, the stone is located and removed. For large stones, some type of energy probe (ultrasonic or electrohydraulic) may be needed to break the stone into small pieces. Generally, patients stay in the hospital for several days and may have a small tube called a nephrostomy tube left in the kidney during the healing process.

One advantage of percutaneous nephrokithotomy over ESWL is that the surgeon removes the stone fragments instead of relying on their natural passage from the kidney.

Ureteroscopic Stone Removal. Although some ureteral stones can be treated with ESWL, urethroscopy may be needed for mid- and lower ureter stones. No incision is made in this procedure. Instead, the surgeon passes a small fiberoptic instrument called a ureteroscope

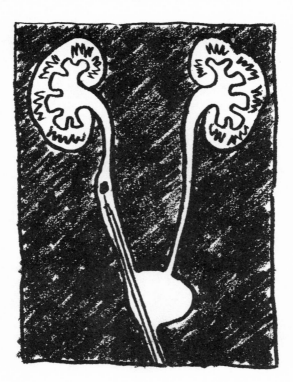

Figure 9.6. Ureteroscopic stone removal.

through the urethra and bladder into the ureter. The surgeon then locates the stone and either removes it with a cage-like device or shatters it with a special instrument that produces a form of shockwave. A small tube or stent may be left in the ureter for a few days after treatment to help the lining of the ureter heal.

Is There Any Current Research on Kidney Stones?

The Division of Kidney, Urologic, and Hematologic Diseases of the National Institutes of Diabetes and Digestive and Kidney Diseases (NIDDK) funds research on the causes, treatments, and prevention of kidney stones. The NIDDK is part of the Federal Government's National Institutes of Health in Bethesda, Maryland.

New drugs and the growing field of lithotripsy have greatly improved the treatment of kidney stones. Still, NIDDK researchers and grantees seek to answer questions such as:

- Why do some people continue to have painful stones?
- How can doctors predict, or screen, who is as risk for getting stones?
- What are the long-term effects of lithotripsy?
- Do genes play a role in stone formation?
- What is the natural substance(s) found in urine that blocks stone formation?

Researchers are also working to develop new drugs with fewer side effects.

Prevention Points to Remember

- People who have a family history of stones or who have had more than one stone are likely to develop another.

- A good first step to prevent any type of stone is to drink plenty of liquids—water is best.

- If a person is at risk for developing stones, the doctor may perform certain blood and urine tests. These tests will determine which factors can be best altered to reduce that risk.

- Some patients will need medicines to prevent stones from forming.

- People with chronic urinary tract infections and stones will often need the stone removed if the doctor determines that the infection results from the stone's presence. Patients must receive careful followup to be sure that the infection has cleared.

Foods and Drinks Containing Calcium and Oxalate

Persons prone to forming calcium oxalate stones may be asked by their doctor to cut back on certain foods on this list.

apples	figs
asparagus	grapes
beer	ice cream
beets	milk
berries, various	oranges
(e.g., cranberries,	parsley
strawberries)	peanut butter
black pepper	pineapples
broccoli	spinach
cheese	Swiss chard
chocolate	rhubarb
cocoa	tea
coffee	turnips
cola drinks	vitamin C
collards	yogurt

Persons should not give up or avoid eating these types of foods without talking to their doctor first. In most cases, these foods can be eaten in limited amounts.

Additional Reading

Prevention and Treatment of Kidney Stones. National Institutes of Health Consensus Development Conference Statement. Available from the National Institutes of Health Consensus Program Clearinghouse, P.O. Box 2577, Kensington, Maryland, 20891. (800) 644-6627.

Understanding Kidney Stones...Management for a Lifetime. Krames Communication, 110 Grundy Lane, San Bruno, CA 94066. (800) 333-3032.

Coe, F.L., et al., "The Pathogenesis and Treatment of Kidney Stones," *New England Journal of Medicine,* Vol. 327, No. 16, pp.1141–1152, 1992.

Curhan, G.C.,etal., "A Prospective Study of Dietary Calcium and Other Nutrients and the Risk of Symptomatic Kidney Stones," *New England Journal of Medicine,* Vol. 328, No. 12, pp. 833–838, 1993.

Jenkins, A.D., "Upgrading Extracorporeal Shock Wave Lithotripsy," *Contemporary Urology,* October 1991, pp. 11–12.

Lawson, R.K., "Smaller Means Safer Intraureternal Eletrohydraulic Lithotripsy," *Contemporary Urology,* October 1991, pp.51–58.

Lingeman, J.E., et al., "Kidney Stones: Acute Management," *Patient Care,* August 15, 1990, pp.20–42.

Lingeman, J.E., et al., "Kidney Stones: Identifying the Causes," *Patient Care,* September 30, 1990, pp.31–46.

O'Brien, W.M., Rotolo, J.E., Pahira, J.J., "New Approaches in the Treatment of Renal Calculi," *American Family Physician,* November 1987, pp. 181–94.

Other Resources

American Foundation for Urologic Disease
300 West Pratt Street
Baltimore, MD 21201-2463
(800) 242-2383; (410) 727-2908

National Kidney Foundation
30 East 33rd Street
New York, NY 10016
(800) 622-9010; (212) 889-2210

National Kidney and Urologic Diseases Information Clearinghouse
Box NKUDIC
9000 Rockville Pike
Bethesda, MD 20892
(301) 654-4415

Oxalosis and Hyperoxaluria Foundation
P.O. Box 1632
Kent, WA 98035
(800) 484-9698 ext: 5100; (206) 631-0386

Chapter 10

Polycystic Kidney Disease

Chapter Contents

Section 10.1

PKD Patient's Manual

An Introduction To ADPKD

The purpose of this chapter is to provide information about autosomal dominant polycystic kidney disease to those who have the disease, those who are at risk for the disease, interested family members and friends.

What Is ADPKD?

Autosomal Dominant Polycystic Kidney Disease or ADPKD is an inherited disorder. It is passed on from affected parent to child and results in the development and growth of cysts in the kidney. Cysts can also form in the liver. There can also be abnormalities of certain blood vessels and in the heart. ADPKD occurs throughout the world. It affects all races but may be less common in blacks. Approximately 500,000 people in the United States have ADPKD.

What Is A Cyst?

A cyst is an outpouching of tissue similar to a blister. It can be filled with clear fluid, blood or white blood cells. Polycystic simply means many cysts.

Where Are My Kidneys?

Each person is born with two kidneys. They are located in the back of the body on each side of the spine. The kidneys are approximately 5½ inches long, three inches wide and two inches thick. They weigh about 10 to 12 ounces each and are protected by the rib cage, fat and muscle. Both kidneys are affected when a person has ADPKD. There may be just a few cysts or many and the cysts may range in size from a pinhead to the size of a grapefruit. If many cysts are present the kidneys can more than double in size and weight.

How Do My Kidneys Work?

Each kidney contains about one million tubes called nephrons. A little over 22% of the blood the heart pumps goes to the kidneys. This blood flows through a filter in the nephron. Red blood cells, white blood cells and larger substances don't pass through the filter but stay in the body. The rest of the fluid and small particles pass through the nephron. There are about 150 quarts (or liters) of fluid filtered by the kidneys each day. The nephrons reabsorb all except one to two quarts (or liters) which comes out as urine.

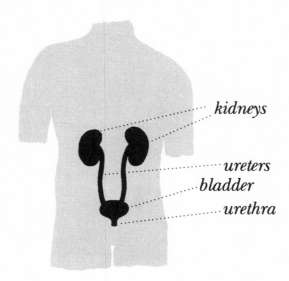

kidneys

ureters

bladder

urethra

Figure 10.1.1. *Normal location of kidneys, ureters, bladder and urethra in abdomen.*

The kidney is a regulating system. It makes sure your chemicals such as sodium, potassium, calcium, phosphorus and other electrolytes are in balance. The kidney regulates the acidity of your body fluid so that it is not too acid or too alkaline. The kidney also filters out and gets rid of the waste products your body makes each day. Some of these waste products are urea nitrogen (BUN) and creatinine. Because the kidney is so efficient at clearing BUN and creatinine, kidney function is measured by the level of these substances in the blood.

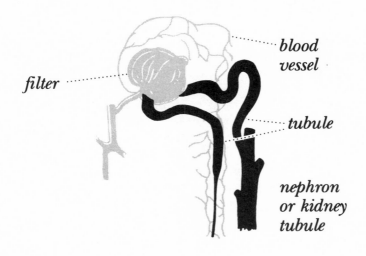

Figure 10.1.2. *The nephron (kidney tubule) is the functional unit of the kidney. It has a filter supplied by blood vessels and a tubule. There are about one million nephrons in each kidney.*

Apart from getting rid of waste products, other functions of the kidneys include making several hormones. One of the hormones called renin helps regulate the body's handling of salt and blood pressure. Another of the hormones, erythropoietin, tells the bone marrow to make red blood cells. When the kidneys are removed, no erythropoietin is made and so there is no message to tell the bone marrow to make red blood cells. This is why people who have had their kidneys removed need blood transfusions every five to seven weeks. The kidney also changes vitamin D to its active form.

What Causes Cysts To Form In My Kidneys?

There is a gene defect on one of the chromosomes in a person who has ADPKD. This gene is now giving an incorrect message to the body to make an abnormal protein. As yet we don't know what the abnormal protein or the message is.

Whatever the mechanism is which causes ADPKD, outpouchings form on the kidney tubules and over time cysts form.

How Do Cysts Cause Loss Of Kidney Function?

No one knows for sure why cysts cause kidney function to decrease especially since only a few of the nephrons have cysts. One way may be that when the cysts get bigger they squeeze out the good nephrons. The result is to have one nephron with a big cyst where there may have been hundreds of good nephrons. With the loss of nephrons, there is a loss of kidney function. There may be other factors involved in loss of kidney function that remain to be found.

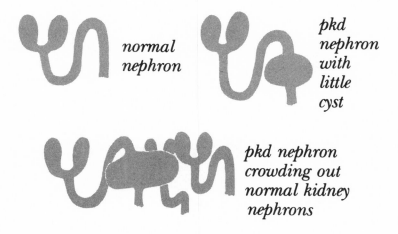

normal nephron

pkd nephron with little cyst

pkd nephron crowding out normal kidney nephrons

Figure 10.1.3. *Nephron with no cyst, with cyst, and with large cyst crowding out normal nephrons.*

How Does A Person Find Out If He Has ADPKD?

Sixty percent of the time there is a family history of ADPKD. Family history helps to see who is at risk to develop cysts. In general, the signs and symptoms of ADPKD are not specific enough to permit a doctor to know if a person has the disease or not. For example, although some people with ADPKD have back pain, so do many other people. A physical exam or a routine blood test alone will not show if a person has the disease.

It appears that ultrasound is one of the best screening tests for ADPKD. Ultrasound can detect nearly all cysts without the injection of dye or radiation. People who are negative on ultrasound but have several symptoms of PKD may be referred for further testing by CT scan. CT scan can pick up some very tiny cysts that cannot be seen by ultrasound. Because of this, some physicians use CT scan as the first test.

Another excellent and highly reliable screening method for PKD is gene linkage analysis. In families where this can be used it is 95 to 99% accurate in telling who in a family carries the PKD gene even before cysts develop.

What Does It Mean To Have ADPKD?

ADPKD is generally a slowly progressive disease. The advance to kidney failure is highly variable. It was once thought that kidney failure occurred at the same age in all family members. This does not seem to be the case. The severity of ADPKD can vary, even in the same family.

Does Everyone With ADPKD Eventually Have To Have Dialysis?

No. A recent study demonstrated that 50% of the people who have ADPKD will not require dialysis or transplantation up to 70 years of age. It is rare for anyone with ADPKD which appeared as an adult to develop kidney failure before age 40. People who have normal blood pressure seem to maintain kidney function longer.

What Kind Of Symptoms Are Associated With ADPKD?

Early in the disease there generally are no symptoms at all. In fact, many people are never diagnosed because they have so few symptoms. Often the first sign of ADPKD is blood in the urine or high blood pressure. Other signs and symptoms include: side or back pain, stomach pain, frequent urination, enlarged kidneys, headache, urinary tract infection, and kidney stones.

Are There Other Problems Associated With ADPKD?

ADPKD is not just a kidney disorder so other organs can be affected. The list that follows looks long and scary but remember most people don't have all of these problems. However, if you have ADPKD you should be aware of the possibilities so you can play a major role in taking care of yourself. It's like being a good driver; by knowing what can happen you can do a lot to prevent problems.

High blood pressure affects 60-70% of those with ADPKD. People with high blood pressure seem to have more and larger cysts than people who have normal blood pressure. The exact reason blood pressure increases is unknown.

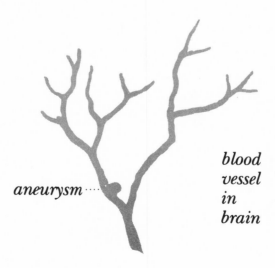

aneurysm

blood vessel in brain

Figure 10.1.4. *Blood vessels in the brain with an aneurysm.*

Urinary tract infection (UTI) can be a problem for those with ADPKD. The infection usually starts in the bladder and can travel up the ureters to the kidney. Women have more of a problem with infection because the tube (urethra) from the bladder to the outside is very short. Sometimes the infection gets into the cysts. This type of infection can be hard to treat and special antibiotics may have to be used.

Berry aneurysms occur in about 10% to 40% of those affected with ADPKD. An aneurysm is an outpouching in a blood vessel. Berry aneurysms occur on the large blood vessels of the brain. These aneurysms can burst or rupture. In that event loss of consciousness, stroke and even death can occur.

Berry aneurysms may run in families. That is if someone in your family had an aneurysm, you may be at a higher risk of having one also.

Not everyone needs to be tested for aneurysm, but if your doctor decides studies should be done, a screening test with a CT scan of the head may be done. In suspicious cases an arteriogram will prove whether or not you have an aneurysm. In some cases your doctor may decide to have the arteriogram done as the first test.

Because this is a potentially serious problem inform your doctor if you are a member of a family that has aneurysms.

Liver cysts occur in 40% to 70% of people with ADPKD. Liver cysts occur as often in men as in women. However, women get liver cysts at a younger age and they have more of them.

The liver can remain fairly normal in size or get to be quite large. Even though there is an increase in liver size, there is still the normal amount of liver tissue. This may be why people with liver cysts continue to have normal liver function.

Mitral valve prolapse (floppy heart valve) occurs in up to 30% of people with ADPKD. Sometimes when a valve is floppy, it may not close tightly between the times the heart beats (pumps). This may cause a small amount of blood to leak backwards before the heart beats again. This is called a heart murmur.

Sometimes a person with mitral valve prolapse feels like he has extra beats in his heart or that his heart is running away. These feelings are called palpitations and are usually not dangerous. Most people with mitral valve prolapse never even know they have it.

If you have mitral valve prolapse and a heart murmur, you may need to take an antibiotic before you have dental work or surgery to prevent the valve from becoming infected. Inform your dentist if you have mitral valve prolapse.

Hematuria (blood in the urine) occurs in 30% to 50% of those with ADPKD at some time. The urine can appear pink, red or the color of Coca-Cola®. The blood may appear only one time or can last days to several weeks.

The bleeding may start because the kidney has been injured; because blood vessels in the cyst wall get so stretched that they break; or because a cyst ruptures. It's more common for people with large kidneys and high blood pressure to have an episode of blood in the urine.

Often the bleeding can be accompanied by pain in the kidney area. It may require bed rest, pain medications and increased fluids. Rarely, a blood transfusion may be needed. Usually the bleeding stops by itself.

Kidney stones occur in about 20% of people with ADPKD and may be the cause of pain and blood in the urine. This kind of pain usually comes in waves and often travels from the back to the groin.

Diverticulae. Some, but not all physicians think that outpouchings called diverticulae can occur in the colon. If this happens in ADPKD it appears to be a problem in older people on dialysis. The main symptom is abdominal pain.

Other Cysts. There has been no association between cysts on the skin, scalp, or the breasts with ADPKD.

How Is ADPKD Passed On?

ADPKD is a hereditary disease. It is passed on from a parent with ADPKD to a child.

Every person has 23 pairs of chromosomes, making a total of 46. Twenty-two pairs are autosomes and one pair determines sex. The most common gene for ADPKD is on chromosome 16 which is an autosome. Because the gene is not on a sex chromosome, men and women have an equal chance of having this disease.

The chromosome pairs split in the formation of female eggs and male sperm. The woman donates 23 of her chromosomes to the baby in the egg and the man donates 23 of his in the sperm. In this way, when the egg is fertilized, the fetus will have the normal number of chromosomes. There are four possible ways the egg and the sperm can combine. In ADPKD two of the possibilities will contain the chromosome with the ADPKD gene and two will not. Therefore, each child of an affected parent has a 50% chance of also having the disease.

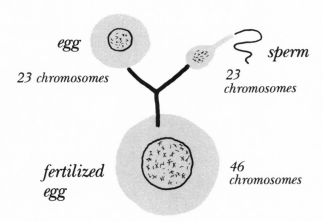

X	JC	‖	‖	X
1	2	3	4	5

K	K	A	H	X	X	H
6	7	8	9	10	11	12

‖	A	‖	A	A	‖
13	14	15	16	17	18

..	K	..		..	i	‖
19	20	21		22	x	y

chromosome 16 has the pkd gene

Figure 10.1.5. *Examples of normal amount of human chromosomes arranged in 23 pairs. Twenty-two of the pairs are called autosomes and one pair determines sex.*

egg

23 chromosomes

sperm

23 chromosomes

fertilized egg

46 chromosomes

Figure 10.1.6. *Female egg with 23 chromosomes (1 of each pair), sperm with 23 chromosomes (1 of each pair) and fertilized egg with 46 chromosomes (2 of each pair).*

If I Have Four Children Does this Mean That Two of My Children Will Have ADPKD and Two Will Not?

In real life it doesn't work out that two children will have the disease and two will not. The risk of a child having the disease is always 50% no matter how many children an affected parent has. It's like the flip of a coin. There is always a 50% chance of getting heads and a 50% chance of getting tails. In some families all of the children are affected and in other families, none are. The most common is to have affected and unaffected children in the same family.

In five to ten percent of affected people there is no ADPKD gene in either parent. This is called a spontaneous mutation. Reasons why these genes change are not known.

Does Everyone Who Has the Gene for ADPKD Have the Disease?

The gene for ADPKD is dominant. This means that if you have the gene you have ADPKD. If you do not have the gene you will not have the disease or pass it on to your children. A dominant gene does not hide or skip a generation. Some people who have the gene for ADPKD have so few symptoms that they may never be diagnosed with the disease.

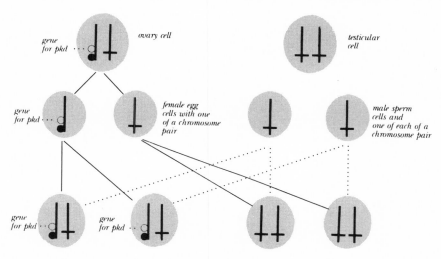

Figure 10.1.7. Example of how PKD is inherited: Two female eggs one with the gene for PKD and one without, two unaffected male sperms and four possible combinations of egg and sperm fertilization. The babies who inherit the PKD gene will have PKD. The babies who don't inherit the gene will not have PKD.

Is There a Blood Test That Will Show If I Have ADPKD?

Although we know that the most common gene for ADPKD is on chromosome 16, as yet we do not have the exact gene location. Therefore, there is no blood test (or other test) that will guarantee 100% you don't have the gene. When we have identified the gene itself, a simple blood test on one person will answer the question, "Do I have ADPKD?" Until then we use a technique called gene linkage analysis. To do this test other family members must be involved. They must also give blood and at least two of them must have the disease.

If you wanted to be tested by gene linkage analysis, blood would be needed from your affected parent and ideally an affected grandparent and perhaps another family member. This test can tell you if you have a 95% chance of having ADPKD, even before you have any symptoms or renal cysts.

This test is done through your doctor who will use a special laboratory to analyze the blood samples.

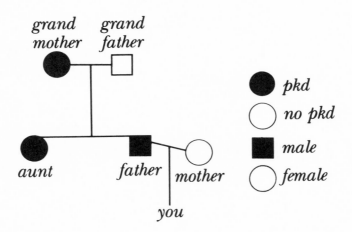

Figure 10.1.8. Gene linkage analysis.

If the Gene Linkage Analysis Is So Accurate and Can Detect the Disease Before Cysts Develop, Shouldn't this Be Used in Everyone Instead of Ultrasonography or CT Scan?

Ultrasonography is cheaper and only requires the person being tested to be involved. If it shows multiple bilateral renal cysts it is likely PKD is present. Ultrasonography also has the advantage of showing how many cysts are in the kidney and liver and how large they are. Cysts may not be present on ultrasonography in up to 50% of people with ADPKD before 20 years of age. Although CT scan is more expensive and has radiation, CT like ultrasonography, requires only the person be tested and also clearly shows kidney and liver cysts. Occasionally even CT scan may not show cysts, then gene linkage is the only way to make the diagnosis of ADPKD.

Should I Have Children If I Have ADPKD?

The decision to have children is a very personal one. Both the husband and wife need to discuss the risks involved and the possibilities of having a child with ADPKD. There is no right or wrong choice. Discussion with your physician or genetic counselor can be helpful in resolving this difficult issue.

Will Pregnancy Make My Kidneys Worse?

Pregnancy does not appear to make kidney function worse if blood pressure and kidney function are normal. However, there is an increased risk of developing new onset high blood pressure during the pregnancy.

Women who have ADPKD and become pregnant should be monitored closely for the development or worsening of high blood pressure, and bladder or kidney infection.

If a Husband or Wife Have ADPKD Can a Baby or Young Child Have Adult Type PKD Also?

Yes. It is now clear that ADPKD can occur as early as fetal life. If gene linkage can be used in your family, amniocentesis can be performed and then it is possible to say if the fetus has the ADPKD gene with less than five percent error rate. This test can also be performed in children. However, prenatal diagnosis or gene testing of children should only be done as part of overall care being given by a physician.

How Will this Affect My Children?

Most children with ADPKD do very well. This is especially true if the child has no symptoms, is diagnosed after one year of age and is identified just because of family screening. Children who present in the first year of life with very large kidneys may require dialysis or transplantation by adolescence or early adulthood. Sometimes children who have or are at risk for ADPKD develop high blood pressure. If they are known to have ADPKD, blood pressure should be checked regularly and treated if it is high for their age.

Should I Limit the Physical Activity of a Child with ADPKD?

There is no information to support limiting physical activity in any child simply because he or she has ADPKD. It is possible that children with really large kidneys or very large cysts might have more episodes of blood in the urine if they play contact sports such as football. However, there is no clear answer to this question and decisions must be made on an individual basis.

Should I Tell My Children They Have or Are at Risk for ADPKD?

To date, no research has been done on the effect such knowledge will have on children.

Generally speaking, there is no need to burden children with information they are too young to understand. They will ask questions as situations arise. However, when they enter reproductive age and/ or consider marriage they should be informed about ADPKD.

What Should I Do To Take Better Care of Myself If I Have ADPKD?

1. Know about ADPKD and have a regular doctor.
2. Don't take any prescribed or over-the-counter medication without checking with your doctor.

Blood Pressure. Blood pressure should be lowered to the normal range of 120/80. This is done with:

- Medication
- Weight loss (if overweight)
- Exercise

If you have ADPKD it may be helpful to have your own blood pressure cuff. Take and record your blood pressure several times a week and bring the readings to your doctor.

There are many different medications to treat high blood pressure. Work with your doctor to find the right one for you. Currently no one blood pressure medicine seems to be better than others for ADPKD.

Although it does not seem that the high blood pressure in ADPKD is caused directly by too much salt, it seems wise to avoid a high salt diet.

Urinary tract infection (UTI). If you have any of the following symptoms consult your doctor. Don't wait several days. Once the infection has started, it may not go away by itself.

- Pain or burning with urination
- Frequency or urgency to urinate
- Back pain associated with fever
- Blood in urine

Headache. Chronic headaches have not been associated with aneurysms in ADPKD. Most people have headaches at some time or other in their lives and some are worse than others.

If you get a headache that occurs all of a sudden and is unbearably painful, go to the emergency room and tell the doctor you may be at risk for aneurysm. A different kind of headache like this may often be associated with:

- Pain on movement of the neck
- Paralysis in moving the eyes

Hematuria (blood in the urine). If you have blood in your urine:

- Let your doctor know
- Drink plenty of fluids

111

- Bed rest if the bleeding continues
- Do not take aspirin or non steroidal anti-inflammatory agents such as Motrin® or Nuprin® as they may prolong the bleeding.

Children. Children at risk of developing ADPKD should be checked yearly for:

- High blood pressure
- White blood cells in urine
- Red blood cells in urine
- Enlarged kidneys

If any of the above occurs, your doctor may wish to have ultrasonography (US) performed. Increased blood pressure should also be treated.

In general children with ADPKD need not have any restrictions placed on their activities.

How Active Can I Be If I Have ADPKD?

Physical fitness has become very important in today's world. With exercise people are enjoying the benefits of greater stamina, improved sense of well being, and perhaps lower blood pressure.

What kinds of exercise are best?

Generally speaking, you can do any exercise you want unless you get blood in the urine or continued back pain. The exercises which are least jarring are:

- Swimming
- Walking
- Biking

The key is to find an activity that is comfortable for you and that you enjoy doing. Also, exercise on a regular basis.

Is There A Special Diet That Will Make My Kidneys Better Or Keep Them From Getting Worse?

At this time there is no specific diet that will make polycystic kidneys better or keep them from getting worse. However, one of the major functions of the kidneys is to remove waste products from the body. The major source of these waste products is the food we eat, especially protein. When kidney function is lost, these waste products back up in the blood and cause the symptoms associated with kidney failure.

When a person has lost a significant amount of kidney function his doctor may put him on a low protein diet. The Polycystic Kidney Research Foundation, 922 Walnut Street, Kansas City, MO 64106 has a diet book, *Your Diet and Polycystic Kidney Disease,* that will help better understand this type of diet.

For those who have a mild to moderate loss of kidney function, a decrease in the amount and type of protein eaten may be better for their kidneys.

Some studies done on both animals and humans show that eating large amounts of protein at one time causes the kidneys to work harder than when eating smaller amounts of protein. Currently the National Institute of Health is conducting a very large study which includes ADPKD patients. This study will seek answers to the question about protein in the diet in kidney disease. In the meantime, it may be wise to avoid excessive meat intake particularly once some impairment of renal function has occurred.

Should I Stop Eating Salt?

High blood pressure in ADPKD does not seem to be caused by salt. However, probably a high salt diet should be avoided.

Can I Drink Alcohol?

There is no information about alcoholic beverages and ADPKD specifically. However, there is data to show that three or more drinks per day can cause high blood pressure. This effect on blood pressure would not be desirable in ADPKD.

How Much Fluid Should I Drink Each Day?

Your body is set up to regulate your water needs. You should drink when you are thirsty. There is no research to suggest that a high fluid intake helps in ADPKD. It makes sense to avoid large amounts of caffeinated beverages such as coffee, tea, and cola drinks.

Should I Take Extra Vitamins to Make Sure I Am Getting All the Nutrients I Need?

A person who eats a fairly regular diet does not need extra vitamins. Unlike food, vitamins are needed only in tiny amounts. Excess amounts of vitamins A, D and E can accumulate in the body and cause medical problems. Generally, if you feel you need extra vitamins, a generic brand one-a-day vitamin is sufficient. Consult your physician before taking extra vitamins of any kind.

What Kind Of Tests Will I Usually Have Done If I Have ADPKD?

Blood tests are often done. The two common tests for kidney function are creatinine and BUN.

Creatinine is a measure of kidney function. As kidney function decreases, blood creatinine values increase. Normal range in adults is 0.6 to 1.4 mg/dl.

Blood urea nitrogen (BUN) is another measure of kidney function. As your kidney function decreases your BUN increases. Normal range is 6 to 15 mg/dl.

A number of factors such as diet and protein intake can affect BUN, but not creatinine. Therefore, creatinine is usually followed more regularly.

Liver function tests (LFT) are also blood tests. Liver function is almost always normal even if there are cysts in the liver.

Urine tests

Red Blood Cells (RBC) in urine. RBC's are not normally in the urine. Sometimes people with ADPKD pass a few RBC. As discussed earlier, sometimes a lot of blood can occur in the urine.

White Blood Cells (WSC) in urine. WBC's are also not present normally in urine although some people with ADPKD do pass a few. However, large numbers can suggest an infection. If your doctor sees large numbers of WBC, the doctor may order a urine culture to determine if an infection is present before you take antibiotics.

Protein in urine. Some people with ADPKD lose small amounts of protein in their urine. Usually this is not a sufficient amount to cause problems.

24 hour urine collection. This test is done in combination with the blood creatinine to determine an aspect of kidney function called creatinine clearance or GFR. This test measures how well your kidneys are working and how much kidney function you have.

Imaging Studies

These are studies to see or image organs and/or blood vessels in your body.

Ultrasonography (US). This is a test done with sound waves. It does not require any dyes to be taken or injected. It has no radiation. It can be done safely in pregnant women, children, and adults. It is often used for screening in ADPKD because it shows the kidneys and liver well. If cysts are very tiny they can occasionally be missed by ultrasonography.

A study similar to ultrasonography, called echocardiography uses sound waves to see the heart valves. This study might be done if your doctor thinks you have mitral valve prolapse.

Computed axial tomography (CT Scan). This is a very sophisticated x-ray. CT scan uses radiation and often dye is injected into the blood to better see the organ. CT scan can be used to examine the kidneys, liver and brain. CT scan will show even small cysts in the kidney or liver. CT scan is also a very helpful test for ADPKD complications such as bleeding into the cysts or kidney stones. CT scan can also see many brain aneurysms.

Magnetic resonance imaging (MRI). MRI takes pictures of your inner organs like CT scan does. However, it doesn't require radiation or contrast media. Although kidney cysts are easily seen, at present

MRI doesn't seem any better for diagnosis of ADPKD than ultrasonography.

Arteriogram. An arteriogram is a study of blood vessels in which an x-ray dye is injected into the blood vessel in order to clearly see the vessel. This test is used in some circumstances to study blood vessels in the brain for aneurysm.

References

1. Dalgaard OZ. Bilateral polycystic disease of the kidneys: a follow-up of two hundred and eighty-four patients and their families. *Acta Med Scand* 1957;158:328–329.
2. Gabow PA, Ikle DW, Holmes JH. Polycystic kidney disease: prospective analysis of nonazotemic patients and family members. *Annals of Internal Medicine*. 1984;101:238–247.
3. Grantham JJ, Gabow PA. Diseases of the kidney. 4th Ed. In Schrier RW and Gottschalk CW. Boston: Little, Brown and CO, 1988; 583–616.
4. Grantham JJ, Gardner KD, Editors. Problems in Diagnosis and Management of Polycystic Kidney Disease—Proceedings of the First International Workshop, Kansas City; PKR Foundation, 1985.

—by Irene Duley, RN, and Patricia Gabow, MD.

Section 10.2

Additional Resources on PKD

Searches-On-File, Topics in Kidney and Urologic Diseases, NKUDIC.

Legend

TI Title
AU Author
CN Corporate Author
SO Source
PD Product
AV Producer/Availability

TI Acquired Renal Cystic Disease.
AU Ishikawa, I.
SO In: Gardner, K.D.; Bernstein, J., eds. *The Cystic Kidney*. Hingham, MA: Kluwer Academic Publishers. 1990. p. 352–377.
AV Available from Kluwer Academic Publishers. P.O. Box 358, Accord Station, Hingham, MA 02018. (617) 871-6600. Price: $166.50. ISBN: 079230392X. Orders must be prepaid.

TI *Advances in the Pathogenesis of Polycystic Kidney Disease: Proceedings of the Conference Held on September 17–18, 1987.*
AU Carone, F.A.; Dobbie, J.W.
SO Kansas City, MO: Polycystic Kidney Research Foundation. 1990. 181 p.
AV Available from Polycystic Kidney Research Foundation, 922 Walnut Street, Suite 411, Kansas City, MO 64106. (816) 421-1869. Price: $35.00 ($29.95 for members) plus $2.50 shipping and handling.

TI **Autosomal Dominant Polycystic Kidney Disease.**
AU Gabow, P.A.
SO In: Gardner. K.D.; Berstein, J., eds. *The Cystic Kidney.*
Hingham, MA: Kluwer Academic Publishers. 1990. p. 296–326.
AV Available from Kluwer Academic Publishers. P.O. Box 358, Accord Station, Hingham, MA 02018. (617) 871-6600. Price: $166.50. ISBN: 079230392X. Orders must be prepaid.

TI **Autosomal Dominant Polycystic Kidney Disease and End Stage Renal Disease.**
AU Barrett, B.J.; Parfrey, P.S.
SO *Seminars in Dialysis.* 4(1): 26–32. January-March 1991.
AV Available from Blackwell Scientific Publications, 238 Main Street, Cambridge, MA 02142. (617) 876-7000.

TI *Autosomal Dominant Polycystic Kidney Disease (ADPKD).*
SO Rochester, MN: Mayo Clinic. 1991. 10 p.
CN Mayo Clinic. Patient and Health Education Center.
AV Available from Mayo Clinic. Patient and Health Education Center, 200 First Street, SW, Rochester, MN 55905. (507) 284-2511. Price: $2.75 plus shipping and handling. Order number MC 102/R391.

TI **Autosomal Dominant Polycystic Kidney Disease: More Than A Renal Disease.**
AU Gabow, P.A.
SO *American Journal of Kidney Diseases.* 16(5): 403–413. November 1990.
AV Available from National Kidney Foundation. 30 East 33rd Street, New York, NY 10016. (212) 889-2210 or (800) 622-9010.

TI **Autosomal Recessive Polycystic Kidney Disease.**
AU Cole, B.R.
SO In: Gardner, K.D.; Bernstein, J., eds. *The Cystic Kidney.*
Hingham, MA: Kluwer Academic Publishers. 1990. p. 327–350.
AV Available from Kluwer Academic Publishers. P.O. Box 358, Accord Station, Hingham, MA 02018. (617) 871-4600. Price: $166.50. ISBN: 079230392X. Orders must be prepaid.

TI *Breakpoint Break for Consortium Studying Adult Polycystic Kidney Disease.*
AU Wunderle, V., et al.
SO Cell. Volume 77: 785–786. June 17, 1994.

TI *Candidate Gene Associated with a Mutation Causing Recessive Polycystic Kidney Disease in Mice.*
AU Moyer, J.H., et al.
SO Science. 264(5163): 1329–1333. May 27, 1994.
AV Available from American Association for the Advancement of Science. 1333 H Street, NW, Washington, DC 20005.

TI **Congenital Multicystic Kidney.**
AU Piel, C.F.
SO In: Gardner, K.D.; Bernstein, J., eds. *The Cystic Kidney.* Hingham, MA: Kluwer Academic Publishers. 1990. p. 393–411.
AV Available from Kluwer Academic Publishers. P.O. Box 358, Accord Station, Hingham, MA 02018. (617) 8714600. Price: $166.50. ISBN: 079230392X. Orders must be prepaid.

TI *Cystic Kidney.*
AU Gardner, K.D.; Bernstein, J., eds.
SO Hingham, MA: Kluwer Academic Publishers. 1990. 453 p.
AV Available from Kluwer Academic Publishers. P.O. Box 358, Accord Station, Hingham, MA 02018. (617) 871-6600. Price: $166.50. ISBN: 079230392X. Orders must be prepaid.

TI *Living with Inherited Kidney Disease: We Asked the Experts.*
AU Smith, B.; Plumridge, D.
SO Renalife. p. 12–14. Fall 1989.
AV Available from American Association of Kidney Patients. 100 South Ashley Drive, Suite 280, Tampa, FL 33602. (813) 223-7099 or (800) 749-2257.

TI **Ethical Issues and Cystic Kidneys.**
AU Weil, W.B.
SO In: Gardner, K.D.; Berstein, J., eds. *The Cystic Kidney.* Hingham, MA: Kluwer Academic Publishers. 1990. p. 278–291.
AV Available from Kluwer Academic Publishers. P.O. Box 358, Accord Station, Hingham, MA 02018. (617) 871-6600. Price: $166.50. ISBN: 079230392X. Orders must be prepaid.

TI   **Genetic Variant of Polycystic Kidney Disease.**
AU   Swyers, J.P.
SO   *Research Resources Reporter*. 13(12): 14, 11–12. December 1989.
AV   Available from Research Resources Information Center. 1601 Research Boulevard, Rockville, MD 20850. (301) 984-2870.

TI   **Genetics of Renal Cystic Disease.**
AU   Reeders, S.E.
SO   In: Gardner, K.D.; Bernstein, J., eds. *The Cystic Kidney*. Hingham, MA: Kluwer Academic Publishers. 1990. p. 117–143.
AV   Available from Kluwer Academic Publishers. P.O. Box 358, Accord Station, Hingham, MA 02018. (617) 871-6600. Price: $166.50. ISBN: 079230392X. Orders must be prepaid.

TI   ***Introduction to Autosomal Dominant Polycystic Kidney Disease of The Adult-Onset Type.***
SO   Kansas City, MO: Polycystic Kidney Research (PKR) Foundation. 1993. 2 p.
CN   PKR Foundation.
AV   Available from PKR Foundation. 922 Walnut Street, Kansas City, MO 64106. (816) 421-869. Single copy free.

TI   **Management of Cystic Kidney Disease.**
AU   Bennett, W.M.; Elzinga, L.W.; Barry, J.M.
SO   In: Gardner, K.D.; Bernstein, J., eds. *The Cystic Kidney*. Hingham, MA: Kluwer Academic Publishers. 1990. p. 247–275.
AV   Available from Kluwer Academic Publishers. P.O. Box 358, Accord Station, Hingham, MA 02018. (617) 871-6600. Price: $166.50. ISBN: 079230392X. Orders must be prepaid.

TI   **Natural History of Autosomal Dominant Polycystic Kidney Disease.**
AU   Fick, G.M.; Gabow, P.A.
SO   In: Coggins, C.H.; Hancock, E.W., eds. *Annual Review of Medicine: Selected Topics in the Clinical Sciences*, Volume 45. Palo Alto, CA: Annual Reviews Inc. 1994. p. 23–29.
AV   Available from Annual Reviews Inc. 4139 El Camino Way, P.O. Box 10139, Palo Alto, CA 94303-0139. (800) 523-8635. Fax: (415) 855-9815. Price: $47.00. ISBN: 0824305450.

TI *Notes from the Baxter PKRF Roundtable on Polycystic Kidney Disease.*
AU Biancarosa, T.
SO Kansas City, MO: Polycystic Kidney Research Foundation. 1989. 2 p.
AV Available from Polycystic Kidney Research Foundation. Suite 411, 922 Walnut Street, Kansas City, MO 64106. (816) 421-1869.

TI *PKD Patient's Manual: Understanding and Living with Autosomal Dominant Polycystic Kidney Disease.*
AU Duley, I.; Gabow, P.
SO Kansas City, MO: Polycystic Kidney Research Foundation. 1989. 24 p.
AV Available from Polycystic Kidney Research Foundation. 922 Walnut Street, Kansas City, MO 64106. (800) PKD-CURE. Price: $4.95 (members) or $7.95 (nonmembers), plus $1.00 shipping and handling.

TI **Polycystic and Acquired Cystic Diseases.**
AU Gabow, P.A.
SO In: Greenberg; A., et al, eds. *Primer on Kidney Diseases*. New York, NY: National Kidney Foundation. 1994. p. 201–206.
AV Available from Academic Press. Order Fulfillment, 6277 Sea Harbor Drive, Orlando, FL 32887. (800) 321-5068. Price: Paperback $49.95 (paper) ISBN: 0122992318, or $99.00 (hardback) ISBN: 012299230X.

TI **Polycystic Kidney Disease I Gene Encodes a 14 kb Transcript and Lies Within a Duplicated Region on Chromosome 16.**
SO *Cell*. Volume 77: 881–894. June 17, 1994.
CN European Polycystic Kidney Disease Consortium.

TI **Polycystic and Acquired Cystic Diseases.**
AU Gabow, P.A.
SO In: Greenberg, A., et al., eds. *Primer on Kidney Diseases*. New York, NY: National Kidney Foundation. 1994. p. 201–206.
AV Available from Academic Press. Order Fulfillment, 6277 Sea Harbor Drive, Orlando, FL 32887. (800) 321-5068. Price: Paperback $49.95 (paper) ISBN: 0122992318, OR $99.00 (hardback) ISBN: 012299230X.

TI **Polycystic Kidney Disease.**
SO New York NY: National Kidney Foundation, Inc. 1990. 2 p.
CN National Kidney Foundation, Inc.
AV Available from the National Kidney Foundation, Inc. 30 East 33rd Street, New York, NY 10016. (800) 622-9010. Price: Single Copy free. Order No. 08–45.

TI **Proceedings of the Fifth International Workshop on Polycystic Kidney Disease.**
AU Gabow, P.A.; Grantham, J.J., eds.
SO Kansas City, MO: PKR Foundation. 1993. 181 p.
AV Available from PKR Foundation. 922 Walnut Street, Suite 411, Kansas City, MO 64106. (800) 753-2873; (816) 421-1869. Price: $33.95 for members; $39.00 for nonmembers, includes shipping and handling. ISBN: 096145671X.

TI **Q and A on PKD**
SO Kansas City, MO: Polycystic Kidney Research Foundation. April 1988. 21 p.
CN Polycystic Kidney Research Foundation.
AV Available from Polycystic Kidney Research Foundation. International Headquarters. 922 Walnut Street, Suite 411, Kansas City, MO 64106. (816) 421-1869. Also available from National Kidney and Urologic Diseases Information Clearinghouse. 3 Information Way, Bethesda, MD 20892-3580; (301) 654-1415.

TI **Renal Cystic Disorders.**
AU Grantham, J.J.; Reekling, J.B.; Slusher, S.L.
SO In: Suki, W.N.; Massry, S.G., eds. *Therapy of Renal Diseases and Related Disorders*, 2nd ed. Hingham, MA: Kluwer Academic Publishers. 1991. p. 543–572.
AV Available from Kluwer Academic Publishers. P.O. Box 358, Accord Station, Hingham, MA 02018. (617) 871-6600. Price: $279.95. ISBN: 0792306767.

TI **Using Watson's Theory to Explore the Dimensions of Adult Polycystic Kidney Disease.**
AU Martin, L.S.
SO *American Nephrology Nurses' Association Journal. (ANNA Journal)*. 18(5): 493–496, 499. October 1991.
AV Available from American Nephrology Nurses' Association. Box 56, North Woodbury Road, Pitman, NJ 08071. (609) 589-2187.

TI *Your Child, Your Family and Autosomal Recessive Polycystic Kidney Disease.*

AU Cole, B.R.; Stapleton, F.B.; Guay-Woodford, L.

SO Kansas City, MO: Polycystic Kidney Research Foundation. 1992. 26 p.

AV Available from Polycystic Kidney Research Foundation. 922 Walnut Street, Suite 411, Kansas City, MO 64106. (800) PKD-CURE. Price: $7.00 plus $1.00 (for members); $10.00 plus $1.00 (for non-members).

TI *Your Diet and Polycystic Kidney Disease.*

AU Fryer, P., et al.

SO Kansas City, MO: Polycystic Kidney Research Foundation. 29 p.

CN Polycystic Kidney Research Foundation.

AV Available from Polycystic Kidney Research Foundation. 922 Walnut Street, Kansas City, MO 64106. (816) 421-1869. Price: $2.00 each plus $1.00 for postage and handling.

Chapter 11

Analgesic-Associated Kidney Disease

Introduction

Ingestion of large amounts of some pain-relieving drugs over long periods of time has been shown to be associated with the development of one type of kidney disease that can lead to kidney failure. Since this problem was first reported in the 1950s, analgesic-associated kidney disease has become recognized as a significant, costly, and potentially preventable and treatable health problem. While research has shown an association of analgesic ingestion with kidney disease, there continues to be debate about the specific drugs that cause it, the mechanisms by which renal damage occurs, and the extent to which this illness may contribute to the overall burden of chronic renal disease in our society. The distributor and prevalence of analgesic-associated kidney disease appear to vary widely in different countries of the world and within the countries where it has been shown to occur.

In an effort to resolve some of the questions about this type of kidney disease, the National Institutes of Health convened a Consensus Development Conference on Analgesic-Associated Kidney Disease on February 27-29, 1984. After a day and a half of scientific presentations by experts of the available data about the problem, a Consensus Panel including representatives of the fields of nephrology, pathology, internal medicine, family medicine, pharmacology, biostatistics, and

NIH Consensus Development Conference Statement, Vol. 5, Number 2, February 1984.

epidemiology, and of the general public considered the scientific evidence and agreed on answers to the following questions:

1. Can analgesics, alone or in combination, cause kidney disease and chronic kidney failure? What evidence supports these conclusions?

2. What are the scope and characteristics of the problem of kidney disease caused excessive use of analgesics in the United States and in other countries?

3. What causes analgesic-associated kidney disease?

4. What factors increase the risk of occurrence of analgesic-associated kidney disease?

5. Can analgesic-associated kidney disease be prevented?

6. What treatment strategies are appropriate?

7. What are the directions for future research?

Panel's Conclusions

Considerable evidence indicates that combinations of antipyretic analgesics, taken in large doses over a long period of time, cause a specific form of kidney disease and chronic renal failure. Persons so exposed may also be more susceptible to the subsequent development of uroepithelial tumors. In contrast, there is little evidence that preparations containing a single analgesic agent have been similarly abused and are similarly harmful.

The occurrence of analgesic-associated nephropathy shows striking geographical differences. Such differences may be related, at least in part, to regional variations in the habitual consumption of antipyretic-analgesic mixtures. The pathogenesis of the condition is uncertain but may involve a direct cytotoxic action of the analgesics on the renal papilla, perhaps enhanced by ischemia.

The sustained use of mixtures of antipyretic analgesics in large doses is not advisable. Serious consideration should be given to limiting over-the-counter products to those containing a single antipyretic-analgesic agent.

Can analgesics, alone or in combination, cause kidney disease and chronic renal failure? What evidence supports these conclusions?

The weight of evidence supports the view that combinations of antipyretic analgesics taken in large doses over long periods of time can cause kidney disease and chronic renal failure.

No evidence has been presented, however, to indicate that single antipyretic-analgesic drugs cause chronic renal disease when taken in the smaller doses usually prescribed by physicians or taken for valid medical reasons in doses recommended by the manufacturer.

Three types of evidence support these conclusions.

Clinical. A characteristic clinical and pathological picture of a chronic tubulo-interstitial disease of the kidneys has emerged from many case reports. It is seen in patients who have consumed large quantities of antipyretic-analgesic mixtures, often in powder form. The disease is slowly progressive and commonly asymptomatic until severe renal failure occurs, although renal damage can be detected earlier by laboratory tests of the kidney's excretory or concentrating abilities. Papillary necrosis and interstitial scarring are characteristic; the disorder may be manifest clinically by urinary passage of necrotic tissue or by urography and signaled by sterile pyuria and low fixed urinary specific gravity.

The condition is seen mainly in women who take large doses of analgesic mixtures daily over long periods of time. Many of them may also exhibit gastrointestinal disorders, anemia, and emotional disturbances.

When persons with analgesic nephropathy stop ingesting analgesic mixtures, progression of the renal disease may be retarded or even reversed. In contrast, if they continue to consume the analgesics, the disease usually progresses.

Epidemiological. Although the epidemiological evidence is limited, certain studies, especially in areas of high consumption outside the United States, support an association between the heavy use of analgesic mixtures and chronic renal disease, particularly papillary necrosis. For example, in one geographic area, the relative risk for developing papillary necrosis was 17 times higher in heavy users than in non-users. In another, prolonged use of phenacetin-containing analgesics by a group of working women studied over a 10-year period was associated with a significant increase in impaired renal function; an increased mortality from cardiovascular and renal disorders was also reported.

Analgesic nephropathy, including papillary necrosis, is most common in regions where the consumption and/or sale of analgesic mixtures is high. Furthermore, where the sale of such compounds has been effectively restricted, the prevalence of the disease appears to have diminished.

Certain evidence also suggests that very heavy and sustained use of some analgesic mixtures may predispose to cancer of the urinary tract, particularly transitional cell carcinoma of the renal pelvis.

Experimental. Large doses of analgesics, including aspirin, phenacetin, acetaminophen, and combinations of these, cause renal papillary necrosis in animals. The period of drug exposure in animal studies has been shorter than that in humans, while the dose necessary to produce injury has often been very high. For these and other reasons, the applicability of animal studies to human disease may be questioned; nevertheless, the demonstration in animals of a type of nephrotoxicity similar to that reported in humans lends weight to a causal association between analgesic abuse and kidney disease. The results of laboratory studies have suggested biochemical mechanisms by which phenacetin or its metabolites, as well as salicylates, may produce tissue damage in the kidney.

What are the scope and characteristics of the problem of kidney disease caused by excessive use of analgesics in the United States and in other countries?

Determining the magnitude and scope of the problem of analgesic-associated nephropathy is difficult. It is relatively easy to identify patients with analgesic nephropathy who have advanced or end-stage renal disease, but earlier or milder cases are difficult to identify. However, the latter must be taken into account to assess fully the potential public health problem.

The magnitude of the problem in its various degrees of severity can be viewed in at least three ways: the frequency of occurrence in the population at large, the frequency of occurrence in persons taking antipyretic analgesics, and the burden that treating the condition imposes on medical and financial resources.

Frequency in the General Population. In the United States, end-stage renal disease due to analgesic nephropathy is rare, occurring roughly on the order of one new case per million population per year. However, in some areas, such as parts of the Southeast, where the use of powders containing combinations of analgesics is more common, the incidence is higher, perhaps on the order of 10 per million per year. The incidence is also higher in areas of Belgium, Australia, and Scotland; in Switzerland, the crude incidence has been estimated to be as high as 15 per million per year.

Data on the incidence or prevalence of less severe analgesic nephropathy in the general population are limited, but its frequency is probably several times that of end-stage analgesic nephropathy.

Frequency in Analgesic Users. The proportion of analgesic users who develop analgesic nephropathy is not known. Evidence of at least moderately impaired kidney function was found to occur in a substantial proportion of a group of working women in Switzerland who took phenacetin-containing analgesics regularly.

There is no evidence that persons taking any antipyretic analgesics occasionally for headaches or other pains develop analgesic nephropathy. Similarly, advanced analgesic nephropathy is rare even among patients for whom regular or frequent use of analgesics is prescribed by physicians. The lack of data about the extent of use of these drugs in the general population, particularly heavy use, makes it very difficult to correlate the occurrence of analgesic nephropathy with the amount of analgesics taken by individuals.

Financial and Medical Care Burden. In most of the United States, analgesic nephropathy accounts for about 2 percent of end-stage renal disease. In northwestern North Carolina, this figure may be as high as 10 percent. If we assume the 2- percent figure, the minimal cost of caring for such patients nationally would be at least $40 million per year, given an estimated annual cost for end-stage renal disease of $2 billion. Thus, even though severe renal failure due to analgesic nephropathy is infrequent in the United States, its financial impact on society is significant.

There are no data to indicate the undoubtedly substantial costs of care for less severe analgesic nephropathy.

What causes analgesic-associated kidney disease?

Four clinical and experimental features are relevant to the pathogenesis of analgesic nephropathy. (1) The disease is most commonly associated with the ingestion of analgesic mixtures in large doses over a prolonged time. (2) The initial lesion occurs in the papilla; changes in the cortex are secondary to papillary damage. (3) Papillary necrosis may be accentuated experimentally and in certain patients by dehydration and low urine volumes. (4) The major phenacetin metabolite, acetaminophen, as well as salicylates, is concentrated on the papilla, particularly during low urine output. These features suggest that the disease results from the effects of a toxic agent or agents in the renal papilla, but the precise pathogenetic mechanisms are still unclear.

Present evidence suggests that acetaminophen causes tissue injury as a result of its conversion to toxic metabolites. By lowering the concentration of glutathione, a substance that protects against such tissue injury, aspirin and other salicylates enhance toxicity. Salicylates and acetaminophen also inhibit prostaglandin synthesis and thus may, by reducing medullary blood flow, potentiate papillary damage. These data offer attractive though yet unproven explanations for the synergistic effects of phenacetin and aspirin in causing papillary necrosis. They also suggest avenues for research into interactions of other analgesic and anti-inflammatory drugs that may lead to renal disease.

What factors increase the risk of its occurrence?

Clinical studies suggest that the risk of developing analgesic nephropathy depends largely on the magnitude and duration of consumption of analgesic mixtures. This in turn is often influenced by cultural acceptance, promotion and availability of the drugs, occupational stress, and regional patterns of overuse of analgesics. Consumption of over-the-counter analgesic mixtures may be enhanced by the inclusion of stimulant drugs such as caffeine and the packaging of the compounds as powder. Additional risk factors, such as hot climate, laxative abuse, and genetic predisposition, have been suggested but not established.

Can it be prevented?

Current evidence suggests that the key to the prevention of analgesic nephropathy is to halt the inappropriate use of analgesics. It should therefore be possible to adopt measures to reduce its incidence substantially, as has already been undertaken in Canada.

In as much as no therapeutic indication has been established for combining antipyretic-analgesic agents, serious consideration should now be given to the withdrawal of such mixed analgesic drugs from over-the-counter use in the United States. Such a measure appears to have reduced the occurrence of analgesic nephropathy in several countries. In Australia, however, when phenacetin in analgesic mixtures was replaced by either salicylamide or acetaminophen, the incidence of end-stage renal disease due to analgesic nephropathy did not fall.

Preparations containing single antipyretic analgesics such as aspirin or acetaminophen should remain available as over-the-counter medications, since there is no evidence that their occasional use is related to analgesic nephropathy. The risk from prolonged use of single-ingredient analgesics appears to be small. Patients who require prolonged high intake of analgesics, however, including nonsteroidal anti-inflammatory drugs, should be observed for the possible appearance of renal dysfunction at an early and potentially reversible stage. A high fluid intake, especially in warm climates, may be helpful in avoiding concentration of salicylates or acetaminophen in the renal papilla.

What treatment strategies are appropriate?

Patients with an established diagnosis of analgesic nephropathy should avoid taking antipyretic analgesics, especially of the mixed variety. If renal insufficiency is not advanced, renal function is likely to stabilize or even improve when analgesics are stopped. Even when renal insufficiency is well advanced, cessation of analgesic intake often slows the rate of loss of renal function.

The main strategies of management must include:

1. Avoidance of antipyretic-analgesic agents, as well as nonsteroidal anti-inflammatory drugs.

2. Prompt treatment of proven urinary tract infections.

3. Awareness that a necrotic papilla may slough and obstruct the urinary tract, sometimes requiring prompt intervention to prevent further loss of renal function.

4. Careful supervision of hypertension.

5. Recognition that tumors of the urinary tract may occur more frequently in patients with analgesic nephropathy. Unexplained episodes of hematuria, including a marked increase in microscopic hematuria, should therefore be evaluated carefully.

6. Consideration of the non-renal manifestations of the analgesic abuse syndrome.

What are the directions for future research?

Epidemiological research is needed in several areas. More data are needed on the prevalence and extent of analgesic use, as well as the characteristics that predispose persons to heavy use and abuse, in each region of the United States. There is a need to evaluate the impact of measures designed to reduce analgesic abuse on the incidence of analgesic nephropathy. Moreover, it is important to establish the incidence of analgesic nephropathy in users of single-ingredient analgesics, as well as of nonsteroidal anti-inflammatory agents. Further basic epidemiological research is needed to elucidate the relationship between analgesic use and mild forms of the disease.

It seems possible that certain people are more susceptible than others to kidney injury from analgesics. Research is needed on the factors that may predispose patients to such injury. These include genetic constitution, variations in drug disposition, physiological factors such as hormonal status or state of hydration, sex, age, and environmental circumstances.

While some of the chemical reactions leading to the formation of cytotoxic metabolites have been characterized, further basic research is needed to study the nature of the toxic metabolites, the ultimate mechanisms of acute and chronic cell injury in various components of the papilla, the role of ischemic versus toxic factors, and the interactions among various drugs in causing papillary damage. More information is required on the relationship between analgesic nephropathy and uroepithelial cancer.

Chapter 12

Diabetes and Kidney Disease

Chapter Contents

Section 12.1

An Overview of Kidney Disease of Diabetes

NIH Publication No. 95–3925, July 1995.

Each year in the United States, more than 50,000 people are diagnosed with end-stage renal disease (ESRD), a serious condition in which the kidneys fail to rid the body of wastes. ESRD is the final stage of a slow deterioration of the kidneys, a process known as nephropathy.

Diabetes is the most common cause of ESRD, resulting in about one-third of new ESRD cases. Even when drugs and diet are able to control diabetes, the disease can lead to nephropathy and ESRD. Most people with diabetes do not develop nephropathy that is severe enough to cause ESRD. About 15 million people in the United States have diabetes, and about 50,000 people have ESRD as a result of diabetes.

ESRD patients undergo either dialysis, which substitutes for some of the filtering functions of the kidneys, or transplantation to receive a healthy donor kidney. Most U.S. citizens who develop ESRD are eligible for federally funded care. In 1994, the Federal Government spent about $9.3 billion on care for patients with ESRD.

African Americans and Native Americans develop diabetes, nephropathy, and ESRD at rates higher than average. Scientists have not been able to explain these higher rates. Nor can they explain fully the interplay of factors

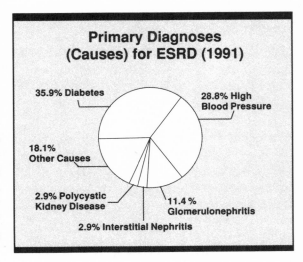

Primary Diagnoses (Causes) for ESRD (1991)

35.9% Diabetes

28.8% High Blood Pressure

18.1% Other Causes

2.9% Polycystic Kidney Disease

11.4% Glomerulonephritis

2.9% Interstitial Nephritis

leading to diabetic nephropathy—factors including heredity, diet, and other medical conditions, such as high blood pressure. They have found that high blood pressure and high levels of blood sugar increase the risk that a person with diabetes will progress to ESRD.

Two Types of Diabetes

In diabetes—also called diabetes mellitus, or DM—the body does not properly process and use certain foods, especially carbohydrates. The human body normally converts carbohydrates to glucose, the simple sugar that is the main source of energy for the body's cells. To enter cells, glucose needs the help of insulin, a hormone produced by the pancreas. When a person does not make enough insulin, or the body is unable to use the insulin that is present, the body cannot process glucose, and it builds up in the bloodstream. High levels of glucose in the blood or urine lead to a diagnosis of diabetes.

NIDDM. Most people with diabetes have a form known as noninsulin-dependent diabetes (NIDDM), or Type II diabetes. Many people with NIDDM do not respond normally to their own or to injected insulin—a condition called insulin resistance. NIDDM occurs more often in people over the age of 40, and many people with NIDDM are overweight. Many also are not aware that they have the disease. Some people with NIDDM control their blood sugar with diet and an exercise program leading to weight loss. Others must take pills that stimulate production of insulin; still others require injections of insulin.

IDDM. A less common form of diabetes, known as insulin-dependent diabetes (IDDM), or Type I diabetes, tends to occur in young adults and children. In cases of IDDM, the body produces little or no insulin. People with IDDM must receive daily insulin injections.

NIDDM accounts for about 95 percent of all cases of diabetes; IDDM accounts for about 5 percent. Both types of diabetes can lead to kidney disease. IDDM is more likely to lead to ESRD. About 40 percent of people with IDDM develop severe kidney disease and ESRD by the age of 50. Some develop ESRD before the age of 30. NIDDM causes 80 percent of the ESRD in African Americans and Native Americans.

The Course of Kidney Disease

The deterioration that characterizes kidney disease of diabetes takes place in and around the glomeruli, the blood-filtering units of the kidneys. Early in the disease, the filtering efficiency diminishes, and important proteins in the blood are lost to the urine. Medical professionals gauge the presence and extent of early kidney disease by measuring protein in the urine. Later in the disease, the kidneys lose their ability to remove waste products, such as creatinine and urea, from the blood.

Symptoms related to kidney failure usually occur only in late stages of the disease, when kidney function has diminished to less than 25 percent of normal capacity. For many years before that point, kidney disease of diabetes exists as a silent process.

Five Stages

Scientists have described five stages in the progression to ESRD in people with diabetes. They are as follows:

Stage I. The flow of blood through the kidneys, and therefore through the glomeruli, increases—this is called hyperfiltration—and the kidneys are larger than normal. Some people remain in stage I indefinitely; others advance to stage II after many years.

Stage II. The rate of filtration remains elevated or at near-normal levels, and the glomeruli begin to show damage. Small amounts of a blood protein known as albumin leak into the urine—a condition known as microalbuminuria. In its earliest stages, microalbuminuria may come and go. But as the rate of albumin loss increases from 20 to 200 micrograms per minute, microalbuminuria becomes more constant. (Normal losses of albumin are less than 5 micrograms per minute.) A special test is required to detect microalbuminuria. People with NIDDM and IDDM may remain in stage II for many years, especially if they have normal blood pressure and good control of their blood sugar levels.

Stage III. The loss of albumin and other proteins in the urine exceeds 200 micrograms per minute. It now can be detected during routine urine tests. Because such tests often involve dipping indicator strips into the urine, they are referred to as "dipstick methods."

Stage III sometimes is referred to as "dipstick-positive proteinuria" (or "clinical albuminuria" or "overt diabetic nephropathy"). Some patients develop high blood pressure. The glomeruli suffer increased damage. The kidneys progressively lose the ability to filter waste, and blood levels of creatinine and urea-nitrogen rise. People with IDDM and NIDDM may remain at stage III for many years.

Stage IV. This is referred to as "advanced clinical nephropathy." The glomerular filtration rate decreases to less than 75 milliliters per minute, large amounts of protein pass into the urine, and high blood pressure almost always occurs. Levels of creatinine and urea-nitrogen in the blood rise further.

Stage V. The final stage is ESRD. The glomerular filtration rate drops to less than 10 milliliters per minute. Symptoms of kidney failure occur.

These stages describe the progression of kidney disease for most people with IDDM who develop ESRD. For people with IDDM, the average length of time required to progress from onset of kidney disease to stage IV is 17 years. The average length of time to progress to ESRD is 23 years. Progression to ESRD may occur more rapidly (5-10 years) in people with untreated high blood pressure. If proteinuria does not develop within 25 years, the risk of developing advanced kidney disease begins to decrease. Advancement to stages IV and V occurs less frequently in people with NIDDM than in people with IDDM. Nevertheless, about 60 percent of people with diabetes who develop ESRD have NIDDM.

Effects of High Blood Pressure

High blood pressure, or hypertension, is a major factor in the development of kidney problems in people with diabetes. Both a family history of hypertension and the presence of hypertension appear to increase chances of developing kidney disease. Hypertension also accelerates the progress of kidney disease where it already exists.

Hypertension usually is defined as blood pressure exceeding 140 millimeters of mercury-systolic and 90 millimeters of mercury-diastolic. Professionals shorten the name of this limit to "140 over 90." The terms systolic and diastolic refer to pressure in the arteries during contraction of the heart (systolic) and between heartbeats (diastolic).

Hypertension can be seen not only as a cause of kidney disease, but also as a result of damage created by the disease. As kidney disease proceeds, physical changes in the kidneys lead to increased blood pressure. Therefore, a dangerous spiral, involving rising blood pressure and factors that raise blood pressure, occurs. Early detection and treatment of even mild hypertension are essential for people with diabetes.

Preventing and Slowing Kidney Disease

Blood Pressure Medicines

Scientists have made great progress in developing methods that slow the onset and progression of kidney disease in people with diabetes. Drugs used to lower blood pressure (antihypertensive drugs) can slow the progression of kidney disease significantly. One drug, an angiotensin-converting enzyme (ACE) inhibitor, has proven effective in preventing progression to stages IV and V. Calcium channel blockers, another class of antihypertensive drugs, also show promise.

An example of an effective ACE inhibitor is captopril, which the Food and Drug Administration approved for treating kidney disease of Type I diabetes. The benefits of captopril extend beyond its ability to lower blood pressure; it may directly protect the kidney's glomeruli. ACE inhibitors have lowered proteinuria and slowed deterioration even in diabetic patients who did not have high blood pressure.

Some, but not all, calcium channel blockers may be able to decrease proteinuria and damage to kidney tissue. Researchers are investigating whether combinations of calcium channel blockers and ACE inhibitors might be more effective than either treatment used alone. Patients with even mild hypertension or persistent microalbuminuria should consult a physician about the use of antihypertensive medicines.

Low-Protein Diets

A diet containing reduced amounts of protein may benefit people with kidney disease of diabetes. In people with diabetes, excessive consumption of protein may be harmful. Experts recommend that most patients with stage III or stage IV nephropathy consume moderate amounts of protein.

Intensive Management

Antihypertensive drugs and low-protein diets can slow kidney disease when significant nephropathy is present, as in stages III and IV. A third treatment, known as intensive management or glycemic control, has shown great promise for people with IDDM, especially for those with early stages of nephropathy.

Intensive management is a treatment regimen that aims to keep blood glucose levels close to normal. The regimen includes frequently testing blood sugar, administering insulin on the basis of food intake and exercise, following a diet and exercise plan, and frequently consulting a health care team.

A number of studies have pointed to the beneficial effects of intensive management. Two such studies, funded by the National Institute of Diabetes and Digestive and Kidney Diseases (NIDDK) of the National Institutes of Health, are the Diabetes Control and Complications Trial (DCCT)2 and a trial led by researchers at the University of Minnesota Medical School.

The DCCT, conducted from 1983 to 1993, involved 1,441 participants who had IDDM. Researchers found a 50-percent decrease in both development and progression of early diabetic kidney disease (stages I and II) in participants who followed an intensive regimen for controlling blood sugar levels. The intensively managed patients had average blood sugar levels of 150 milligrams per deciliter—about 80 milligrams per deciliter lower than the levels observed in the conventionally managed patients.

In the Minnesota Medical School trial, researchers examined kidney tissues of long-term diabetics who received healthy kidney transplants. After 5 years, patients who followed an intensive regimen developed significantly fewer lesions in their glomeruli than did patients not following an intensive regimen. This result, along with findings of the DCCT and studies performed in Scandinavia, suggests that any program resulting in sustained lowering of blood glucose levels will be beneficial to patients in the early stages of diabetic nephropathy.

Dialysis and Transplantation

When people with diabetes reach ESRD, they must undergo either dialysis or a kidney transplant. As recently as the 1970's, medical experts commonly excluded people with diabetes from dialysis and transplantation, in part because the experts felt damage caused by diabetes would offset benefits of the treatments. Today, because of better control of diabetes and improved rates of survival following treatment, doctors do not hesitate to offer dialysis and kidney transplantation to people with diabetes.

Currently, the survival of kidneys transplanted into diabetes patients is about the same as survival of transplants in people without diabetes. Dialysis for people with diabetes also works well in the short run. Even so, people with diabetes who receive transplants or dialysis experience higher morbidity and mortality because of coexisting complications of the diabetes—such as damage to the heart, eyes, and nerves.

Good Care Makes a Difference

If you have diabetes:

- Ask your doctor about the DCCT and how its results might help you.

- Have your doctor measure your glycohemoglobin regularly. The HbA1c test averages your level of blood sugar for the previous 1-3 months.

- Follow your doctor's advice regarding insulin injections, medicines, diet, exercise, and monitoring your blood sugar.

- Have your blood pressure checked several times a year. If blood pressure is high, follow your doctor's plan for keeping it near normal levels.

- Ask your doctor whether you might benefit from receiving an ACE inhibitor.

- Have your urine checked yearly for microalbumin and protein. If there is protein in your urine, have your blood checked for elevated amounts of waste products such as creatinine.

- Ask your doctor whether you should reduce the amount of protein in your diet.

Looking to the Future

The incidences of both diabetes and ESRD caused by diabetes have been rising. Some experts predict that diabetes soon might account for half the cases of ESRD. In light of the increasing morbidity and mortality related to diabetes and ESRD, patients, researchers, and health care professionals will continue to benefit by addressing the relationship between the two diseases. The NIDDK is a leader in supporting research in this area.

Several areas of research supported by NIDDK hold great potential. Discovery of ways to predict who will develop kidney disease may lead to greater prevention, as people with diabetes who learn they are at risk institute strategies such as intensive management and blood pressure control. Discovery of better anti-rejection drugs will improve results of kidney transplantation in patients with diabetes who develop ESRD. For some people with IDDM, advances in transplantation—especially transplantation of insulin-producing cells of the pancreas—could lead to a cure for both diabetes and the kidney disease of diabetes.

Reference

National Kidney and Urologic Diseases Information Clearinghouse
3 Information Way
Bethesda, MD 20892-3580
(301) 654-4415

The National Kidney and Urologic Diseases Information Clearinghouse is a service of the National Institute of Diabetes and Digestive and Kidney Diseases, part of the National Institutes of Health, under the U.S. Public Health Service. Authorized in 1987, the clearinghouse provides information about diseases of the kidneys and urologic system to people with such afflictions and to their families, health care professionals, and the public. The clearinghouse answers inquiries; develops, reviews, and distributes publications; and works closely with professional and patient organizations and government agencies to coordinate resources about kidney and urologic diseases.

Section 12.2

Additional Resources on Kidney Disease of Diabetes

Searches-On-File, Topics in Kidney and Urologic Diseases, NKUDIC.

Legend

TI   Title
AU   Author
CN   Corporate Author
SO   Source
PR   Product
AV   Producer/Availability

TI   ACE in the Hole.
AU   Roberts, S.S.
SO   *Diabetes Forecast*. 46(11): 24, 26–27. November 1993.
AV   Available from American Diabetes Association. 1660 Duke Street, Alexandria, VA 22314. (800) 232-3472.

TI   Before the Dawn of Kidney Disease.
AU   Dinsmoor, R.S.
SO   *Juvenile Diabetes Foundation International Countdown. (JDF International Countdown)*. 15(2):37–40. Spring 1994.
AV   Available from Juvenile Diabetes Foundation, International. 432 Park Avenue South, New York, NY 10016-8013. (800) 223-1138; (212) 889-7575.

TI   Black Americans: Diabetes and Obesity.
SO   *Diabetes Forecast*. 43(2):74–75. February 1990.

TI **Causes and Symptoms of Kidney Failure.**
AU Gabriel, R.
SO In: Gabriel, R. *Patient's Guide to Dialysis and Transplantation.* 4th ed. Hingham, MA: Kluwer Academic Publishers. 1990. p. 32–45.
AV Available from Kluwer Academic Publishers. P.O. Box 358, Accord Station. Hingham, MA 02018. (617) 871-6600. Price: $24.50. ISBN: 0792389506.

TI *Complications.*
SO Indianapolis, IN: Eli Lilly and Company. 1991. 4 p.
CN Eli Lilly and Company.
AV Available from Eli Lilly and Company. Indianapolis, IN 46285. (317) 276-2000. Single copy free. Order Number 60-HI-2727-0. Available only to health professionals through Lilly sales representatives. Contact the above for referral to a local representative.

TI *Diabetes and Kidney Disease.*
SO Bethesda, MD: Virgil Smirnow Associates. 199x. 12 p.
CN Virgil Smirnow Associates.
AV Available from Virgil Smirnow Associates. Health Information Library, P.O. Box 55109, Lexington, KY 40555. (301) 469-7933. Price: $1.95 plus $.25 shipping and handling for single copies.

TI *Diabetes and Kidney Disease.*
SO New York, NY: Juvenile Diabetes Foundation International. 1990. 4 p.
CN JDF International.
AV Available from the Juvenile Diabetes Foundation International. 432 Park Avenue South, New York, NY 10016. (800) JDF-CURE. Single copy free.

TI *Diabetes and Kidney Disease.*
SO New York, NY: National Kidney Foundation. 1992. 6 p.
CN National Kidney Foundation.
AV Available from National Kidney Foundation. 30 East 33rd Street, New York, NY 10016. (212) 889-2210 or (800) 622-9010. Single copy free Order Number 02-09-PP.

TI *Diabetes and the Kidney.*
AU Juneja, V.
SO Hamilton, Ontario: St. Joseph's Hospital. 1991. 41 p.
AV Available from Veena Juneja. Renal Nutritionist, St. Joseph's Hospital, 50 Charlton Avenue East, Hamilton, Ontario L8N 4A6 CANADA. (905) 5224941. Price: $10.00. Make checks payable to Veena Juneja, M.Sc., R.D.

TI *Diabetes and the Kidneys: Patient's Guide to Therapy.*
AU Friedman, M.; Friedman, E.A.
SO Rockville, MD: American Kidney Fund. 1991. 12 p.
AV Available from American Kidney Fund. 6110 Executive Boulevard, Suite 1010, Rockville, MD 20852. (301) 881-3052 or (800) 638-8299 or (800) 492-8361 (in Maryland). Price: Single copy free; bulk copies $.25 each.

TI *Diabetes and Your Kidneys.*
SO Seattle, WA: Northwest Kidney Foundation. 199x. 2 p.
CN Northwest Kidney Foundation.
AV Available from Northwest Kidney Foundation. P.O. Box 3035, Seattle WA 98114. (206) 292-5351. Free.

TI *Diabetes and The Kidneys* (**Large Print Edition**).
AU Friedman, M.; Friedman, E.A.
SO Rockville, MD: American Kidney Fund. 1994. 21 p.
AV Available from American Kidney Fund. 6110 Executive Boulevard, Suite 1010, Rockville, MD 20852. (800) 638-8299 or (301) 881-0898 (fax). Price: Single copy free, $0.40 each for additional copies; postage/shipping.

TI *Diabetes Control and Complications Trial: How Will the Result Affect Your Treatment?*
AU Hazlett, J.
SO Diabetes Self-Management. p. 6–8. September-October 1993.

TI **Diabetes Definitions: Diabetic Nephropathy; Sulfonylureas; Neuropathy.**
AU Dinsmoor, R.S.
SO *Diabetes Self-Management*. 8(4): 46–47. July-August 1991.
AV Available from R.A. Rapaport Publishing Company. 150 West 22nd Street, New York, NY 10011. (212) 989-0220.

TI   **Dialysis.**
AU   Copley, J.B.
SO   *Diabetes Forecast*. p. 30–35. June 1990.

TI   *Diet for Hemodialysis.*
AU   Buntjer, K.; Edelstein, L.; Ostergren, C., eds.
SO   West Linn, OR: Oregon Council on Renal Nutrition. 1991. 28 p.
CN   Oregon Council on Renal Nutrition.
AV   Available from Oregon Council on Renal Nutrition. Nancy Frazeur, R.D., 5431 Windsor Terrace, West Linn, OR 97068. Price: $5.00 (bulk prices available). Also available as one of three books in a series for $10.00.

TI   *Diet for Peritoneal Dialysis.*
AU   Buntjer, K.; Edelstein, L.; Ostergren, C., eds.
SO   West Linn, OR: Oregon Council on Renal Nutrition. 1991. 32 p.
CN   Oregon Council on Renal Nutrition.
AV   Available from Oregon Council on Renal Nutrition. Nancy Frazeur, R.D., 5431 Windsor Terrace, West Linn, OR 97068. Price: $5.00 (bulk prices available). Also available as one of three books in a series for $10.00.

TI   *Do You Know Where Your Kidneys Are?*
SO   New York, NY: National Kidney Foundation.: 1992. (poster).
CN   National Kidney Foundation of the National Capital Area, Inc.
PR   Poster (11½ in x 17 in), 2-color, glossy paper.
AV   Available from National Kidney Foundation. 30 East 33rd Street, New York, NY 10016. (800) 622-9010 or (202) 337-6600. Single copy free.

TI   **Early Detection, Treatment May Prevent, Slow Kidney Failure.**
AU   Weaver, M.
SO   *Diabetes in the News*. 10(6): 42–43. December 1991.

TI   *Eating Right: A Nutritional Guide for the Diabetic Dialysis Patient* (3rd ed.).
SO   Minneapolis, MN Minneapolis Medical Research Foundation, Inc. 1993. 21 p.
CN   Education Department of the Regional Kidney Disease Program, Minneapolis Medical Research Foundation, Inc.

AV   Available from Dialyrn Renal Education System. 914 South Eighth Street, Minneapolis, MN 55404. (612) 347-5949. Price: $3.50 per copy for 1-9 copies; $3.00 per copy for 10 or more. Order No. 330.

TI   *End-Stage Renal Disease: Choosing a Treatment That's Right For You,* **September 1991.**

SO   National Diabetes Information Clearinghouse.

AV   Available from National Diabetes Information Clearinghouse. Box NDIC, 9000 Rockville Pike, Bethesda, MD 20892. (301) 654-3327. Single copy free.

TI   **Exercise Okay Even When You Have Complications.**

AU   Harper, P.; Hornsby, W.G., JR.

SO   *Diabetes In The News.* 12(5): 10–12. October 1993.

TI   **Exercises For People With Complications.**

AU   Graham, C.

SO   *Diabetes Self-Management.* 8(6): 26–28. November-December 1991.

AV   Available from R.A. Rappaport Publishing Company. 150 West 22nd Street, New York, NY 10011. (212) 989-0220.

TI   *Fighting Long-term Complications.*

AU   Beaser, R.S.; Aho, C.

SO   Boston, MA: Joslin Diabetes Center. 1992. 19 p.

AV   Available from Joslin Diabetes Center. Publications Department, One Joslin Place, Boston, MA 02215. (617) 732-2695, FAX (617) 732-2664. Price: $29.50 for package of 10. ISBN: 1879091127.

TI   *Handbook for Transplant Patients*

AU   Bartell, L.

SO   Minneapolis, MN: University of Minnesota Hospital and Clinic. September 1990. 195 p.

CN   University of Minnesota Hospital and Clinic

AV   Available from University of Minnesota Hospital and Clinic. Nursing Professional Services, Box 603, University of Minnesota Hospital and Clinic, Minneapolis, MN 55455. (612) 626-3354. Price: Free to patients at the Transplant Center. $40.00 plus 7% shipping and handling for nonpatients.

TI   *Healthy Food Guide: Diabetes and Kidney Disease.*
SO   Chicago, IL: American Dietetic Association. 1993. 31 p.
CN   American Dietetic Association.
AV   Available from American Dietetic Association. 216 West Jackson Boulevard, Chicago, IL 60606-6995. (312) 899-0440. Price: $19.95 for 10 copies for American Dietetic Association members; $23.50 for non-members; plus shipping and handling. ISBN: 0880911182.

TI   **Hope for Prevention of Diabetic Kidney Disease Increasing.**
AU   Hostetter, T.H.
SO   *Kidney '90.* 7(5): 4–5. September-October 1990.

TI   *How Well Are Your Kidneys? An Important Question for People with Type I Insulin-Dependent Diabetes.*
SO   Princeton, NJ: Bristol-Myers Squibb Company. 1994. 17 p.
CN   Bristol-Myers Squibb.
AV   Available from Becton-Dickinson Consumer Products. 1 Becton Drive, Franlin Lakes, NJ 07417. (800) 237-4554. Single copy free.

TI   **Independent, Home Self-Care Dialysis Possible for Blind Persons with Kidney Failure.**
AU   Schmidt, L.M.
SO   *Voice of the Diabetic.* 6(1): 4. Winter, 1991.

TI   **Independent, Home, Self-Care Dialysis Possible for Blind Persons With Kidney Failure.**
AU   Schmidt, L.M.
SO   *Voice of the Diabetic.* 9(1): 11–12. Winter 1994.

TI   **Indiana Conducts Model Hypertension Screening Program.**
SO   *Affiliate Update.* 4(2): 10, 13. Summer 1991.
CN   National Kidney Foundation.
AV   Available from National Kidney Foundation. 30 East 33rd Street, New York, NY 10016.

TI   **Intensive Treatment of Diabetes Prevents Complications.**

AU   Moon, M.A.

SO   *NCRR Reporter*. National Center for Research Resources Reporter. 18(1): 8–10. January-February 1994.

AV   Available from Superintendent of Documents. U.S. Government Printing Office, Washington, D.C. 20402. (202) 783-3238.

TI   *Kidney Complications (Nephropathy).*

SO   Alexandria, VA: American Diabetes Association, Diabetes Information Service Center. 4 p

CN   American Diabetes Association.

AV   Available from American Diabetes Association, Diabetes Information Service Center. 1660 Duke Street, Alexandria, VA 22314. (800) 232-3472 or (703) 549-1500. Single copy free. Also available from local ADA affiliates.

TI   *Kidney Damage: "Nephropathy".*

SO   Albuquerque, NM: Indian Health Service Diabetes Program. October 1991. 13 p.

CN   Indian Health Service Diabetes Program.

AV   Available from Indian Health Service Diabetes Program. 2401 12th Street, N.W., Room 211N, Albuquerque, NM 87102. (505) 766-3980. Available only to health providers serving the Native American population. Single copy free.

TI   **Kidney-Pancreas Transplantation: New Hope for Diabetics With End-Stage Renal Failure.**

AU   Sollinger, H.W.

SO   *NKF Family Focus*. 2(1): 11. March 1991.

AV   Available from National Kidney Foundation, Inc. Medical Department, 30 East 33rd Street, New York, NY 10016. (800) 622-9010 or (212) 889-2210.

TI   **Kidneys Produce a Special Enzyme Which Regulates Your Blood Pressure.**

AU   Moss, E.

SO   *21st Century Health Letter*. p. 8. Winter 1993.

TI *Low Protein Cookery: Recipes, Helpful Hints and Information Relating to Protein-Restricted Diets.*
SO Edmonton, Alberta: University of Alberta Hospitals, Nutrition and Food Services. February 1992. 50 p.
CN University of Alberta Hospitals, Nutrition and Food Services.
AV Available from University of Alberta Hospitals. Nutrition and Food Services, 8440-112 Street, Edmonton, Alberta T6G 2B7. (403) 492-6882, (403) 492-8645 (fax). Price: $8.00 includes shipping and handling.

TI **Magnificent Seven.**
AU Ryan, C.
SO *Diabetes Forecast.* 47(1): 37–39. January 1994.
AV Available from American Diabetes Association, Inc. 1660 Duke Street, Alexandria, VA 22314. (800) 232-3472.

TI *Managing Your Diabetes: Kidneys.*
SO Indianapolis, IN: Eli Lilly and Company. 1991. 4 p.
CN Eli Lilly and Company.
AV Available from Eli Lilly and Company. Lilly Corporate Center, Indianapolis, IN 46285. (317) 276-2000. Free.

TI **Medical Tests Explained: Interpreting Test Results.**
AU Dinsmoor, R.S.
SO *Diabetes Self-Management.* 7(4): 12–16. July-August 1990.

TI *NKF Science Writers News Briefing: News Briefing for Science Writers on Transplantation, Dialysis, and Kidney Research* **(press packet).**
SO New York, NY: National Kidney Foundation, Inc. August 1990. 55 p.
CN National Kidney Foundation, Inc.
AV Available from the National Kidney Foundation, Inc. 30 East 33rd Street, New York, NY 10016. (212) 889-2210 or (800) 622-9010. Single copy free.

TI *Nutrition and Changing Kidney Function.*
SO New York, NY: National Kidney Foundation, Inc. 1990. 2 p.
CN National Kidney Foundation, Inc.
AV Available from the National Kidney Foundation, Inc. 30 East 33rd Street, New York, NY 10016. (800) 622-9010. Single copy free. Order No. 08-55.

TI **Please Pass (Up) the Salt.**
AU Reader, D.
SO *Diabetes Forecast*. 43(10): 56, 58, 60, 62. September 1990.

TI **Pregnancy in End Stage Renal Disease.**
AU Hou, S.H.
SO *NKF Family Focus. National Kidney Foundation Family Focus*. 4(2): 13. Spring 1993.
AV Available from National Kidney Foundation, Inc. 30 E. 33rd Street, New York, NY 10016. (800) 622-9010; (212) 889-2210.

TI **Preventing Diabetic Kidney Disease**
AU Laffel, L.
SO *JDF International Countdown*. 13(4): 21. Fall 1992.
AV Available from Juvenile Diabetes Foundation International. 432 Park Avenue South, New York, NY 10016. (212) 889-7575 or (800) 223-1138.

TI ***Renal Diabetic Diet Instruction Guide.***
SO Iowa City, IA: University of Iowa Hospitals and Clinics.
CN University of Iowa Hospitals and Clinics.
AV Available from University of Iowa Hospitals and Clinics. Publications, Dietary Department, Iowa City, IA 52242. (319) 356-2692. Price: $4.00

TI **Renal Failure, Dialysis, and Transplantation.**
AU Bryant, E.
SO *Voice of the Diabetic*. 9(1): 3–4,8,13. Winter 1994.

TI ***Renal Lifestyles Manual and Diet Guide.***
AU Harum, P., ed.
SO Marina del Rey, CA: R and D Laboratories, Inc. 1992. 176 p.
AV Available from R and D Laboratories, Inc. 4204 Glencoe Avenue, Marina del Rey, CA 90292. (213) 305-8053 or (800) 338-9066. Price: $55.00.

TI ***Sample Menus for Your Diabetic Low Protein Diet.***
SO Minneapolis, MN: Dialyrn Renal Education System. 1991. 24 p.
CN Dialyrn Renal Education System.
AV Available from Dialyrn Renal Education System. Regional Kidney Disease Program, 900 South Eighth Street, Minneapolis,

MN 55404. (612) 347-5949. Price: $3.00 (bulk prices available). Order Number 310-C.

TI **Smart Operators: Your Kidneys Work Hard for You, Learn How to Protect Them.**
AU Friedman, E.A.
SO *Diabetes Forecast*. 47(6): 34, 36–39. June 1994.
AV Available from American Diabetes Association, Inc. 1660 Duke Street, Alexandria, VA 22314. (800) 232-3472.

TI *Take Charge of Your Diabetes, A Guide for Patients, 1991.*
SO National Diabetes Information Clearinghouse.
AV Available from Division of Diabetes Translantion Centers for Disease Control and Prevention, 4770 Buford Hwy, N.E. Mail Stop K-13, Atlanta, GA 30341 3724. (404) 488-5080. Single copy free.

TI *Taking Care of Your Kidneys: Prevent and Treat Infections.*
SO Albuquerque, NM: Indian Health Service Diabetes Program. 1991. 11 p.
CN Indian Health Service Diabetes Program.
AV Available from Indian Health Service Diabetes Program. 2401 12th Street, N.W., Room 211N, Albuquerque, NM 87102. (505) 766-3980. Available only to health care professionals working with Native American populations. Free.

TI **Travel? Yes You Can!**
AU Cobb, R.F.
SO *NKF Family Focus. National Kidney Foundation Family Focus*. 2(2): 3–4 June 1991.
AV Available from National Kidney Foundation, Inc. 30 East 33rd Street, New York, NY 10016.

TI *Understanding the Complications of Diabetes Mellitus.*
AU Ross, S.; Hunt, J.; Lillie, D.
SO Toronto, Ontario: Canadian Diabetes Association. 1992. 8 p.
AV Available from Canadian Diabetes Association. National Office, 15 Toronto Street, Suite 1001, Toronto, Ontario MSC 2E3. (416) 363-3373. Price: $0.25 each.

TI   *Using Fast Foods on Your Diabetic Low Protein Diet.*

SO   Minneapolis, MN: Dialyrn Renal Education System. 1991. 2 p.

CN   Dialyrn Renal Education System.

AV   Available from Dialyrn Renal Education System. Regional Kidney Disease Program, 900 South Eighth Street, Minneapolis, MN 55404. (612) 347-5949. Price: $5.00 for reproducible master. Order Number 310-A.

TI   *Using Prepared Entrees on Your Diabetic Low Protein Diet.*

SO   Minneapolis, MN: Dialyrn Renal Education System. 1991. 2 p.

CN   Dialyrn Renal Education System.

AV   Available from Dialyrn Renal Education System. Regional Kidney Disease Program, 900 South Eighth Street, Minneapolis, MN 55404. (612) 347-5949. Price: $5.00 for reproducible master. Order Number 310-B.

TI   *What's Left To Eat? Meal Planning for Diabetes and Kidney Problems.*

AU   Barry, B.

SO   International Diabetes Center. 6(2): 18–21. Spring 1991.

AV   Available from Chronimed Publishing. 13911 Ridgedale Drive, Suite 250, Minnetonka, MN 55305. (800) 848-2793.

TI   **You Can Prevent Many Diabetes Complications.**

AU   Hinnen, D.

SO   *Diabetes In The News.* 12(5): 26–27. October 1993.

TI   *Your Nutrition Plan: To Help You Take Care of Your Kidneys.*

AU   Hill, L., ed.

SO   Lexington, KY: Dialysis Clinic, Inc. l99x. 20 p.

AV   Available from Dialysis Clinic, Inc. 1353 Leestown Road, Lexington, KY 40508. Price: $4.00 (bulk prices available).

TI   *Your Renal Diet (Diabetic Diet).*

SO   Cleveland, OH: Community Dialysis Center, Inc. 1992. 7 p.

CN   Community Dialysis Center.

AV   Available from Community Dialysis Center, Inc. P.O. Box 12220, East Cleveland, OH 44112. (216) 229-1100. Price: $1.50 each plus $2.50 shipping and handling per order.

TI *Your Renal Diet: Diabetes Edition.*
AU Hill, L.; Nally, L.
SO Lexington, KY: Dialysis Clinic Inc. 26 p.
CN Central Baptist Hospital. Humana Hospital. Dialysis Clinic, Inc. Good Samaritan Hospital. Saint Joseph Hospital. Veteran's Administration Medical Center.
AV Available from Renal Dietitian, Dialysis Clinic, Inc. 1353 Leestown Road, Lexington, KY 40508. Price: $4.00 each; 10% discount for more than 10 copies.

For Additional Information

CHID is available on-line through CDP Online. If you would like references to materials on other topics, you may request a special literature search of CHID from a library that subscribes to CDP Online or from the National Kidney and Urologic Diseases Information Clearinghouse, 3 Information Way, Bethesda, MD 20892-3580; (301) 654-4415.

Chapter 13

High Blood Pressure and Kidney Disease

Chapter Contents

Section 13.1

High Blood Pressure and Your Kidneys

"High Blood Pressure and Your Kidneys," © 1986, revised 1995,
by The National Kidney Foundation, and excerpts from "Ten Facts You
Should Know about High Blood Pressure and Your Kidneys."

Did you know these facts about high blood pressure?

- 50 million Americans have high blood pressure; the only way you can tell if you are one of them is to have your blood pressure checked.

- High blood pressure is called a silent killer because you can have it for years without knowing it.

- High blood pressure is a leading cause of heart attacks, strokes and kidney disease.

- If high blood pressure is controlled by treatment, the risk of these complications is reduced greatly.

- Making changes to a healthier lifestyle—such as losing weight, exercising more and cutting down on salt—often helps to control blood pressure.

- High blood pressure can affect anyone at any age. Even children can have high blood pressure, although it is less common. Regular high blood pressure checkups should begin in childhood and continue throughout life.

- High blood pressure is a more serious problem among black Americans. Not only do more black Americans develop high blood pressure (it affects 38 percent of the black population compared with 24 percent of the white population), but they tend to develop earlier, more severe cases of the disease. This is related to the fact that more black Americans have strokes, heart failure and kidney failure. About 30 percent of the people who need dialysis or a kidney transplant due to kidney failure are black.

- Many effective drugs are available for treating high blood pressure. Scientific evidence also points to a role for lifestyle changes such as weight loss and regular exercise in regulating blood pressure. In some cases, a healthier lifestyle may be sufficient to regulate blood pressure; in other instances, combining drug therapy with lifestyle changes may permit smaller doses of medication to be used.

- Many of the drugs used to treat high blood pressure are associated with side effects, including fatigue, insomnia, increased frequency of urination, depression, drowsiness, dry mouth, nasal congestion, dizziness, headaches, and decreased sexual function. Patients should report any side effects to their doctors. The doctor may be able to change to medications that eliminate intolerable side effects.

What is blood pressure?

Blood pressure is the force of your blood pushing against the walls of your arteries. This pressure moves blood from the heart to organs like the brain, kidneys and the gut.

How is blood pressure measured?

Blood pressure is measured with a blood pressure cuff around your upper arm. This cuff is pumped up and then let down while listening for the pulse sound. The top number of your blood pressure reading is called the systolic pressure and the bottom number is called the diastolic pressure—for example, 120/80.

What is high blood pressure (hypertension)?

High blood pressure (also known as hypertension) occurs when the force of blood against your artery walls increases. For adults, blood pressures that stay at 140/90 or more are considered high. A diagnosis of high blood pressure is not made on the basis of one high reading, but must be confirmed on follow-up visits to your doctor or clinic. High blood pressure should be watched by your doctor.

How often should I have my blood pressure checked?

Your blood pressure should be checked at least once a year. If your blood pressure is too high, you should have it checked as often as your doctor advises.

What causes high blood pressure?

The causes of high blood pressure are not known in many cases. However, some people may have a greater chance of developing high blood pressure. These include:

- older people
- people who have a family history of high blood pressure
- African-Americans
- people who are overweight
- people who have an inactive lifestyle
- people who use a lot of salt in their food
- women who use oral contraceptives (the pill)

Men are also more likely to develop high blood pressure than women.

How are African-Americans affected by high blood pressure?

High blood pressure is a major health problem among African-Americans. Not only do they have a higher rate of high blood pressure than whites, but they develop high blood pressure at an earlier age and more severely than whites. As a result, African-Americans have a greater rate of strokes, heart disease and chronic kidney failure. African-Americans need to have regular blood pressure check-ups and to follow their doctor's advice carefully if high blood pressure is detected.

How can high blood pressure hurt my body?

Uncontrolled high blood pressure can damage important organs in your body like your heart, brain and kidneys. It can also cause heart attacks, strokes and kidney failure.

How are high blood pressure and kidney disease related?

High blood pressure and kidney disease are closely related. Some kidney diseases may cause high blood pressure, but more commonly, high blood pressure may cause kidney disease. The working units of the kidneys (called nephrons) are damaged after years of stress from the high pressure. Kidney disease caused by high blood pressure is a leading cause of kidney failure in the United States. If high blood pressure is controlled, however, your chances of developing kidney disease and other complications can be reduced.

What are the symptoms of high blood pressure?

You will probably have no symptoms of high blood pressure. Most people with high blood pressure do not feel ill. However, if high blood pressure has damaged your body organs, you may have:

* headaches
* nose bleeds
* shortness of breath
* blurred vision
* chest pain

How is high blood pressure treated?

Although high blood pressure cannot be cured, it can be controlled. If you have high blood pressure, your doctor may ask you to make some of the following lifestyle changes:

* lose weight
* exercise more
* cut down on salt
* cut back on alcohol

If these steps do not control your blood pressure well enough, your doctor may order medicines for you. Sometimes, more than one medicine may be needed to get your blood pressure under control. If you are a smoker, your doctor will advise you to quit. Smoking increases your risk of complications such as heart attacks and strokes.

What should I do if my medicine causes side effects?

Sometimes, high blood pressure medicine may cause problems like:

- dizziness
- tiredness
- headaches
- problems with your sex life

If you have any side effects, you should report them to your doctor. The doctor may be able to change the amount of your medicine or switch you to another medicine that works better for you. Never stop your medicine on your own because that can be very damaging to your body and can cause strokes and heart attacks.

What can I do about high blood pressure?

Make sure you go to your doctor or clinic regularly to have your blood pressure checked. Early detection and long-term treatment are the keys to a longer and healthier life by preventing the complications of high blood pressure. If high blood pressure is detected, you will need to work with your doctor to get your blood pressure under control. Follow your doctor's advice about any lifestyle changes you may need to make. If you have questions about diet, your doctor or clinic can refer you to a registered dietitian who will help you learn more about the right foods to eat in the right amounts to help control your blood pressure.

If you need to take medicine to control your blood pressure, you should take it faithfully, even when you are feeling fine, because high blood pressure may not cause any symptoms at all. Remember to take your medicine at the time of day you are told. If you have trouble remembering when to take your medicine, special pill boxes are available that have small compartments labeled with the days of the week as well as the time of day. Watches with alarms or beepers may also be helpful.

How can my family help me win the fight against high blood pressure?

If you have high blood pressure, it's a good idea to get your whole family involved in your care. Since high blood pressure often runs in families, some of your family members may also be at risk of developing high blood pressure. You should encourage them to learn all they can about high blood pressure and to have their blood pressure checked at least once a year. It's also helpful if your family members join you in making changes to a healthier lifestyle. It's much easier (and can even be fun) doing things like following a healthy diet, exercising and stopping smoking if you do them together.

What if I have more questions?

If you have more questions, speak to your doctor. You may also get additional information by contacting your local National Kidney Foundation office.

Things you should remember...

- High blood pressure is a leading cause of heart attacks, strokes and kidney disease.

- Controlling high blood pressure reduces the chance of having these complications.

- Have your blood pressure checked at least once a year. Don't wait until your body organs are damaged.

- Spread the word about high blood pressure to your family and friends and encourage them to have their blood pressure checked too.

Section 13.2

Additional Resources on Kidney Disease and High Blood Pressure

Searches-On-File, Topics in Kidney and Urologic Diseases, NKUDIC.

Legend

TI   Title
AU   Author
CN   Corporate Author
SO   Source
PR   Product
AV   Producer/Availability

TI   Aging Kidney.
AU   Oreopoulos, D.G.
SO   *Advances in Peritoneal Dialysis* (Toronto, Canada). Volume 6 (Supplement): 2–5. 1990.
AV   Available from the Peritoneal Dialysis International Bulletin, Inc. Toronto Western Hospital, Edith Cavel Wing, Room 525, 399 Bathhurst Street, Toronto, Ontario M5T 2S8, CANADA. (416) 369-5189.

TI   Angiotensin-I Converting Enzyme Inhibition: Clinical Effects in Chronic Renal Disease.
AU   DeJong, P.E., et al.
SO   *American Journal of Kidney Diseases*. 17(5 Supplement 1): 85–88. May 1991.
AV   Available from National Kidney Foundation. 30 East 33rd Street, New York, NY 10016. (212) 889-2210 or (800) 622-9010.

TI Are Newer Antihypertensive Agents Really More Effective Than Traditional Drugs in Progressive Renal Disease?

AU Ritz, E., et al.

SO *American Journal of Kidney Diseases*. 17(5 Supplement 1): 76–80. May 1991.

AV Available from National Kidney Foundation. 30 East 33rd Street, New York, NY 10016. (212) 889-2210 or (800) 622-9010.

TI Baseline Characteristics in the Modification of Diet in Renal Disease Study.

AU Greene, T., et al.

SO *JASN. Journal of the American Society of Nephrology*. 3(11): 1819–1834. May 1993.

AV Available from Williams & Wilkins, 428 E. Preston Street, Baltimore, MD 21202. (800) 638-6423.

TI Basic Research in Renal Mechanisms and Pathophysiology of Hypertension.

AU Ploth, D.W.

SO *Nephrology News and Issues*. 4(2): 38, 40. February 1990.

AV Available from Nephrology News and Issues. 13901 N. 73rd Street, Suite 214, Scottsdale, AZ 85260-9804. (602) 443-4635.

TI Blacks Struck by High Rate of Kidney Disease: High Blood Pressure is Major Culprit.

AU Harris, M.

SO *The NIH Record*, Vol. XLII No. 24, US Dept. of HHS, NIH. Page 8, 10. November 27, 1990.

AV Available from NIH Record Office, Building 31, Room 2B-03, 9000 Rockville Pike, Bethesda, MD 20892. (301) 496-1485.

CN National Institute of Diabetes and Digestive and Kidney Diseases.

TI Blood Pressure Control: Special Role of the Kidneys and Body Fluids.

AU Guyton, A.C.

SO *Science*. 252(5014): 1813–1816. June 28, 1991.

AV Available from American Association for the Advancement of Science. 1333 H Street, NW, Washington, DC 20005.

TI Calcium Channel Blockers: A Unique Group of Antihypertensives

AU Constantin, P.

SO *Contemporary Dialysis and Nephrology: For Patients Only.* 6(4): 16–17. July/August 1993.

AV Available from Contemporary Dialysis, Inc. 6300 Variel Avenue, Suite I, Woodland Hills, CA 91367. (818) 704-5555.

TI Calcium Channel Blockers: Effects on Progressive Renal Disease.

AU Zucchelli, P.; Zuccala, A.; Gaggi, R.

SO *American Journal of Kidney Diseases.* 17(5 Supplement 1): 94–97. May 1991.

AV Available from National Kidney Foundation. 30 East 33rd Street, New York, NY 10016. (212) 889-2210 or (800) 622-9010.

TI Can Intravenous Urography be Replaced by Sonography?

AU Tomei, E.; Hricak, H.

SO In: Andreucci, V.E. *International Yearbook of Nephrology 1990.* Hingham, MA: Kluwer Academic Publishers. 1990. p. 265–286.

AV Available from Kluwer Academic Publishers. P.O. Box 358, Accord Station, Hingham, MA 02018-0358. (617) 871-6600.

TI Care of the Organ Transplant Recipient.

AU Bromberg, J.S.; Grossman, R.A.

SO *JABFP. Journal of the American Board of Family Practice.* 6(6): 563–576. November-December. 1993.

TI Causes, Consequences, and Treatment of Hyperlipidemia in Patients with Renal Disease.

AU Kasiske, B.L.; Keane, W.F.

SO In: Andreucci, V.E.; Fine, L.G., eds. *International Yearbook of Nephrology 1991.* Hingham, MA: Kluwer Academic Publishers. 1990. p. 179–196.

AV Available from Kluwer Academic Publishers. P.O. Box 348, Accord Station, Hingham, MA 02018-0358. (617) 871-6600. PRICE: $110.00. ISBN: 0792310020.

TI Controlled Trials of Antihypertensive Drugs in Pregnancy.

AU Redman, C.W.

SO *American Journal of Kidney Diseases.* 17(2): 149–153, February 1991.

AV Available from National Kidney Foundation. 30 East 33rd Street, New York, NY 10016. (212) 889-2210 or (800) 622-9010.

TI Current Issues in Nutrition and Metabolism: Symposium Highlights, Part II.

AU Nuttall, F.Q.; Hollenbeck, C.B.

SO *Diabetes Spectrum.* 2(3): 145–151. May-June 1989.

AV Available from American Diabetes Association, Inc. 1660 Duke Street, Alexandreia, VA 22314. (800) 232-3472.

TI Current Recommendation for First Line Therapy of Uncomplicated Hypertension.

AU Schmieder, R.E.; Rockstroh, J.K.; Messerli, F.H.

SO In: Andreucci, V.E.; Fine, L.G., eds. *International Yearbook of Nephrology 1991.* Hingham, MA: Kluwer Academic Publishers. 1990. p. 141–157.

AV Available from Kluwer Academic Publishers. P.O. Box 348, Accord Station, Hingham, MA 02018-0358. (617) 871-6600. Price: $110.00. ISBN: 0792310020.

TI Current Trends in the Treatment of Hypertensive Syndromes: Progression of Chronic Renal Disease; Role of Systemic and Glomerular Hypertension.

AU Anderson, S.

SO *American Journal of Kidney Diseases.* 13(6 Supplement 1): 8–12. June 1989.

AV Available from National Kidney Foundation. 30 East 33rd Street, New York, NY 10016. (212) 889-2210 or (800) 622-9010.

TI Current Trends in the Treatment of Hypertensive Syndromes: Current Concepts in the Management of Renovascular Hypertension and Ischemic Renal Failure.

AU Novick, A.C.

SO *American Journal of Kidney Diseases.* 13(6 Supplement 1): 33–37. June 1989.

AV Available from National Kidney Foundation. 30 East 33rd Street, New York, NY 10016. (212) 889-2210 or (800) 622-9010.

TI **Diabetic Renal Disease in Blacks: Inevitable or Preventable?**

AU Rostand, S.G.

SO *New England Journal of Medicine.* 321(16): 1121–1122. October 19, 1989.

TI **Diagnosis and Treatment of Renal Vascular Disease.**

AU Pohl, M.

SO *Nephrology News and Issues.* 4(1): 34–38. January 1990.

AV Available from Nephrology News and Issues. 13901 N. 73rd Street, Suite 214, Scottsdale, AZ 85260-9804. (602) 443-4635.

TI *Diseases of the Kidney, the Lower Urinary Tract, and the Male Genital System.*

SO Geneva, Switzerland: Council for International Organizations of Medical Sciences, World Health Organization. 1992. 191 p.

CN Council for International Organizations of Medical Sciences, World Health Organization.

AV Available from World Health Organization. Distribution and Sales, 1211 Geneva 27, Switzerland. Price: $18.00 plus shipping and handling. ISBN: 924154414 (WHO) or 929036050X (CIOMS).

TI **A Perspective on Converting Enzyme Inhibitors and Calcium Channel Antagonists in Diabetic Renal Disease.**

AU Valentino, V.A., et al.

SO *Archives of Internal Medicine.* 151(12): 2367–2372. December 1991.

TI **Effect of Angiotensin-Converting-Enzyme Inhibition on Diabetic Nephropathy.**

AU Lewis, E.J., et al.

SO *New England Journal of Medicine.* 329(20): 1456–1462. November 11, 1993.

TI **Effects of Antihypertensive Therapy on Renal Function.**

AU Bauer, J.H.; Reams, G.P.

SO In: Kaplan, N.M.; Brenner, B.M.; Laragh, J.H., eds. *New Therapeutic Strategies in Hypertension.* New York, NY: Raven Press. 1989. p. 253–287.

AV   Available from Raven Press. 1185 Avenue of the Americas, New York, NY 10036. (212) 930-9541. Price: $104.00 plus $3.00 shipping and handling. ISBN: 0881675288.

TI   ***High Blood Pressure and Your Kidneys.***
SO   New York: National Kidney Foundation. 1990. 4 p.
CN   National Kidney Foundation, Inc.
AV   Available from National Kidney Foundation, Inc. 30 East 33rd Street, New York, NY 10016. (800) 622-9010. Price: Free.

TI   ***Hypertension (Alta Tension Arterial). Hypertension (High Blood Pressure).***
SO   Alexandria, VA: American Diabetes Association, Diabetes Information Service Center. April 1989. 4 p.
CN   American Diabetes Association.
AV   Available from American Diabetes Association, Diabetes Information Service Center. 1660 Duke Street, Alexandria, VA 22314. (800) 232-3472 or (703) 549-1500. (Also available from local Chapters). Price: $.13 per copy.

TI   ***Hypertension (High Blood Pressure).***
SO   Alexandria, VA: American Diabetes Association, Diabetes Information Service Center. March 1989. 4 p.
CN   American Diabetes Association.
AV   Available from American Diabetes Association, Diabetes Information Service Center. 1660 Duke Street, Alexandria, VA 22314. (800) 232-3472 or (703) 549-1500. (Also available from local Chapters). Price: $.13 per copy.

TI   ***Hypertension and Chronic Renal Failure: National High Blood Pressure Education Program (NHBPEP) Working Group Report.***
SO   Bethesda, MD: National Institutes of Health. August 1990. 28 p.
CN   National Institutes of Health
AV   Available from Information Center for the National Heart, Lung and Blood Institute. 7200 Wisconsin Avenue, Box 329, Bethesda, MD 20814. (301) 951-3260. Price: Single copy free. Order Number 90-3032.

TI **Hypertension and Diabetes.**
AU Wilcox, C.S.
SO *Nephrology News and Issues.* 4(11): 24–27. November 1990.
AV Available from Nephrology News and Issues. 13901 N. 73rd Street, Suite 214, Scottsdale, AZ 85260-9804. (602) 443-4635.

TI **Hypertension and Renal Insufficiency: Recognition and Management.**
AU Moore, M.A.; Porush, J.G.
SO *American Family Physician.* 45(3): 1248–1256. March 1992.

TI **Hypertension in the Black Population: Revisited.**
AU Baskin, S.
SO *Nephrology News and Issues.* 4(11): 24–27. November 1990.
AV Available from Nephrology News and Issues. 13901 N. 73rd Street, Suite 214, Scottsdale, AZ 85260-9804. (602) 443-4635.

TI **Hypertension.**
AU Seikaly, M.G.; Arant, B.S.
SO In: Barakat, A.Y. *Renal Disease in Children: Clinical Evaluation and Diagnosis.* Secaucus, NJ: Springer-Verlag. 1990. p. 307–328.
AV Available from Springer-Verlag. Order Department, 44 Hartz Way, Secaucus, NJ 07094. (800) 777-4643 or (212) 460-1500 ext. 599. Price: $85.00. ISBN: 0387970363.

TI **Hypertension: Racial Differences.**
AU Eisner, G.M.
SO *American Journal of Kidney Diseases.* 16(4 Supplement 1): 35–40. October 1990.
AV Available from National Kidney Foundation. 30 East 33rd Street, New York, NY 10016. (212) 889-2210 or (800) 622-9010.

TI **Hypertensive Nephropathy: Re-Examined.**
AU Rosansky, S.J.
SO *Kidney.* 24(2): 1–8. October 1991.
AV Available from National Kidney Foundation, Inc. Medical Department, 30 East 33rd Street, New York, NY 10016. (800) 622-9010.

TI *International Yearbook of Nephrology 1990.*
AU Andreucci, V.E., ed.
SO Hingham, MA: Kluwer Academic Publishers. 1990. 298 p.
AV Available from Kluwer Academic Publishers. P.O. Box 358, Accord Station, Hingham, MA 02018-0358. (617) 871-6600.

TI *Investigating Hypertension in Children.*
AU Ingelfinger, J.R.
SO Nephrology News and Issues. 3(2): 29. February 1989.
AV Available from Nephrology News and Issues. 13901 N. 73rd Street, Suite 214, Scottsdale, AZ 85260-9804. (602) 443-4635.

TI **Kidney in Hypertensive Pregnancies: Victim and Villain.**
AU Brown, M.A.; Whitworth, J.A.
SO *American Journal of Kidney Diseases.* 20(5): 427–442. November 1992.
AV Available from National Kidney Foundation. 30 East 33rd Street, New York, NY 10016. (212) 889-2210 or (800) 622-9010.

TI **Kidneys Produce a Special Enzyme Which Regulates Your Blood Pressure.**
AU Moss, E.
SO *21st Century Health Letter.* p. 8. Winter 1993.

TI *Managing Your Diabetes: Kidneys.*
SO Indianapolis, IN: Eli Lilly and Company. 1991. 4 p.
CN Eli Lilly and Company.
AV Available from Eli Lilly and Company. Lilly Corporate Center, Indianapolis, IN 46285. (317) 276-2000. Price: Free.

TI **Modality Selection for the Elderly: Medical Factors.**
AU Maiorca R., et al.
SO *Advances in Peritoneal Dialysis* (Toronto, Canada). Volume 6 (Supplement): 18–25. 1990.
AV Available from the Peritoneal Dialysis International Bulletin, Inc. Toronto Western Hospital, Edith Cavel Wing, Room 525, 399 Bathhurst Street, Toronto, Ontario MST 2S8, CANADA. (416) 369-5189.

TI   **National High Blood Pressure Education Program Working Group Report on Hypertension and Chronic Renal Failure.**
SO   *Archives of Internal Medicine.* 151(7): 1280–1287. July 1991.
CN   National High Blood Pressure Education Program.

TI   *Noninflammatory Vascular Diseases of the Kidney.*
AU   Eknoyan, G.
SO   In: Suki, W.N.; Massry, S.G., eds. Therapy of Renal Diseases and Related Disorders, 2nd ed. Hingham, MA: Kluwer Academic Publishers. 1991. p. 425–441.
AV   Available from Kluwer Academic Publishers. P.O. Box 358, Accord Station, Hingham, MA 02018. (617) 871-6600. Price: $279.95. ISBN: 0792306767.

TI   *Nutrition in the Pathogenesis and Treatment of Hypertension.*
AU   Krishna, G.G.
SO   Bethlehem, PA: St. Luke's Hospital. 1991.
PR   Audiocassette (60 min).
AV   Available from St. Luke's Hospital. Nutrition Services-Renal, 801 Ostrum Street, Bethlehem, PA 18015. (215) 954-4000. Price: Contact directly for details.

TI   **Pregnancy and Birth Control in Dialysis Patients.**
AU   Hou, S.
SO   *Dialysis and Transplantation.* 23(1): 22–23,26. January 1994.
AV   Available from Creative Age Publications, Inc. 7628 Densmore Avenue, Van Nuys, CA 91406-2088. (818) 782-7328.

TI   **Pregnancy in End-Stage Renal Disease.**
AU   Hou, S.H.
SO   *NKF Family Focus. National Kidney Foundation Family Focus.* 4(2): 13. Spring 1993.
AV   Available from National Kidney Foundation, Inc. 30 E. 33rd Street, New York, NY 10016. (800) 622-9010; (212) 889-2210.

TI   **Preventing Diabetic Kidney Disease.**
AU   Laffel, L.
SO   *JDF International Countdown.* 13(4): 21. Fall 1992.

AV   Available from Juvenile Diabetes Foundation International. 432 Park Avenue South, New York, NY 10016. (212) 889-7575 or (800) 223-1138.

TI   **Progression of Kidney Disease May Be Preventable.**
AU   Klahr, S.
SO   *Kidney '90* [National Kidney Foundation]. 7(4): 6–7. July-August 1990.
AV   Available from National Kidney Foundation. 30 East 33rd Street, New York, NY 10016. (800) 622-9010.

TI   **Renal and Ocular Manifestations of Hypertensive Diseases of Pregnancy.**
AU   Seidman, D.S.; Serr, D.M.; Ben-Rafael, Z.
SO   *Obstetrical and Gynecological Survey.* 46(2): 71–76. February 1991.

TI   **Renal Disease and Hypertension in Pregnancy.**
AU   Umans, J.G.; Lindheimer, M.D.
SO   In: Levine, D.Z. *Care of the Renal Patient.* Orlando, FL: W.B. Saunders Company. 1991. p. 85–96.
AV   Available from W.B. Saunders Company. 6277 Sea Harbor Drive, Orlando, FL 32887. (800) 782-4479. Price: $40.00 plus shipping and handling. ISBN: 0721630561.

TI   **Renal Disease in Hypertensive Adults: Effect of Race and Type II Diabetes Mellitus.**
AU   Tierney, W.M.; McDonald, C.J.; Luft, F.C.
SO   *American Journal of Kidney Diseases.* 13(6): 485–493. 1989.
AV   Available from National Kidney Foundation. 30 East 33rd Street, New York, NY 10016. (212) 889-2210 or (800) 622-9010.

TI   **Risk Factors for Progression of Renal Insufficiency in Diabetic Nephropathy: Therapeutic Implications.**
AU   Nyberg, G.
SO   In: Andreucci, V.E.; Fine, L.G., eds. *International Yearbook of Nephrology 1991.* Hingham, MA: Kluwer Academic Publishers. 1990. p. 161–175.
AV   Available from Kluwer Academic Publishers. P.O. Box 348, Accord Station, Hingham MA 02018-0358. (617) 871-6600. Price: $110.00. ISBN: 0792310020.

TI   **Role of Hypertension in the Progression of Renal Diseases.**

AU   Campese, V.M.; Bigazzi, R.

SO   *American Journal of Kidney Diseases*. 17(5 Supplement 1): 43–47. May 1991.

AV   Available from National Kidney Foundation. 30 East 33rd Street, New York, NY 10016. (212) 889-2210 or (800) 622-9010.

TI   **Solitary Kidney: A Risky Situation for Progressive Renal Damage?**

AU   Oldrizzi, L., et al.

SO   *American Journal of Kidney Diseases*. 17(5 Supplement 1): 57–61. May 1991.

AV   Available from National Kidney Foundation. 30 East 33rd Street, New York, NY 10016. (212) 889-2210 or (800) 622-9010.

TI   **Systolic Hypertension in the Elderly: Reasons Not to Treat.**

AU   Michelis, M.F.

SO   *American Journal of Kidney Diseases*. 16(4): 332–334. October 1990.

AV   Available from National Kidney Foundation. 30 East 33rd Street, New York, NY 10016. (212) 889-2210 or (800) 622-9010.

For Additional Information

CHID is available on-line through CDP Online. If you would like references to materials on other topics, you may request a special literature search of CHID from a library that subscribes to CDP Online or from the National Kidney and Urologic Diseases Information Clearinghouse, 3 Information Way, Bethesda, MD 20892-3580; (301) 654-4415.

Chapter 14

Resources on Pyelonephritis

Legend

TI   Title
AU   Author
CN   Corporate Author
SO   Source
PR   Product
AV   Producer/Availability
AB   Abstract

TI   **Acute Pyelonephritis: Preventing Complications Through Prompt Diagnosis and Proper Therapy.**
AU   Tenner, S.M.; Yadven, M.W.; Kimmel, P.L.
SO   *Postgraduate Medicine*. 91(2): 261–268. February 1, 1992.
AB   This article reviews acute pyelonephritis, the most serious form of urinary tract infection. Topics covered include distinguishing pyelonephritis from acute cystitis, how to treat a patient outside of the hospital setting, and antibiotic therapy. The authors address these and other issues of concern to primary care physicians in this review of the diagnosis, treatment, and potential complications of acute pyelonephritis. The authors stress that elderly, diabetic, immunocompromised hospitalized patients, and patients subject to instrumentation

present a more complex diagnostic challenge and require more intense parenteral treatment.

TI   **Etiology and Pathophysiology of Pyelonephritis.**
AU   Roberts, J.A.
SO   *American Journal of Kidney Diseases.* 17(1): 1–9. January 1991.
AB   This article explores the etiology and pathophysiology of pyelonephritis. Escherichia coli (E coli) is the most frequent cause of pyelonephritis. Its possible virulence factors include the ability to adhere and colonize the urinary tract, an important initiating factor in all urinary tract infections (UTIs). Topics discussed include bacterial adhesion; fimbrial adhesion; host receptor density; the bacterial effect on ureteral physiology; ischemic events; damage from oxygen radicals during phagocytosis; and the prevention of chronic pyelonephritis. The authors note that acute pyelonephritis during the first 3 years of life more often produced the renal damage that could lead to end-stage renal disease. Thus, the prevention of end-stage renal diseases that may occur from acute pyelonephritis during infancy depends on early diagnosis and rapid, effective antibiotic treatment. Such treatment will eradicate the bacteria and stop the destructive reperfusion damage and that associated with the inflammatory response.

TI   *Pyelonephritis.*
SO   Port Washington, NY: Romaine Pierson Publishers, Inc. September 1983.
PR   Chart (7 3/8 in x 10 3/4 in), col, three-hole punched.
AV   Available from Romaine Pierson Publishers, Inc., 80 Shore Road, Port Washington, NY 11050. (516) 883-6350. PRICE: $0.60 each; bulk discount available.
AB   This chart shows a color drawing of pyelonephritis, a disease of the kidney. The drawing shows a cross-section of the renal duct, an internal portion of the kidney, and the growth of nodules on the kidney surface. The chart is designed to aid physicians in explaining the disease to patients.

TI   **Recognizing and Treating Acute Pyelonephritis.**
AU   Johnson, J.R.
SO   *Emergency Medicine.* 24(3): 25–27, 30–31. February 29, 1992.

AB   Acute pyelonephritis, infection of the renal pelvis or paren-
chyma, is one of the most common serious infectious diseases
of adult women, causing as many as 100,000 hospitalizations
a year in the United States. This article discusses recognizing
and treating acute pyelonephritis, focusing on prompt diagnosis and careful selection of antimicrobial agents to prevent
permanent kidney damage. Topics covered include risk factors
and etiology, clinical presentation, diagnostic evaluation,
pathogenesis, and treatment of acute pyelonephritis. Specific
treatment issues covered include inpatient versus outpatient
treatment, choice of initial IV therapy, management during
pregnancy, duration of IV therapy, delayed response to therapy,
choice of initial oral therapy, and total duration of therapy. A
final section discusses follow-up.

TI   *Understanding Urinary Tract Infections: Treatment and
Prevention for Men and Women.*

SO   San Bruno, CA: Krames Communications. 1988. 8 p.

AV   Available from Krames Communications. 1100 Grundy Lane,
San Bruno, CA 94066-3030. (415) 742-0400. PRICE: $1.10
each; bulk discounts available. Order No. 1283.

AB   This booklet explains the pathogenesis, symptoms and treatment of urinary tract infection (UTI) in men and women in a
colorfully illustrated text. An early medical evaluation of UTI
is encouraged because it can lead to successful treatment and
prevent development of more serious diseases. Types of UTIs
such as cystitis, pyelonephritis, urethral syndrome in women,
and prostatitis and urethritis in men are distinguished. UTIs
are caused by bacteria entering the urogenital system due to
poor hygiene, lowered resistance or reduced immune response,
or sexual intercourse. Treatment consists predominantly of
medications. It is extremely important to adhere to the prescribed treatment plan (e.g., drug therapy, drinking lots of water,
etc.) to prevent recurrence.

TI   **Urinary Tract Infections in Women Diagnosis and
Treatment.**

AU   Johnson, J.R; Stamm, W.E.

SO   *Annals of Internal Medicine.* 111(11): 906–917. December 1,
1989.

AB This paper reviews recent developments in the diagnosis and treatment of acute urinary tract infections among women. In acute lower urinary tract infection, empiric short-course therapy (single dose or 3-day therapy) with one of several antibiotics is recommended in the absence of complicating factors. When complications are present, the antibiotic susceptibility profile of the infecting organism should be determined and therapy with an appropriate agent should be given for 7 days. Ampicillin and related drugs are probably inferior to trimethoprim-sulfamethoxazole in treating occult renal infection. In acute pyelonephritis, most patients need hospitalization and treatment with intravenous antibiotics until they can take oral medications. In uncomplicated cases, a single broad spectrum intravenous agent can be initially used, followed by an oral agent selected on the basis of antibiotic-susceptibility test results. Patients with uncomplicated acute pyelonephritis who are less ill can be managed with oral therapy as outpatients, based on such susceptibility test results. Complicated acute pyelonephritis needs more aggressive diagnostic and therapy measures. Therapy for uncomplicated acute pyelonephritis should be given for 14 days. The role of post-therapy cultures in managing urinary tract infections is not well defined, but cultures probably can be safely omitted in most cases of uncomplicated acute cystitis.

TI **Urinary Tract Infections in Women.**
AU Johnson, M.G.
SO *American Family Physician*. 41(2): 565–571. February 1990.
AB This article discusses urinary tract infections in women and notes that the clinical conditions that cause dysuria in women can usually be differentiated by the history and selected physical and laboratory examinations. Cystitis can be treated with short-course therapy in uncomplicated cases. Pretreatment cultures are usually not necessary, since most infections are caused by 'Escherichia coli.' Outpatient treatment of pyelonephritis is appropriate in selected patients. Follow-up culture after treatment of either cystitis or pyelonephritis is indicated to identify those patients requiring longer treatment or urologic evaluation. The article recounts research that suggests that recurrent urinary tract infections can be managed with postcoital antibiotics, long-term prophylaxis or

patient self-administration of short-course therapy. The article stresses that bacteriuria and pyelonephritis in pregnancy must be aggressively diagnosed and treated.

TI **Urinary Tract Infections.**
SO *Medical Times*. 199x. 2 p.
PR Chart (7 3/8 in x 10 3/4 in), col, two sided, 3-hole punched.
AV Available from Romaine Pierson Publishers, Inc., 80 Shore Road, Port Washington, NY 11050. (516) 883 6350. Price: $0.60, bulk discount available.
AB This color anatomical chart educates patients about urinary tract infections. It illustrates acute pyelonephritis, urethritis, cystitis, and prostatitis. It also shows how bacteria spread from the site of colonization into the bladder.

For Additional Information

CHID is available on-line through BRS Online, a division of InfoPro Technologies. If you would like references to materials on other topics, you may request a special literature search of CHID from a library that subscribes to BRS or from the National Kidney and Urologic Diseases Information Clearinghouse, Box NKUDIC, 9000 Rockville Pike, Bethesda, MD 20892; (301)654-4415.

Chapter 15

Lupus and Kidney Disease

Chapter Contents

Section 15.1

Lupus and Kidney Disease

Kidney and Urology Facts, National Kidney Foundation ©1992.
Used by permission.

Lupus can harm your kidneys as well as other organs and tissues in your body. This fact sheet will give you information about lupus in general and about how it can affect your kidneys. It also offers suggestions about how you can live with your disease and keep feeling your best.

What is lupus?

Lupus is a short name for a disease called "lupus erythematosus." The word lupus means wolf in Latin. The skin rash that some patients get can form a butterfly pattern over the bridge of the nose, resembling the bite of a wolf. Lupus is called an "autoimmune" disease because the immune system, which usually protects the body from disease, turns against the body, causing harm to organs and tissues.

There are two types of lupus. Systemic lupus erythematosus can harm your skin, joints, kidneys and brain and may be fatal. The other type, called "discoid" lupus erythematosus, affects only your skin.

What causes lupus?

No one knows what causes the disease. Your family history and things in your environment such as infections, viruses, toxic chemicals or pollutants (car fumes, factory smoke) may play a role in causing the disease.

People of all ages, races and both sexes get lupus. However, it is about ten times more common in women than men. About 500,000 Americans have lupus.

What are the symptoms of lupus?

Different people get different symptoms. These may include: skin rashes, joint pain, hair loss, sun sensitivity, tiredness, weight loss, fever, swelling of lymph glands, chest pain and nerve involvement.

How can lupus harm the kidneys?

Lupus can harm your kidneys a little or a lot. It can cause a lot of damage to the filtering units (glomeruli) of the kidney. Since these filtering units clear your blood of waste, damage to them can cause your kidneys to work poorly or not at all. About 90 percent of lupus patients will have some kidney damage but only 2 to 3 percent actually develop kidney disease severe enough to require treatment.

The kidney disease may be "silent" and not cause any symptoms. However, you may have dark urine, flank pain, high blood pressure, weight gain from extra fluid, and swelling around your eyes and or your hands and feet.

How do I know if I have lupus?

Your doctor will do a physical examination, get your medical history, and do special tests such as x-rays and a blood test for "antinuclear" antibody.

How is lupus treated?

Lupus is treated with drugs that block your body's immune system. Some of these are prednisone, azathioprine, cyclophosphamide or cyclosporine.

Do these treatments have side effects?

Yes. These drugs have some side effects, such as weight gain and increased susceptibility to infections and tumors. Fortunately, these side effects usually are manageable for most patients.

Do I need to follow a special diet?

Sometimes. All patients should follow a well-balanced diet. When the disease is active, you may have to follow some restrictions. You need to talk with your doctor or dietitian about the best diet for you.

If you have kidney disease, you may need to eat less protein and sodium (salt). If you have high blood pressure, you should be sure to take the drugs prescribed to control your pressure. If you are overweight, losing weight may help to control your blood pressure.

How can I tell if the disease has hurt my kidneys?

The doctor can tell if lupus has harmed your kidneys by finding protein or blood in your urine. Also, the levels of urea and creatinine in your blood will be high because your kidneys are not getting rid of these waste products as well as usual. Your doctor may want to collect a 24 hour urine sample.

What happens if my kidneys fail?

If your kidneys fail, you can be treated with dialysis or a kidney transplant. Lupus patients do as well with these treatments as people who have other types of kidney disease.

Many patients with lupus kidney disease have received a kidney transplant. The drugs used to prevent your body from rejecting the new kidney are the same or like those used to treat lupus. It is unusual for lupus to come back in the new kidney. Most of the time, the lupus stays inactive. Lupus patients with new kidneys do as well as any other patients with transplanted kidneys.

What is my long-term outlook?

Most patients do well long-term. You may need to take drugs over many years. Even patients who have less involvement should have periodic checkups.

What can I do to help myself?

You should learn more about the disease and the factors that cause it to flare up. One of these factors is sun exposure. You should avoid outdoor activities between 10 a.m. and 4 p.m. If you must go out, you should wear strong sunscreens, wide-brimmed hats and long-sleeved shirts. You need to follow your doctor's orders carefully and take your medicines as directed.

Tiredness also can cause the disease to flare up. You should plan your physical activities and schedule rest periods. Planned exercise is helpful.

Chronic illness requires coping as well as understanding and support from family members. When the disease is active, lupus patients may have decreased ability to handle household or job-related tasks. The ability to cope and to be flexible will go a long way toward learning to live with lupus.

What if I have more questions?

If you have more questions, you should speak to your doctor. You also can get additional information by contacting your local National Kidney Foundation Affiliate and the Lupus Foundation of America.

What is The National Kidney Foundation and how does it help?

Twenty million Americans have some form of kidney or urologic disease. Millions more are at risk. The National Kidney Foundation, Inc., a major voluntary health organization, is working to find the answers through prevention, treatment and cure. Through its 50 Affiliates nationwide, the Foundation conducts programs in research, professional education, patient and community services, public education and organ donation. The work of The National Kidney Foundation is funded entirely by public donations.

Section 15.2

Additional Resources on Lupus Nephritis

NKUDIC, Topics in Kidney and Urologic Diseases, December 1994.

Legend

TI   Title
AU   Author
CN   Corporate Author
SO   Source
AV   Producer/Availability

TI   *Glomerulonephritis.*
SO   New York, NY: National Kidney Foundation, Inc. 6 p. 1987.
CN   National Kidney Foundation, Inc.
AV   Available from the National Kidney Foundation, Inc., 30 East 33rd Street, New York, NY 10016. (800) 622-9010.

TI   *Lupus and Kidney Disease: How Does Lupus Affect Your Kidneys?*
SO   Ann Arbor, MI: National Kidney Foundation of Michigan, Inc. 1986. 6 p.
CN   National Kidney Foundation of Michigan, Inc.
AV   Available from National Kidney Foundation of Michigan, Inc., 2350 South Huron Parkway, Ann Arbor, MI 48104. (313) 971-2800 or (800) 482-1455.

TI   **Plasmapheresis in Glomerulonephritis.**
AU   Pusey, C.D.
SO   In: Catto, G.R.D. *New Clinical Applications-Nephrology: Glomerulonephritis*. Hingham, MA: Kluwer Academic Publishers. p. 139–162. 1990.

AV   Available from Kluwer Academic Publishers. P.O. Box 358, Accord Station, Hingham, MA 02018-0358. (617) 871-6600. PRICE: $54.00. ISBN: 0746201095.

TI   **Lupus Nephritis.**
AU   Ballardie, F.W.
SO   In: Catto, G.R.D., ed. *Multisystem Diseases*. Boston, MA: Kluwer Academic Publishers. p. 49–76.
AV   Available from Kluwer Academic Publishers. P.O. Box 358, Accord Station, Hingham, MA 02018-0358. (617) 871-6600. PRICE: $50.00 plus shipping and handling. ISBN 0746200609.

TI   **Development of Immunopathologic Investigation of Kidney Disease.**
AU   Dixon, F.J.; Wilson, C.B.
SO   *American Journal of Kidney Disease*. 16(6): 574–578. December 1990.
AV   Available from National Kidney Foundation. 30 East 33rd Street, New York, NY 10016. (212) 889-2210 or (800) 622-9010.

TI   *Renal Disease and Lupus.*
SO   Washington, DC: Lupus Foundation of America. 1988. 4 p.
CN   Lupus Foundation of America.
AV   Available from the Lupus Foundation of America. 1717 Massachusetts Avenue, NW, Suite 203, Washington, DC 20036. (800) 558-0121. PRICE: Single copy free.

TI   **Maternal and Fetal Complications in Pregnant Women with Systemic Lupus Erythematosus.**
AU   Hayslett, J.P.
SO   *American Journal of Kidney Diseases*. 17(2): 123–126. February 1991.
AV   Available from National Kidney Foundation. 30 East 33rd Street, New York, NY 10016. (212) 889-2210 or (800) 622-9010.

TI   **Systemic Lupus Erythematosus.**
AU   Andrew, S.L.; Huston, D.P.
SO   In: Suki, W.N.; Massry, S.G., eds. *Therapy of Renal Diseases and Related Disorders*, 2nd ed. Hingham, MA: Kluwer Academic Publishers. 1991. p. 395–411.

AV   Available from Kluwer Academic Publishers. P.O. Box 358, Accord Station, Hingham, MA 02018. (617) 871-6600. PRICE: $279.95. ISBN: 0792306767.

TI   Renal Transplantation in Systemic Inherited and Metabolic Disease.
AU   Lederer, E.D.; Suki, W.N.
SO   In: Suki, W.N.; Massry, S.G., eds. *Therapy of Renal Diseases and Related Disorders*, 2nd ed. Hingham, MA: Kluwer Academic Publishers. 1991. p. 921–941.
AV   Available from Kluwer Academic Publishers. P.O. Box 358, Accord Station, Hingham, MA 02018. (617) 871-6600. PRICE: $279.95. ISBN: 0792306767.

TI   Pregnancy in Women with Renal Disease.
AU   Hou, S.
SO   *American Kidney Fund Nephrology Letter*. 8(1): 1–12. February 1991.
AV   Available from American Kidney Fund. 6110 Executive Boulevard, Suite 1010, Rockville, MD 20852. (800) 638-8299 or (301) 881-3052.

TI   Glomerular Diseases.
AU   Makker, S.P.
SO   In: Kher, K.K.; Makker, S.P., eds. *Clinical Pediatric Nephrology*. Blue Ridge Summit, PA: McGraw-Hill. 1992. p. 175–276.
AV   Available from McGraw-Hill, Inc. 13311 Monterey Avenue, Blue Ridge Summit, PA 17294. (800) 262-4729. PRICE: $85.00 plus $3.00 for shipping and handling. ISBN: 0070345430.

TI   Being On the Other Side.
AU   Allegra, K.
SO   *For Patients Only*. 4(2): 21–23, 26. March-April 1991.
AV   Available from Contemporary Dialysis, Inc. 6300 Variel Avenue, Suite 1, Woodland Hills, CA 91367. (818) 704-5555.

TI   Course and Treatment of Lupus Nephritis.
AU   Appel, G.B.; Valeri, A.

SO   In: Coggins, C.H.; Hancock, E.W., Eds. *Annual Review of Medicine: Selected Topics in the Clinical Sciences*, Volume 45. Palo Alto, CA: Annual Reviews Inc. 1994. p. 525–537.

AV   Available from Annual Reviews Inc. 4139 El Camino Way, P.O. Box 10139, Palo Alto, CA 94303-0139. (800) 523-8635. Fax: (415) 855-9815. PRICE: $47.00. ISBN: 0824305450.

Chapter 16

Alport Syndrome

What is Alport Syndrome? What are its symptoms?

Alport Syndrome is an inherited disease that affects the glomeruli, the tiny blood vessels within the kidneys that filter the blood of its wastes. An English doctor, A. Cecil Alport, described many of the important features of the disease in the *British Medical Journal* in 1927, and his name has been associated with the disorder ever since.

Because of the way Alport Syndrome is inherited, the disease tends to be more severe in men than in women. The central feature of the disease is the presence of blood in the urine. Boys with Alport Syndrome develop this symptom in infancy, while girls who carry the Alport gene may or may not have it.

Another important symptom of Alport Syndrome is hearing loss. In boys with the disease, hearing loss is usually detectable by 8-10 years of age, and it may be severe enough to require the use of hearing aids. Hearing loss in girls tends to be much milder, rarely resulting in the need for hearing aids.

Some boys with Alport Syndrome lose large amounts of protein in the urine, resulting in retentions of fluid and body swelling. This condition is called the "nephrotic syndrome." With the passage of years, boys with Alport Syndrome develop the typical signs and symptoms

Sections from Kidney and Urology Facts, National Kidney Foundation ©1991 and Searches on File, Topics in Kidney and Urologic Diseases, NKUDIC. Copyrighted material used by permission.

of kidney failure—high blood pressure, swelling, and in some cases, impaired growth.

Some people with Alport Syndrome have an eye problem called anterior lenticonus, in which the shape of the lens becomes distorted. This can interfere with the sharpness of vision.

How serious is Alport Syndrome?

Alport Syndrome causes progressive kidney damage. This means that the glomeruli undergo a gradual but persistent process of destruction, leading to kidney failure in many cases. Boys with Alport Syndrome inevitably develop kidney failure, but kidney failure in girls is unusual. The age at which boys with Alport Syndrome develop kidney failure varies from family to family. It may occur as early as 15-20 years of age, but in some families, kidney failure does not develop until the men are 40-50 years of age.

How is Alport Syndrome diagnosed?

Absolute diagnosis of Alport Syndrome can be difficult because its symptoms are similar to those of other kidney diseases, particularly benign familial hematuria (BFH). BFH is another inherited disease that causes many members of a family to have blood in the urine. However, it does not lead to kidney failure.

The diagnosis of Alport Syndrome is done by a careful family history and a kidney biopsy (examination of a small piece of tissue taken from the kidney). Characteristic changes occur in the walls of the capillaries that make up the glomeruli, which are seen only in people with Alport Syndrome. Recently, a group of researchers at the University of Utah School of Medicine in Salt Lake City isolated the gene that is responsible for Alport Syndrome. This discovery will permit the development of a simpler and more precise test for the disease.

How is Alport Syndrome treated?

Currently, there is no specific therapy for Alport Syndrome. Treatment of the kidney disease consists of controlling high blood pressure and restricting dietary phosphorus. Men with Alport Syndrome eventually require replacement of kidney function with dialysis or kidney transplantation. In most cases, Alport Syndrome does not recur in transplanted kidneys, so successful transplantation essentially cures the kidney component of the disease. In about 5-10 percent of transplanted patients, inflammation develops in the glomeruli of the transplanted kidney, which usually leads to failure of the transplant. This is different from rejection, and is caused by a specific immunologic reaction against the transplanted kidney.

Kidney specialists currently are evaluating new approaches designed to preserve kidney function in people with chronic kidney disease. Methods such as dietary protein restriction and the use of a specific blood pressure medication called angiotensin converting enzyme inhibitors may eventually prove useful in delaying, if not preventing, the development of kidney failure in people with Alport Syndrome.

How is Alport Syndrome inherited?

The gene for Alport Syndrome generally is located on the X chromosome, which is one of the chromosomes that determines an individual's sex. The disease is less severe in women because they have two X chromosomes. A normal gene on one of the X chromosomes limits the effects of the Alport gene. Since men only have one X chromosome, there is no normal gene to oppose the effects of the Alport Syndrome, resulting in more severe disease.

About 15-20 percent of the people who have Alport Syndrome do not have a family history of the disease. In these cases, Alport Syndrome results from new mutations in the gene that is affected in Alport Syndrome. In this case, the affected person is the first member of the family to develop the disease.

What research is being done? What is the future outlook for Alport Syndrome?

The isolation of the gene for Alport Syndrome at the University of Utah is an important breakthrough. The Utah team identified three mutations of the gene. These mutations are associated with defects in a protein known as collagen type IV, which is an integral part of the glomerular basement membrane, a structure that plays a key role in the filtering of blood by the kidney. This discovery not only will permit more precise diagnosis of Alport Syndrome, but it opens the possibility for future gene therapy for this disorder.

What is The National Kidney Foundation and how does it help?

Twenty million Americans have some form of kidney or urinary tract diseases. Millions more are at risk. The National Kidney Foundation, Inc., a major voluntary health organization, is working to find the answers through prevention, treatment and cure. Through its 50 Affiliates nationwide, the Foundation conducts programs in research, professional education, patient and community services, public education and organ donation. The work of The National Kidney Foundation is funded entirely by donations from the public.

Citations on Alport Syndrome

Legend

TI   Title
AU   Author
CN   Corporate Author
SO   Source
AV   Producer/Availability

TI   Alport Syndrome, Basement Membranes and Collagen.
AU   Kashtan, C.E., et al.
SO   *Pediatric Nephrology*. 4(5): 523–532. September 1990.

**TI   *Alport Syndrome.*
SO   New Fairfield, CT: National Organization for Rare Disorders, Inc. 1989. 7 p.
CN   National Organization for Rare Disorders, Inc.
AV   Available from National Organization for Rare Disorders, Inc. P.O. Box 8923, New Fairfield, CT 06812. (203) 746-6518.

**TI   *Alport Syndrome.*
SO   New York, NY: National Kidney Foundation, Inc. 1991. 3 p.
CN   National Kidney Foundation, Inc.
AV   Available from National Kidney Foundation, Inc. 30 East 33rd Street, New York, NY 10016. (800) 622-9010. Order Number KU-4. Single copy free.

TI   **Glomerular Diseases.**
AU   Makker, S.P.
SO   In: Kher, K.K.; Makker, S.P., eds. *Clinical Pediatric Nephrology*. Blue Ridge Summit, PA: McGraw-Hill. 1992. p. 175–276.
AV   Available from McGraw-Hill, Inc. 13311 Monterey Avenue, Blue Ridge Summit, PA 17294. (800) 262-4729. $85.00 plus $3.00 for shipping and handling. ISBN: 0070345430.

TI   **Inherited Renal and Genitourinary Disorders.**
AU   Chesney, R.W.
SO   In: Thoene, J.G.; Smith, D.C., eds. *Physicians' Guide to Rare Diseases*. Montvale, NJ: Dowden Publishing Company, Inc. 1992. p. 833–855.
AV   Available from Dowden Publishing Company, Inc. 110 Summit Avenue, Montvale, NJ 07645. (201) 391-9100. $69.50 plus $6.95 shipping and handling. ISBN: 0962871605.

TI   **Research Profile: Spotlight on Alport Syndrome.**
SO   *Kidney*. January-February 1989.

TI   **Utah Researchers Announce Discovery of Gene that Causes Severe Kidney Disease.**
SO   *Nephrology News and Issues*. 4(7): 12–13. July 1990.

Chapter 17

Focal Glomerulosclerosis

What is Focal Glomerulosclerosis?

Focal sclerosis is a common form of kidney disease that may cause permanent kidney failure in children and adults. In children who have nephrotic syndrome (large amounts of protein in the urine), 7 to 16 percent will be found to have focal sclerosis. About 15 percent of adults with large amounts of protein in the urine will be found to have focal sclerosis. Focal sclerosis is one of more than 20 different types of glomerulonephritis, a disease that affects the kidney's filtering units. Focal sclerosis in adults usually develops between 15 and 30 years of age.

What are the symptoms?

The symptoms are the same as those of other causes of kidney failure. These include fatigue, nausea and headache. If very large amounts of protein are lost in the urine, swelling of the ankles and of the belly may occur.

What causes focal sclerosis?

Although the cause is not know in most cases, focal sclerosis sometimes occurs in patients with reflux nephropathy or chronic kidney infections. IV drug abuse also can lead to focal sclerosis. This may be

Excerpts from Kidney and Urology Facts, National Kidney Foundation ©1986; and Searches-On-File, Topics in Kidney and Urologic Diseases, NKUDIC. Copyrighted material used by permission.

caused by a toxic substance used to "cut" the drugs. Focal sclerosis may also occur in patients with AIDS.

How is focal sclerosis diagnosed?

The diagnosis is usually made by a kidney biopsy—a tiny piece of the kidney is removed with a special needle and examined under a microscope.

What can I expect?

Most patients with focal sclerosis progress to kidney failure and require dialysis treatments or kidney transplant. This may take from one to 20 years to happen, but generally, it happens within 10 years.

How is focal sclerosis treated?

Drugs that affect the body's immune system, such as prednisone or immunosuppressants, have been used to treat the disorder, but it is not certain whether these drugs have a definite benefit. Treatment is usually aimed at slowing the rate of loss of kidney function by controlling high blood pressure with medicine and reducing the intake of protein in the diet.

What is my long term outlook? Can I get a kidney transplant?

Patients who progress to kidney failure generally are young and good candidates for kidney transplants. Focal sclerosis can recur in the transplanted kidney. This may be more common when the kidney comes from a blood relative. However, you should not be discouraged about trying a transplant since the majority of patients do not develop recurrent disease.

What is The National Kidney Foundation and how does it help?

Twenty million Americans have some form of kidney or urologic disease. Millions more are at risk. The National Kidney Foundation, Inc., a major voluntary health organization, is working to find the answers through prevention, treatment and cure. Through its 50 Affiliates nationwide, the Foundation conducts programs in research, professional education, patient and community services, public education and organ donation. The work of The National Kidney Foundation is funded entirely by public donations.

Additional Resources on Focal Glomerulosclerosis

Legend

TI   Title
AU   Author
CN   Corporate Author
SO   Source
PD   Product
AV   Availability

TI   **Renal Disease in Children with the Acquired Immuno-deficiency Syndrome.**
AU   Strauss, J., et al.
SO   *New England Journal of Medicine*. 321(10): 625–630. September 7, 1989.

TI   **AIDS and Renal Disease: Clinical and Pathological Features.**
AU   Bauer, F.; Cutler, R.E.; Pettis, J.L.
SO   *Dialysis and Transplantation*. 17(1): 37–38. January 1988.

TI   **Recurrence of Glomerulonephritis After Renal Transplantation.**
AU   Walker, R.G.; Kincaid-Smith, P.
SO   In: Andreucci, V.E. *International Yearbook of Nephrology 1990*. Hingham, MA: Kluwer Academic Publishers. 1990. p. 37–51.
AV   Available from Kluwer Academic Publishers. P.O. Box 358, Accord Station, Hingham, MA 02018-0358. (617) 871-6600.

TI   **Histological Patterns of Glomerulonephritis.**
AU   Sweny, P.; Farrington, K.; Moorhead, J.F.
SO   In: Sweny, P., Farrington, K., and Moorhead, J.F. *The Kidney and Its Disorders*. St. Louis, MO: Mosby Yearbook, Inc. 1989. p. 243–256.

TI   **Clinical Role of Proteinuria.**
AU   D'Amico, G.
SO   *American Journal of Kidney Diseases*. 17(5 Supplement 1): 48–52. May 1991.

TI   *Problems in Pediatric Nephrology.*
AU   Gauthier, B.
SO   Chapel Hill, NC: Health Sciences Consortium. 1991. (computer-assisted instruction program).
PD   Computer assisted instruction program for IBM and Apple II computers, 8 diskettes (5 1/4 in or 3 ½ in), with instructions. IBM format requires IBM PC, PC/XT, PC/AT, PS/2 or 100 percent compatibles, running IBM/MS DOS 2.0 and higher. Apple format requires AppleII plus, Apple IIe, or 100 percent compatible computers with 48K bytes of RAM and at least two floppy disk drives.
AV   Available from Health Sciences Consortium (HSC). 201 Silver Cedar Court, Chapel Hill, NC 27514. (919) 942-8731. Price: $1,056.00 (non-members) or $748.00 (HSC members) plus $5.00 shipping and handling for IBM version. Order Number: IBM A890-MC-020I. Contact HSC for price and ordering information for Apple format software.

TI   **Nephrotic Syndrome.**
AU   Jennette, J.C.; Mandal, A.K.
SO   In: Mandal, A.K.; Jennette, J.C., eds. *Diagnosis and Management of Renal Disease and Hypertension*. Baltimore, MD: Williams and Wilkins. 1988. p. 238–280.
AV   Available from Williams and Wilkins. 428 East Preston Street, Baltimore, MD 21202. (800) 638-0672. Price: $67.50 plus $3.50 shipping and handling. ISBN: 081211129X.

TI   **Nephrotic Syndrome.**
AU   Kher, K.K.
SO   In: Kher, K.K.; Makker, S.P., eds. *Clinical Pediatric Nephrology*. Blue Ridge Summit, PA: McGraw-Hill. 1992. p. 137–174.
AV   Available from McGraw-Hill, Inc. 13311 Monterey Avenue, Blue Ridge Summit, PA 17294. (800) 262-4729. Price: $85.00 plus $3.00 for shipping and handling. ISBN: 0070345430.

TI *Focal Glomerulosclerosis.*
SO New York, NY: The National Kidney Foundation, Inc. 1993. 2 p.
CN The National Kidney Foundation, Inc.
AV Available from The National Kidney Foundation, Inc. 30 East 33rd Street, New York, NY 10016. (800) 622-9010. Single copy free from State Affiliates. Order Number 02-28NN.

TI *Problems in Pediatric Nephrology.*
AU Gauthier, B.
SO Chapel Hill, NC: Health Sciences Consortium. 199x. (computer program).
PD MED-CAPS is available in IBM and Apple II formats; IBM format is available on 5 1/4" and 3 ½" disks; Apple II format is available on 3 ½" disks and requires 48 KB RAM and two floppy disk drives; case driver disk is needed to run diagnostic problem disks.
AV Available from Health Sciences Consortium. 201 Silver Cedar Court, Chapel Hill, NC 27514-1517. (919) 942-8731, (919) 942-3689 (fax). Price: $1,056.00, HSC members $739.20. Catalog number A890-MC-0201.

Chapter 18

Other Rare Kidney Disorders

Chapter Contents

Section 18.1

IgA Nephropathy

Kidney and Urology Facts, National Kidney Foundation,
Publication No. 02–16NN, ©1991. Used by permission

What is IgA Nephropathy?

In many parts of the world, IgA Nephropathy is the most common form of glomerulonephritis—a disease that damages the tiny filtering units of the kidney, called glomeruli. The damage caused by IgA Nephropathy results from abnormal deposits of a protein called "IgA" in the glomeruli.

One of the kidney's most important jobs is to filter toxic waste products from the blood, and the glomeruli play a key role in this process. As more glomeruli are damaged by the IgA protein, the kidney progressively loses its ability to clear wastes from the body. In some patients with IgA Nephropathy, this loss of kidney function progresses to chronic kidney failure, which requires dialysis treatment or a kidney transplant to maintain life.

IgA Nephropathy is sometimes called "Berger's Disease," because a French physician named Berger was one of the first to describe the disease.

What are the signs and symptoms of IgA Nephropathy?

The most common sign is blood in the urine. The amount of blood may be so small that it is only visible with the aid of a microscope. Another common sign is protein in the urine, which may be associated with swelling of the feet.

As more loss of kidney function occurs, symptoms may include: pain in the back below the ribs, increased need to urinate especially at night, fatigue, nausea, swelling of hands and feet, and high blood pressure.

What causes IgA Nephropathy?

The causes of IgA Nephropathy are not known exactly. The disease seems to cluster in certain families and in certain areas of the world. In addition, it is rare in blacks. These facts suggest that genetic influences may play a role in the development of the disease.

How is IgA Nephropathy diagnosed?

The presence of blood and/or protein in the urine may suggest a diagnosis of IgA Nephropathy. However, to confirm this diagnosis, it is necessary to remove a small piece of tissue from the kidney (biopsy) and examine it microscopically for the presence of the characteristic IgA deposits in the glomeruli.

How is IgA Nephropathy treated?

To date, no specific treatment has been proven to be effective. Efforts to slow the progression of kidney damage may include: limiting the amount of protein in the diet and careful control of high blood pressure if present. For patients who develop progressive kidney failure, treatment may consist of dialysis or a kidney transplant. The success rate of transplants is good in these patients. Even though the IgA deposits reappear in the transplanted kidney in about half the patients within one year after the operation, the signs and symptoms of the disease remain mild. Loss of a transplanted kidney to recurrent IgA Nephropathy is uncommon. The milder form of the disease seen after transplantation may be due to the use of anti-rejection drugs such as cyclosporine.

What is the outlook for patients with IgA Nephropathy?

About 20-40 percent of the patients develop end stage kidney failure about 20 years after the disease becomes apparent. Those patients who have an increased level of creatinine in their blood at the time of their diagnosis are more likely to develop chronic kidney failure. It is harder to predict which of the patients who have normal levels of creatinine at the time of diagnosis will develop kidney failure. In general, a poor prognosis is expected for those patients who have high blood pressure, a loss of more than 2 grams of protein a day in their urine, and a significant amount of damage present in their biopsy specimen.

What research is being done?

Several centers in the United States and other countries are studying IgA Nephropathy. Researchers are investigating the chemical composition of the IgA protein, the rate of production of this protein, possible genetic influences on the expression of the disease, analysis of the long-term clinical outcome, and development of animal models to study the disease. Cooperative treatment trials on the effectiveness of the drug, prednisone, and diets rich in fish oils in the treatment of IgA Nephropathy have begun in the United States. However, these studies have not been completed as yet, and these treatments are considered experimental.

What is The National Kidney Foundation and how does it help?

Twenty million Americans have some form of kidney or urinary tract diseases. Millions more are at risk. The National Kidney Foundation, Inc., a major voluntary health organization, is working to find the answers through prevention, treatment and cure. Through its 50 Affiliates nationwide, the Foundation conducts programs in research, professional education, patient and community services, public education and organ donation. The work of The National Kidney Foundation is funded entirely by donations from the public.

Section 18.2

Medullary Sponge Kidney

Excerpts from *Professional Guide to Diseases*, Fourth Edition,
©Springhouse Corporation; and *Physician's Guide to Rare Diseases*,
©Dowden Publishing Company. Used by permission.

In medullary sponge kidney, the collecting ducts in the renal pyramids dilate, and cavities, clefts, and cysts form in the medulla. This disease may affect only a single pyramid in one kidney or all pyramids in both kidneys. The kidneys are usually somewhat enlarged but may be of normal size; they appear spongy.

Since this disorder is usually asymptomatic and benign, it's often overlooked until the patient reaches adulthood. Although medullary sponge kidney may be found in both sexes and in all age-groups, it primarily affects men aged 40 to 70. It occurs in about 1 in every 5,000 to 20,000 persons. Prognosis is generally very good. Medullary sponge kidney is unrelated to medullary cystic disease; these conditions are similar only in the presence and location of the cysts.

Causes

Medullary sponge kidney may be transmitted as an autosomal dominant trait, but this remains unproven. Most nephrologists still consider it a congenital abnormality.

Signs and Symptoms

Symptoms usually appear only as a result of complications and are seldom present before adulthood. Such complications include formation of calcium oxalate stones, which lodge in the dilated cystic collecting ducts or pass through a ureter, and infection secondary to dilation of the ducts. These complications, which occur in about 30%

205

of patients, are likely to produce severe colic, hematuria, lower urinary tract infection (burning on urination, urgency, frequency), and pyelonephritis.

Secondary impairment of renal function from obstruction and infection occurs in only about 10% of patients.

Diagnosis

Intravenous pyelography is usually the key to diagnosis, often showing a characteristic flowerlike appearance of the pyramidal cavities when they fill with contrast material. Retrograde pyelography or excretory urography may show renal calculi, but these tests are usually avoided because of the risk of infection.

Urinalysis is generally normal unless complications develop; however, it may show a slight reduction in concentrating ability or hypercalciuria.

Diagnosis must distinguish medullary sponge kidney from renal tuberculosis, renal tubular acidosis, and papillary necrosis.

Treatment

Treatment focuses on preventing or treating complications caused by stones and infection. Specific measures include increasing fluid intake and monitoring renal function and urine. New symptoms necessitate immediate evaluation.

Since medullary sponge kidney is a benign condition, surgery is seldom necessary, except to remove stones during acute obstruction. Only serious, uncontrollable infection or hemorrhage requires nephrectomy.

Special Considerations

- Explain the disease to the patient and his family. Stress that the condition is benign and the prognosis good.

- To prevent infection, instruct the patient to bath often and use proper toilet hygiene. Such hygiene is especially important for a female patient, since the proximity of the urinary meatus and the anus increases the risk of infection.

- If infection occurs, stress the importance of completing the pre-scribed course of antibiotic therapy.

- Emphasize the need for fluids.

- Explain all diagnostic procedures, and provide emotional support. Demonstrate how to collect a clean-catch urine specimen for culture. Check for allergy to intravenous pyelography dye.

- When the patient is hospitalized for a stone, drain all urine, administer analgesics freely, and force fluids. Before discharge, tell the patient to watch for and report any signs of stone passage and urinary tract infection.

Resources

For more information on medullary sponge kidney: National Organization for Rare Disorders (NORD); National Kidney and Urologic Diseases Information Clearinghouse; The National Kidney Foundation.

For genetic information and genetic counseling referrals: March of Dimes Birth Defects Foundation; National Center for Education in Maternal and Child Health.

Section 18.3

Primary Hyperoxaluria

Physician's Guide to Rare Diseases, ©Dowden Publishing Co.
Used by permission.

Description. PH is an inherited disorder characterized by an excess of oxalic acid, which forms oxalate crystals and urine stones. Two forms are presently recognized, types I and II.

Synonyms. Lepoutre's Syndrome, Oxalosis and Oxaluria.

Signs and Symptoms. Manifestations usually first appear in childhood, but the onset of symptoms can occur during infancy or occasionally in adulthood. Calcium oxalate crystals and stones can cause renal colic, urinary tract obstruction, and damage and eventual renal failure. Some patients present in endstage renal disease with oliguria or anuria. Calcium oxalate deposition (oxalosis) can occur in the eyes, bones, joints, heart, and other organs.

Prenatal diagnosis has been obtained by fetal liver biopsy at the 17th week of pregnancy.

Etiology. Type I PH, the most common form of the disorder, is inherited as an autosomal recessive trait. Type I is due to a deficiency of peroxisomal alanine: glyoxalate aminotransferase.

Type II PH, also autosomal recessive, is due to a deficiency of D-glycerate dehydrogenase.

Epidemiology. Males and females are affected in equal numbers.

Treatment—Standard. The principal treatment for types I and II consists of high fluid intake, large daily doses of pyridoxine (vitamin B6), and supplements of phosphate and magnesium. A low oxalate diet is helpful, one that omits foods high in oxalic acid such as spinach, rhubarb, soybeans, tofu, beets, greens, plantain, Swiss chard, collards, gooseberries, leeks, okra, wheat germ, raspberries, sweet potatoes, peanut butter, and tea.

In patients who still have kidney function, a greatly increased fluid intake helps keep the kidneys flushed out and limits crystal formation. In patients who have lost kidney function, aggressive dialysis is an appropriate treatment until kidney transplantation can be performed. This should be done as soon as possible, since dialysis does not adequately remove oxalate. Previously, kidney transplants were considered inappropriate for patients with PH, but transplantation with therapy to help prevent recurrence is now a successful method of treatment.

Genetic counseling is helpful to families. However, the severity of the disease may be impossible to predict because it varies widely even in the same family.

Treatment—Investigational. For type I PH, liver transplantation provides the normal enzyme and corrects the metabolic defect. Combined liver and kidney transplantation alone has been performed on one patient with adequate residual kidney function.

Please contact the agencies listed under Resources, below, for the most current information.

Resources

For more information on primary hyperoxaluria: National Organization for Rare Disorders (NORD); The Oxalosis and Hyperoxaluria Foundation; National Institute of Diabetes, Digestive and Kidney Diseases Information Clearinghouse; Research Trust for Metabolic Diseases in Children.

For genetic information and genetic counseling referrals: March of Dimes Birth Defects Foundation; National Center for Education in Maternal and Child Health (NCEMCH).

Part Five

Cancer of the Kidney

Chapter 19

Kidney Cancer

Chapter Contents

Section 19.1

What You Need to Know about Kidney Cancer

DHHS, National Institutes of Health, Pub. No. 91–1569.
For more information on cancer and its treatment see:
The Cancer Sourcebook for Women (Health Reference Series Vol. 10),
The New Cancer Sourcebook (Health Reference Series Vol. 12).

Each year, more than 23,000 Americans find out they have cancer of the kidney. The following chapter has been prepared by the National Cancer Institute (NCI) to help patients and their families and friends better understand kidney cancer. We also hope it will encourage all readers to learn more about this disease.

This chapter has information on the symptoms, diagnosis, and treatment of kidney cancer. Other NCI booklets about cancer, its treatment, and living with the disease are listed at the end of the chapter. However, no booklet can answer all questions or take the place of talks with doctors, nurses, and other members of the health care team.

Throughout this chapter, words that may be new to readers are printed in italics. Definitions of these and other terms related to kidney cancer are also found at the end of the chapter.

Knowledge about kidney cancer is increasing. Research is leading to better ways to detect and treat this disease. For up-to-date information about kidney cancer, call the NCI-supported Cancer Information Service (CIS) at 1-800-4-CANCER.

The Kidneys

The kidneys are part of the *urinary tract*. They are a pair of organs found just above the waist on each side of the spine. The kidneys remove waste products from the blood and produce *urine*. As blood flows through the kidneys, they filter waste products, chemicals, and unneeded water from the blood. Urine collects in the middle of each kidney, an area called the *renal pelvis*. Urine then drains from the kidney through a long tube, the *ureter*, to the *bladder,* where it is stored.

The kidneys also make substances that help control blood pressure and regulate the formation of red blood cells.

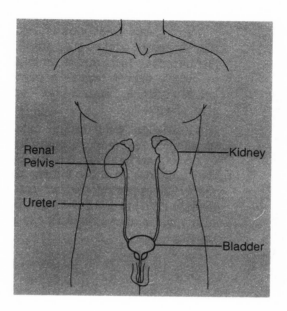

Figure 19.1.1.

What is Cancer?

Cancer is a group of diseases. More than 100 different types of cancer are known—and there are several types of kidney cancer. They all have one thing in common: cells become abnormal. These abnormal cells grow and destroy body tissue and can spread to other parts of the body.

Healthy cells that make up the body's tissues grow, divide, and replace themselves in an orderly way. This process keeps the body in good repair. If cells lose the ability to control their growth, they grow too rapidly and without any order. They form too much tissue. The mass of extra tissue is called a *tumor*. Tumors can be *benign* or *malignant*.

215

- Benign tumors are not cancer. They do not spread to other parts of the body and are seldom a threat to life. Benign tumors can usually be removed, and they are not likely to return.

- Malignant tumors are cancer. They can invade and destroy nearby healthy tissues and organs. Cancer cells can also break away from the tumor and enter the bloodstream and *lymphatic system*. That is how cancer can spread to other parts of the body. This spread is called *metastasis*. Cancer that spreads is the same disease, and the new tumors have the same name as the original, or primary, cancer.

In adults, most kidney cancers develop in the tissues that filter blood and produce urine. This type of cancer is called *renal cell cancer*. Cancer of the renal pelvis is called *transitional cell carcinoma*. This disease is very much like the type of cancer that occurs in the bladder, and it is often treated like bladder cancer.

Childhood kidney cancer is different from kidney cancer in adults. The most common type of kidney cancer in children is Wilms' tumor. This disease is discussed in the NCI booklet, *Young People With Cancer.*

Symptoms

The most common symptom of kidney cancer is blood in the urine. In some cases, a person can actually see the blood. It may be present one day and not the next. Also, traces of blood may be found in urinalysis, a urine test done as part of a regular medical checkup.

Another symptom of kidney cancer is a lump or mass that can be felt in the kidney area. The tumor may cause a dull ache or pain in the back or side. Less often, signs of a kidney tumor include high blood pressure or an abnormal number of red blood cells.

Symptoms may develop suddenly. However, as with other types of cancer, kidney cancer can cause a general feeling of poor health. People with this disease may feel tired, lose their appetite, and lose weight. Some have a fever that comes and goes.

These symptoms may be caused by cancer or by other, less serious problems such as an infection or a fluid-filled *cyst*. Only a doctor can tell for sure.

Diagnosis

To diagnose kidney cancer, the doctor asks about the patient's personal and family medical history and does a complete physical exam. In addition to checking temperature, pulse, blood pressure, and other general signs of health, the doctor usually orders blood and urine tests and may do one or more of the exams described below. (If the doctor thinks the patient might have transitional cell carcinoma, other tests may be used.)

- An *IVP* (*intravenous pyelogram*) is a test that lets the doctor see the kidneys, ureters, and bladder on x-rays. The x-rays are taken after an injection of dye that shows up on the x-ray film.

- A *CT* or *CAT* scan is another x-ray procedure that gives detailed pictures of cross sections of the body. The pictures are created by a computer.

- *Ultrasound* is a test that sends high-frequency sound waves, which cannot be heard by humans, into the kidney. The pattern of echoes produced by these waves creates a picture called a sonogram. Healthy tissues, cysts, and tumors produce different echoes.

- An *arteriogram* is a series of x-rays of blood vessels. Dye is injected into a large blood vessel through a narrow tube called a *catheter.* X-rays show the dye as it moves through the network of smaller blood vessels around and in the kidney.

- *MRI* (*magnetic resonance imaging*) uses a very strong magnet linked to a computer to create pictures of cross sections of the kidney.

- A *nephrotomogram* is a series of x-rays of cross sections of the kidney. The x-rays are taken from several angles before and after injection of a dye that outlines the kidney.

If these tests suggest that a tumor is present, the doctor may confirm the diagnosis with a *biopsy.* A thin needle is inserted into the tumor to withdraw a sample of tissue. The tissue is examined under a microscope by a *pathologist* to check for cancer cells.

When a diagnosis of kidney cancer is made, the doctor needs to know the extent, or stage, of the disease. Because kidney cancer may spread to the bones, lungs, liver, or brain, *staging* procedures may include special x-rays and tests to check these organs.

Treatment

Treatment for kidney cancer depends on the location and size of the tumor and whether the cancer has spread to other organs. The doctor also considers the person's age and general health to develop a treatment plan to fit the patient's needs.

Planning Treatment

Before starting treatment, the patient might want a second doctor to review the diagnosis and treatment plan. There are a number of ways to get a second opinion:

- The patient's doctor can discuss the case with other doctors who treat kidney cancer. Names of doctors and up-to-date treatment information are available from NCI's computerized resource called PDQ. Many of these doctors conduct *clinical trials* (treatment studies) and have a special interest in kidney cancer.

- Patients can get the names of doctors to talk with from the local medical society or a nearby hospital or medical school.

- The Cancer Information Service, at 1-800-4-CANCER, can answer questions about kidney cancer and its treatment and also may be able to help patients locate doctors for a second opinion.

Treatment Methods

Kidney cancer is treated with *surgery, embolization, radiation therapy, hormone therapy, biological therapy, or chemotherapy*. The doctor may use just one treatment method or combine them, depending on the patient's needs. In many cases, the patient is referred to doctors who specialize in different kinds of cancer treatment. Sometimes, several specialists work together as a team.

Most kidney cancer patients have surgery, an operation called *nephrectomy*. In some cases, the surgeon removes the whole kidney or just the part of the kidney that contains the tumor. More often, the surgeon removes the whole kidney along with the adrenal gland and the fat around the kidney. Also, nearby lymph nodes may be removed because they are one of the first places where kidney cancer spreads. Finding cancer cells in the lymph nodes means there may be cancer elsewhere in the body.

In embolization, a substance is injected to clog the renal blood vessels. The tumor shrinks because it does not get the blood supply it needs to grow. In some cases, embolization makes surgery easier. When surgery is not possible, this treatment may help reduce pain and bleeding.

Radiation therapy (also called radiotherapy) uses high-powered rays to damage cancer cells and stop them from growing. Radiation therapy may be used to shrink a tumor before surgery or to kill cancer cells that may remain in the body after surgery. For patients who cannot have surgery, radiation therapy may be used instead. Also, radiation may be used to treat kidney cancer that has spread to the bones or other parts of the body.

The radiation comes from a large machine. The patient receives radiation therapy 5 days a week for 5 to 6 weeks. This schedule helps protect normal tissue by spreading out the total dose of radiation. The patient doesn't need to stay in the hospital for radiation therapy.

Surgery, embolization, and radiation therapy are forms of *local therapy*. They affect only the cells in the treated area. Hormone therapy, biological therapy, and chemotherapy are types of *systemic therapy*. The substances travel through the bloodstream and affect cells all over the body.

Some kidney cancers may be treated with *hormones* to control the growth of cancer cells. Some hormones are taken by mouth; others are given by injection. Patients do not need to be in the hospital for their treatment. This kind of treatment helps a small number of patients with advanced kidney cancer, especially when the disease has spread to the lungs.

Biological therapy is a new way of treating kidney cancer. This treatment attempts to improve the way the body's *immune system* fights disease. Interleukin-2 and interferon are two forms of biological therapy being studied to treat advanced kidney cancer. Doctors are also exploring the benefits of using biological therapy after surgery for early stage kidney cancer. This additional treatment is called *adjuvant therapy*. Doctors are trying to find out whether adjuvant biological therapy can prevent the cancer from recurring by killing undetected cancer cells that may remain in the body. Most patients having biological therapy must stay in the hospital so that the effects of their treatment can be watched.

Chemotherapy uses drugs to kill cancer cells. Chemotherapy has not been very effective against kidney cancer, but researchers are studying new drugs and new drug combinations that may prove to be useful.

Side Effects of Treatment

The methods used to treat kidney cancer are very powerful. It is hard to limit the effects of treatment so that only cancer cells are destroyed; healthy cells may also be damaged. That's why treatment often causes unpleasant side effects. Side effects depend on the type of treatment and the part of the body being treated.

Nephrectomy is major surgery. For a few days after the operation, most patients need medicine to relieve pain. Discomfort may make it difficult to breathe deeply, and patients have to do special coughing and breathing exercises to help keep their lungs clear. Patients may need *IV (intravenous)* feedings and fluids for several days before and after the operation. Nurses will keep track of the amount of fluid the patient takes in and the amount of urine produced. The remaining kidney takes over the work of the one that was removed.

Embolization can cause pain, fever, nausea, or vomiting. These problems are treated with medicine. Often, patients also need intravenous fluids.

During radiation therapy, the patient may become very tired as the treatment continues. Resting as much as possible is important. Skin reactions (redness or dryness) in the treated area are also common, and the skin should be protected from the sun. Good skin care is important at this time, but the patient should not use any lotion or cream on the skin without the doctor's advice. Radiation therapy may cause nausea, vomiting, and diarrhea. Usually, the doctor can suggest certain foods and medicines to ease these problems.

The side effects of hormone therapy are usually mild. *Progesterone* is the hormone most often used to treat kidney cancer. Drugs containing progesterone generally cause few side effects, though some patients may retain fluid and gain weight.

The side effects caused by biological therapies vary with the type of treatment. Often, these treatments cause flu-like symptoms such as chills, fever, muscle aches, weakness, loss of appetite, nausea, vomiting, and diarrhea. Sometimes patients get a rash with dry, itching skin. Patients often feel very tired after treatment. In addition, interleukin-2 can cause the patient to retain fluid. These problems can be severe, and most patients need to stay in the hospital during treatment.

Loss of appetite can be a serious problem for patients during their treatment for cancer. Patients who eat well may be better able to withstand the side effects of their treatment, so good nutrition is an important part of the treatment plan. Eating well means getting enough calories to prevent weight loss and having enough protein to regain strength and rebuild normal tissues. Many patients find that eating several small meals and snacks during the day works better than trying to have three large meals.

The side effects that patients have during cancer treatment vary for each person. They may even be different from one treatment to the next. Doctors try to plan therapy to keep problems to a minimum. Fortunately, most side effects are temporary. Doctors, nurses, and dietitians can explain the side effects of cancer treatment and can suggest ways to deal with them. Helpful information about cancer treatment and coping with side effects is given in the NCI publications *Radiation Therapy and You, Managing Interleukin-2 Therapy, and Eating Hints*.

Followup Care

Regular followup is very important after treatment for kidney cancer. The doctor will continue to check the patient closely to be sure that the cancer has not returned. Checkups may include exams, chest x-rays, and lab tests. The doctor sometimes orders scans (special x-rays) and other tests, too.

Living With Cancer

The diagnosis of kidney cancer can change the lives of cancer patients and the people who care about them. These changes can be difficult to handle. It's natural for patients and their families and friends to have many different and sometimes confusing emotions.

At times, patients and their loved ones may feel frightened, angry, or depressed. These are normal reactions when people face a serious health problem. Others in the same situation have found that they cope with their emotions better if they can talk openly about the illness and their feelings with those close to them. Sharing feelings

221

can help everyone feel more at ease, opening the way for others to show their concern and offer their support.

Concerns about what the future holds—as well as worries about tests, treatments, a hospital stay, and medical bills—are common. Talking with doctors, nurses, or other members of the health care team may help to calm fears and ease confusion. Patients can take an active part in decisions about their medical care by asking questions about kidney cancer and their treatment choices. Patients often find it helpful to write down questions to ask the doctor as they think of them. Taking notes during visits to the doctor helps them remember what was said. It also helps to take a family member or friend along to the physician. Patients should ask the doctor to explain anything that is not clear.

Patients have many important questions, and the doctor is the best person to answer them. Most people ask about the extent of their cancer, how it can be treated, and how successful the treatment is likely to be.

Doctors often talk about "surviving" cancer, or they may use the term "remission" rather than "cure." They use these terms because cancer can recur. It is natural for patients to be concerned about their future. Sometimes they use statistics to try to figure out their chance of being cured.

It is important to remember, however, that statistics are averages. They are based on the experiences of large numbers of patients, and no two cancer patients are alike. Only the doctor who takes care of the patient knows enough about his or her case to discuss the chance of recovery *(prognosis)*.

These are some other important questions to ask the doctor:

- What are my treatment choices?
- What are the benefits of treatment?
- What are the risks and side effects of treatment?
- If I have pain, how will you help me?
- Will I need to change my normal activities? For how long?
- Can I keep working during treatment?
- How often will I need to have checkups?

The doctor is the best person to give advice about treatment, working, or limiting daily activities. Patients may also want to discuss concerns about the future, family relationships, and finances. If it is hard to talk with the doctor about feelings or other personal matters, it may be helpful to speak with a nurse, social worker, counselor, or member of the clergy.

Sometimes patients who have been treated for cancer are concerned that the changes in their lives and the changes to their bodies will affect the way other people feel about them. They may worry about holding a job, caring for their family, or starting new relationships.

Learning to live with the changes brought about by kidney cancer is easier for patients and those who care about them when they have helpful information and support services. Many patients feel that it also helps to talk with others who are facing problems like theirs. They can meet other cancer patients through self-help and support groups. Often, a social worker at the hospital or clinic can suggest local and national groups that will help with rehabilitation, emotional support, financial aid, transportation, or home care.

The American Cancer Society (ACS), for example, is a nonprofit organization that has many services for patients and their families. Local ACS offices are listed in the white pages of the telephone directory.

Living with any serious disease can be difficult and challenging. The public library is a good source of books and articles on living with cancer. Cancer patients and their families can also find helpful suggestions in the NCI booklet *Taking Time.*

Information about other programs and services is available through the Cancer Information Service. The toll-free number is 1-800-4-CANCER.

The Promise of Cancer Research

Scientists at hospitals and medical centers all across the country are studying this disease. They are trying to learn what causes kidney cancer and how to prevent it. They also are looking for better ways to diagnose and treat it.

Cause and Prevention

Kidney cancer affects men about twice as often as women. Most people who get this disease are over the age of 50.

At this time, the causes of kidney cancer are not well understood. Doctors can seldom explain why one person gets this disease and another doesn't. Kidney cancer is not contagious; no one can "catch" any type of cancer from another person.

Although scientists do not know exactly why kidney cancer develops, they have learned that some things *(risk factors)* increase a person's chance of getting this disease. For example, we know that smoking is a major risk factor for kidney cancer. Smokers are twice as likely to get this disease as nonsmokers. Scientists think cigarette smoking causes more than one-fourth of all kidney cancers in the United States. People who smoke are also more likely to get cancers of the lung, mouth, throat, larynx (voice box), esophagus, bladder, and pancreas.

Some people have developed kidney cancer after heavy, long-term use of a painkilling drug called phenacetin. This drug is no longer sold in the United States.

Several studies suggest that the risk of developing kidney cancer may be higher than average among people with certain jobs. Groups with increased risk include coke oven workers and those who work with asbestos. Scientists are trying to learn more about these workers, and they are studying other occupations as well.

Although scientists cannot yet explain why, research shows that being overweight can increase the chance of getting some types of cancer. Kidney cancer may be one of them. Maintaining ideal weight may reduce the risk of cancer and other diseases, including heart disease, diabetes, and high blood pressure.

Detection and Diagnosis

Scientists are trying to find better ways to detect kidney cancer in an early stage, before it has begun to spread. For example, they are studying tumor markers, substances that may be present in abnormal amounts in the blood or urine of a person with kidney cancer. Several of these markers have been studied, but no reliable marker has been found.

Treatment

The NCI is supporting many studies of new treatments for kidney cancer. When laboratory research shows that a new treatment method has promise, it is used to treat cancer patients in clinical trials. These trials are designed to answer scientific questions and to find out whether a new treatment is both safe and effective. Patients who take part in clinical trials make an important contribution to medical science and may have the first chance to benefit from improved treatment methods.

A person with kidney cancer who is interested in taking part in a trial should discuss this option with his or her doctor. *What Are Clinical Trials All About?* is an NCI booklet about treatment studies.

Doctors can learn about clinical trials through PDQ, a computerized resource of cancer treatment information. Developed by NCI, PDQ contains the latest information on studies being done around the country for most types of cancer. Doctors can use an office computer or the services of a medical library to get PDQ information. Cancer Information Service (CIS) offices also provide PDQ information and can tell doctors how to use PDQ on a regular basis. Patients and the public can also get PDQ information by calling the CIS.

Medical Terms

Adjuvant therapy: Treatment given in addition to the primary treatment.

Adrenal glands (a-DREE-nal): A pair of small glands, one located on top of each kidney. The adrenal glands produce hormones that help control heart rate, blood pressure, the way the body uses food, and other vital functions.

Arteriogram (ar-TEER-ee-o-gram): An x-ray of blood vessels, which can be seen after an injection of a dye that shows up in the x-ray pictures.

Benign (bee-NINE): Not cancer; does not spread to other parts of the body.

Biological therapy: Treatment that stimulates the body's immune system to fight disease more effectively. Also called immunotherapy.

Biopsy (BY-op-see): The removal of a sample of tissue for examination under a microscope. This tells the doctor whether cancer cells are present. Removing tissue or fluid with a needle is called needle biopsy.

Bladder: The hollow organ that stores urine.

Cancer: A term for more than 100 diseases that have uncontrolled growth of abnormal cells. These abnormal (cancerous) cells can spread through the bloodstream and lymphatic system to other parts of the body.

Carcinoma (kar-sin-O-mah): Cancer that begins in the tissues that line or cover an organ.

Catheter: A slender, flexible tube used for draining or injecting fluids.

225

Chemotherapy (kee-mo-THER-a-pee): Treatment with anticancer drugs.

Clinical trials: Studies of new cancer treatments. Each study is designed to answer scientific questions and to find better ways to treat patients.

CT or CAT scan. An x-ray procedure that uses a computer to produce detailed pictures of cross sections of the body.

Cyst (sist): An abnormal sac within a tissue or organ, usually filled with fluid.

Embolization (em-bo-li-ZAY-shun): A treatment that clogs small blood vessels and blocks the flow of blood to a tumor. Also called infarction.

Hormones: Chemicals produced by glands in the body. Hormones control the way certain cells or organs act.

Hormone therapy: Treatment of cancer by removing, blocking, or adding hormones.

Immune system (I-MYOON): The complex group of organs and cells that defend the body against infection or disease.

IV(intravenous) (in-tra-VEE-nus): Injected in a vein.

IVP (intravenous pyelogram) (in-tra-VEE-nus PY-e-lo-gram): An x-ray study of the urinary tract.

Local therapy: Treatment that affects a tumor and the cells in the area close to it.

Lymph (limf): The almost colorless fluid that bathes body tissues and carries cells that help fight infection.

Lymph nodes: Small, bean-shaped organs located along the lymphatic system. Nodes filter bacteria or cancer cells from lymph. Also called lymph glands.

Lymphatic system (lim-FAT-ik): The tissues and organs that produce, carry, and store cells that fight infection. This system includes the bone marrow, spleen, thymus, lymph vessels, and lymph nodes.

MRI (magnetic resonance imaging) (magNET-ik REZo-nans IM-ajing): A diagnostic test that uses a magnet linked to a computer to create pictures of cross sections of the body.

Malignant (ma-LIG-nant): Cancerous; can spread to other parts of the body.

Metastasis (me-TAS-ta-sis): The spread of cancer from one part of the body to another. Cells in the metastatic (second) tumor are like those in the original (primary) tumor.

Nephrectomy (nef-REK-to-mee): Surgery to remove the kidney. Radical nephrectomy removes the kidney, the adrenal gland, nearby lymph nodes, and other surrounding tissue. Simple nephrectomy removes just the affected kidney. Partial nephrectomy removes the tumor, but not the entire kidney.

Nephrotomogram (nef-ro-TOE-mo-gram): A series of special x-rays of the kidneys. The x-rays are taken from different angles. They show the kidneys clearly, without the shadows of the organs around them.

Oncologist (on-KOL-ojist): A doctor who specializes in treating cancer.

Pathologist (path-OL-ojist): A doctor who identifies diseases by studying cells and tissues under a microscope.

Progesterone (pro-JES-ter-own): A female hormone.

Prognosis (prog-NO-sis): The probable outcome of a disease; the prospect of recovery.

Radiation therapy (ray-dee-AY-shun THER-a-pee): Treatment with high-energy rays from x-rays or other sources to kill cancer cells.

Renal capsule: The fibrous connective tissue that surrounds each kidney.

Renal cell cancer: Cancer that develops in the lining of the renal tubules, which filter the blood and produce urine.

Renal pelvis: The area at the center of the kidney. Urine collects here and is funneled into the ureter.

Risk factor: Something that increases a person's chance of getting a particular type of cancer.

Staging: The process of learning the extent of the tumor and whether the disease has spread from its original site to other parts of the body.

Surgery: An operation.

Systemic therapy: Treatment that reaches and affects cells all over the body.

Transitional cell carcinoma: Cancer that develops in the lining of the renal pelvis. This type of cancer also occurs in the ureter and the bladder.

Tumor: An abnormal mass of tissue.

Ultrasound: A test that bounces sound waves off tissues and changes the echoes into pictures (sonograms). The pictures are shown on a monitor like a TV screen. Different types of tissue reflect sound waves differently. This makes it possible to find abnormal growths and to tell a fluid-filled cyst from a solid mass.

Ureter (YURe-ter): The tube that carries urine from each kidney to the bladder.

Urethra (yur-EE-thra): The tube that empties urine from the bladder

Urinalysis: A test that determines the content of the urine.

Urinary tract (YUR-in-air-ee): The organs of the body that produce and discharge urine. These include the kidneys, ureters, bladder, and urethra.

Urine (YUR-in): Fluid containing water and waste products. Urine is made by the kidneys, stored in the bladder, and leaves the body through the urethra.

Urologist (yur-OL-ojist): A doctor who specializes in diseases of the urinary organs in females and the urinary and sex organs in males.

X-ray: High-energy radiation. It is used in low doses to diagnose diseases and in high doses to treat cancer.

Resources

General information about cancer is widely available. Some helpful resources and booklets are listed below. Others may be available at a local library or from support groups in the community.

Cancer Information Service
1-800-4-CANCER

The NCI-supported Cancer Information Service (CIS) is a nationwide telephone service that answers questions from cancer patients and their families, health care professionals, and the public. Information specialists can answer questions and provide booklets on all aspects of cancer. They also may know about cancer-related services in local areas. Spanish-speaking staff members are available during daytime hours. By dialing the toll-free CIS number, callers will be connected to the CIS office that serves their area.

American Cancer Society
1599 Clifton Road NE
Atlanta, GA 30329
404-319-3333

The American Cancer Society (ACS) is a national voluntary organization that provides free printed materials, offers a range of services to patients and their families, and carries out programs of research and education. Additional information about these services and activities can be obtained from the national headquarters or a local chapter (listed in the white pages of the telephone book under American Cancer Society).

National Kidney Foundation
30 East 33rd Street
New York, NY 10016
1-800-622-9010

The National Kidney Foundation is a voluntary agency concerned with the prevention and treatment of diseases of the kidneys and urinary tract. It supports research, support groups and other services for patients, and public education. Information is available from the national headquarters or a local chapter (listed in the white pages of the telephone book under National Kidney Foundation).

For Further Information

Cancer patients, their families and friends, and others may find the following booklets useful. They are available free of charge by calling 1-800-4-CANCER or writing:

Office of Cancer Communications
National Cancer Institute
Building 31, Room 10A24
Bethesda, MD 20892

- *Advanced Cancer: Living Each Day*
- *Answers to Your Questions About Metastatic Cancer*
- *Eating Hints: Recipes and Tips for Better Nutrition During Cancer Treatment*
- *Managing Interleukin-2 Therapy*

- *Questions and Answers About Pain Control* (also available from the American Cancer Society)
- *Radiation Therapy and You: A Guide to Self-Help During Treatment*
- *Research Report: Adult Kidney Cancer and Wilms' Tumor*
- *Taking Time: Support for People With Cancer and the People Who Care About Them*
- *What Are Clinical Trials All About?*
- *When Cancer Recurs: Meeting the Challenge Again*

Section 19.2

Kidney Cancer Fact Sheet

National Kidney Cancer Association, © 1995.

In 1993, there were an estimated 27,200 new cases of kidney cancer diagnosed in the United States. Males accounted for 16,800 new cases with females accounting for the other 10,400 cases.

An estimated 11,000 Americans died from kidney cancer in 1993. These deaths were split 6,500 males and 4,500 females.

- Approximately 917 Americans die of kidney cancer in an average month, about 1 every 45 minutes.
- During the ten years of war in Vietnam, 483 Americans died in an average month.

1,170,000 new cases of cancer were estimated for 1993. Kidney cancer is the eleventh most common form of cancer. While only 2 percent of all cancer cases, kidney cancer causes more deaths than melanoma, rectal, and uterine cancer.

The cost of cancer to the U.S. economy was about $110 billion in 1992, an amount growing by 9.8 percent annually. Cancer is the single most expensive disease in the U.S. economy. On a pro rata basis, kidney cancer cost $2.4 billion in 1992, or about $95,000 for each new kidney cancer case diagnosed.

There are over 8 million cancer patients in the U.S. today, people who have "tested positive" for cancer. By comparison, there are about 1.5 million Americans who have tested positive for the HIV antibody with about 75 percent of these developing AIDS. During the 1980's, many more people died of kidney cancer than died of AIDS. Until 1987, there were more cases of kidney cancer.

Kidney cancer is often "curable" by removal of the kidney when the tumor is localized. In about 35 percent of newly diagnosed cases, the disease has spread beyond the kidney with over 15 percent of patients showing Stage IV disease, spread to distant organs, at time of diagnosis. Once it has spread, kidney cancer is difficult to stop because it is resistant to chemotherapy. Early diagnosis is, therefore, critical.

Symptoms include: blood in the urine, abdominal mass, back or flank pain, weight loss, low blood counts, tumor calcification on x-ray, and fever. Kidney cancer is often misdiagnosed due to its varied symptoms.

Radiation is not commonly used except for metastatic disease of the bone or brain. Conventional chemotherapy has proven to be ineffective with single digit response rates being common. New combination therapies are better.

Immunotherapy to stimulate the immune system is often the best therapy such as combination with alpha-interferon, interleukin-2 and 5FU. While only about 22 percent of patients respond to IL-2 alone, new experimental therapies are now achieving response rates as high as 65 percent. Gene therapy and radioactive monoclonal antibody trials are also underway.

Section 19.3

IL-2 Treatment with Kidney Cancer Patients

National Cancer Institute, CancerNet online information service.

A long-term followup of cancer patients receiving high-dose interleukin-2 (IL-2) a natural factor that bolsters immunity demonstrates for the first time that this immunologic approach can bring dramatic and long-lasting antitumor responses in some patients, according to researchers at the National Cancer Institute (NCI).

In the March 23 issue of the Journal of the American Medical Association (JAMA), NCI's Steven A. Rosenberg, M.D., Ph.D., the study's principal investigator, and his colleagues reported on 283 cancer patients given IL-2 from September 1985 through December 1992. Of the 283 patients with metastatic melanoma or kidney cancer, 7 percent achieved complete tumor regression and another 12 percent experienced partial tumor regression, for an overall response rate of 19 percent.

"This study provides the best available evidence we have that immunotherapy can impact on bulky cancers in some patients to produce long-term, meaningful, disease-free survival," said Dr. Rosenberg, who is chief of NCI's Surgery Branch.

Of particular interest, noted Dr. Rosenberg, is that of the 19 patients who had complete regressions following IL-2 therapy, 15 are still in complete remission today, up to 8 years after treatment. Of these, roughly one-half are more than 3 years out from therapy, while four patients have been disease free for more than 5 years.

The durability of partial responses in the study was more variable, with a median duration of 22 months for patients with renal cell cancer and 8 months for patients with melanoma. There were no statistical differences in response based on age or gender.

Immunotherapy or biological therapy relies on stimulating the patient's immune response against a growing cancer, rather than giving treatments such as surgery, radiotherapy, or chemotherapy that attack the cancer directly. While several biologic agents have modest therapeutic antitumor effects, Dr. Rosenberg said, IL-2 is unique in that it is the only immunotherapy with no direct impact on cancer cells. Instead, IL-2 works indirectly to enhance host immunity, presumably by stimulating the body's T cells, white blood cells that orchestrate key immune responses, and by stimulating the production of lymphokine-activated killer (LAK) cells that can target tumors, but not normal cells.

In the IL-2 study, 134 patients had widespread metastatic melanoma, a type and stage of skin cancer, while 149 patients had metastatic kidney cancer. All of the patients had failed standard treatment for their cancers.

In 1992, after reviewing the clinical trial data from 21 institutions using the regimen developed by Dr. Rosenberg and described in the JAMA article, the U.S. Food and Drug Administration approved IL-2 for the treatment of patients with advanced kidney cancer. IL-2 is currently the only approved drug treatment for this disease in the United States.

As a treatment for human cancers, IL-2 has been used alone, in combination with other cytokines, with systemically administered chemotherapeutic agents, and in combination with LAK and other immune system cells. In the most recent experimental studies, Dr. Rosenberg and his colleagues, who were the first to use gene therapy in cancer treatments, have used the IL-2 gene in a novel vaccine attempt to immunize terminally ill patients against their own cancers. The studies also involve augmenting patients' tumors with a gene for tumor necrosis factor, another powerful immune substance with proven antitumor activity, and genetically altering the body's lymphocytes to enhance their cancer-fighting ability.

While these investigations proceed, the current review underscores the importance of immunotherapy in cancer treatment today, Dr. Rosenberg believes. Along with surgery, radiation, and chemotherapy, physicians may soon be using these "purely immunologic maneuvers" to help rid selected patients of established malignancies, he said.

In an editorial accompanying the JAMA article, Samuel Hellman, M.D., Department of Radiation and Cellular Oncology, University of Chicago, described Dr. Rosenberg's work as "a significant advance in cancer therapy" as well as "first and foremost . . . proof of the principle of the immunotherapy of cancer."

Additional Information

The Cancer Information Service (CIS), a program of the National Cancer Institute, provides a nationwide telephone service for cancer patients and their families, the public, and health care professionals. CIS information specialists have extensive training in providing up-to-date and understandable information about cancer. They can answer questions in English and Spanish and can send free printed material. In addition, CIS offices serve specific geographic areas and have information about cancer-related services and resources in their region. The toll-free number of the CIS is 1-800-4-CANCER (1-800-422-6237).

Chapter 20

Kidney Cancer and Von Hippel-Lindau Disease

Von Hippel-Lindau disease is a hereditary condition involving the deactivation of one tumor-suppressor gene, the VHL gene. This flaw in the body's normal tumor-suppression system causes a series of tumors in various parts of the body throughout a person's life. One of the kinds of tumors which may be involved are tumors of the kidney, which are cancer.

Deactivation of the VHL gene has been shown to be involved in the majority of cases of sporadic renal cell carcinoma (RCC) as well. But in VHL, an inherited form of kidney cancer, there are three important differences:

- it is normal to see cysts and tumors on both sides in VHL;
- the tumors follow a different behavior pattern than sporadic RCC, and
- there may be other tumors in other parts of the body which also need attention.

If the patient in fact has VHL, not sporadic RCC, then this treatment might be less aggressive, other family members may be at risk, and this patient and other at-risk family members might be screened proactively to avoid the worst consequences of other tumors in the body.

A diagnosis of VHL is normally assumed to require evidence of two types of tumors in this same patient, or another of the typical VHL

VHL Family Alliance, *VHL Family Forum*, Revised April 1995.

tumors in another closely related person. The treatment pattern for VHL must take into account that the tumor(s) that present now are probably not the last kidney tumors this patient will experience. The challenge is to avoid metastasis while keeping this patient on his or her own kidney power as long as possible.

Further information is available from the VHL Family Alliance, vhl@pipeline.com.

When to Watch; When to Act?

Both the panel in Kansas City [April 1994] and the Symposium in Freiburg (May 1994) addressed this key question: When to watch a kidney tumor, and when to act? With today's better diagnostic methods, we are able to see tumors when they are very small, but at what point should action be taken?

There is no simple formula on which all physicians agree. But the evidence is mounting that VHL tumors have different behavioral characteristics than sporadic renal cell carcinoma: they tend to grow more slowly, are less aggressive, are more numerous, and have a 50% chance that there will be more after some years in the future.

There are no definite rules to guide patients or physicians, and our speakers were divided on this subject. Dr. Mark J. Noble of the University of Kansas Medical Center said that most urologists familiar with VHL now agree that you need not remove kidney tumors less than 2-3 cm. in size. He then removes the tumors and saves as much functioning kidney as possible. Dr. Craig Hawkins shared that in the experience of the Mayo Clinic they did have one patient who seemed to have a metastatic cancer from a tumor smaller than 2 cm. While they also practice renal sparing surgery whenever possible, they tend to operate on smaller tumors and cysts. Dr. Hartmut Neumann and his colleagues at the University of Freiburg do not operate for cysts alone, but only for larger tumors. His experience is that the safety limit may be higher than 3 cm. He generally waits until 4 cm.

Because no one can be sure, it is important that the patient be involved in making the decision about when to remove the tumors. With today's surgical techniques it is unlikely that the kidney can be operated upon more than 3 times before it will need to be completely removed, so operating too soon may result in loss of the kidney earlier in life. On the other hand, waiting too long may result in the cancer spreading to another place in the body. Dr. Neumann works with his patients to evaluate the position of the tumors, their tissue densities and growth patterns, the family kidney history, and the risk the patient is willing to live with. He has ten patients with tumors ranging up to 4 cm. without metastasis.

New kidney treatments may make it possible to operate more often on the kidney with less damage to kidney function, but they still entail surgery. The best hope is that research such as Dr. Linehan's work on the genetics of kidney cancer will lead to non-surgical therapies which will constrain the growth of kidney tumors and prevent or reverse the spread of kidney cancer.

VHL Gene Linked to Kidney Cancer

Reviewing "Mutations of the VHL Tumor Suppressor Gene in Renal Carcinoma"[1]

A study published in the May issue of *Nature Genetics* shows that the VHL gene plays a role not only in the formation of tumors in people who inherit a flaw in the VHL gene, but also in 85% of the kidney cancers in the general population as well. The cancer, called sporadic (non-familial) clear cell carcinoma, accounts for about 23,500 newly diagnosed cases of kidney cancer each year in the U.S. alone.

"With identification of this kidney cancer gene, it will be possible to develop new methods to improve the diagnosis and treatment of the disease and potentially to find ways to prevent it," said W. Marston Linehan, M.D., of the Surgery Branch, National Cancer Institute (NCI). "The finding also will make it possible to develop a blood or urine test that can detect kidney cancer early when it is most treatable." When detected in its earliest stages, the survival rate is 86%.

The damaged or mutated gene responsible for sporadic clear cell carcinoma of the kidney is a tumor suppressor gene located on the short arm of chromosome 3. The protein produced by the gene appears to normally restrain growth. The researchers found that this gene is mutated (inactivated) in a high percentage of tumors (57%) from patients with sporadic, non-familial cancer.

This is the same gene that was identified last year as the cause of the inherited cancer syndrome Von Hippel-Lindau (VHL) disease. "The disease appears to fit the two-hit model for development of cancer, where both copies of the critical gene are damaged or mutated," said co-investigator Berton Zbar, M.D., chief of NCI's Laboratory of Immunobiology.

Everyone has two copies of the VHL gene, as they do of every gene, one from the mother and one from the father. When we say that a

237

person has VHL, that means that they inherited the faulty copy of the VHL gene from the parent who has VHL. One normal copy of a gene is sufficient to prevent development of a tumor. If both copies are damaged or mutated, the two-hit model cancer may develop.

In people in the general population, the two copies of the VHL gene they inherit are both healthy. In order for a tumor to form, both copies of this gene must become deactivated. There are numerous theories of how genes get changed: environmental factors, water pollution, cigarette smoke, radiation, free radicals, etc., we don't understand just what happens, but step by step the process is becoming clearer.

From the work on the VHL gene previously reported by Latif, Lerman, Bar, et al.[2] we know that the VHL gene is on chromosome 3p. This article reports that the gene has been cloned by the same team[3] and that an article reporting the cloning has been submitted for publication. Now that the gene has been cloned, scientists can make greater headway in understanding how the gene operates. The gene appears to be important in encoding a functional protein. The next step is to understand what this protein does in the body, and what occurs when it is not present.

It is as if it takes two occurrences for a tumor to grow and become cancerous. First, the brakes have to be off; second the accelerator has to be on. The disabling of the VHL gene takes off the brakes. But what puts the accelerator on?

The researchers also found that the kidney cancer gene is affected early in the development of the disease. This finding is important, Dr. Linehan explained, because its early presence makes it possible to consider development of treatments to halt or reverse the progression of the disease in its early stages.

All this implies that exposure of the kidney to environmental carcinogens may lead to mutation of the VHL gene and subsequent tumor formation. This demonstration that mutations in the VHL gene foster tumor growth in renal cell carcinoma "should lead to a better understanding of how renal epithelial cell growth is regulated and should aid in methods of diagnosis and treatment of patients with this malignancy."[4]

For people with VHL, what do we learn from this? We learn that VHL kidney tumors are indeed closely related to renal cell carcinoma. But we also learn that there is more to be learned. Dr. Linehan tells us, for example, that while he can get 80% of sporadic renal cell carcinoma tissue to grow in the lab, he has been unable to get VHL kidney tumor tissue to grow there. He still does not understand why. We know that VHL takes the brakes off, but what presses the accelerator? The same environmental factors which cause the VHL gene to change affect both people with VHL and people with sporadic kidney cancers.

World Focuses Attention on VHL

"In the last ten years, Von Hippel-Lindau disease has gone from an obscure medical curiosity to a condition with far-reaching implications in oncology," said Dr. Alfred G. Knudson of Philadelphia, originator of the now widely accepted theory of tumor-suppressor genes, delivering the keynote address at the First International Symposium on Von Hippel-Lindau (VHL) in Freiburg, Germany. He noted that study of VHL is helping scientists to understand the mechanisms of many kinds of cancer.

Eighty respected physicians and scientists gathered from Japan, the United States, England, Germany, France, Italy and the Netherlands. They shared the results of their research on the molecular genetics and clinical management of VHL. Dr. Knudson lauded the presentation of urologist Dr. Gyula Kovacs of Heidelberg, saying that he "has made an enormous contribution" to the field. Honored American attendees included Dr. Y. Edward Hsia of the University of Honolulu, and Dr. Nuzhet O. Atuk of the University of Virginia, whose studies of large VHL kindreds have provided key pieces of the VHL puzzle.

In the May issue of Nature Genetics, the VHL gene has been shown to play a role in 85% of kidney cancer cases which occur in the general population, affecting 23,000 people each year in the United States alone.

The meeting was hosted by Dr. Otmar Wiestler of Bonn, and Dr. Hartmut P.H. Neumann of Freiburg, who has spent the last twelve years concentrating on improving diagnosis and treatment of patients with Von Hippel-Lindau disease. Dr. Neumann recently completed a tour of the United States, sponsored by the VHL Family Alliance, where he spoke on VHL in five cities.

The principal questions for this symposium concerned diagnosis and therapy: how to improve diagnosis through clinical findings and/or through molecular genetics; how to reduce exposure to radiation in diagnostics; how to reduce the complexity of the diagnostic process. In the area of therapy, Dr. Neumann posed the question how to find the right balance between undertreatment and overtreatment. With improvements in diagnostics, tumors are now found at very early stages, but at what point should action be taken? The goal of the symposium was to make recommendations to physicians and to inform the decisions of the patients regarding their treatment. Joyce Graff of Brookline, Massachusetts, and Peggy Graham of Warren, Michigan, attended the Symposium, representing the VHL Family Alliance. Both Joyce and Peggy have children affected with VHL. They met with families from Germany, and were interviewed on German television. They spent most of Saturday with Peter and Sylvine Z. from East Berlin, who send their best greetings to all the members of the VHL Family Alliance. Nearly thirty talks and posters were presented.

The French National VHL Registry project under Dr. Stephane Richard found hundreds of previously misdiagnosed cases of VHL. They found that 30% of all cases of cerebellar hemangioblastoma and 58% of cases of spinal hemangioblastoma were in fact VHL. Among patients under the age of thirty, the percentages rose to 47% and 77% respectively. When tumors occur in young people, they are more likely caused by a hereditary condition.

On the last day, Dr. Neumann summarized the recommendations of the symposium regarding cerebellar hemangioblastomas. Screening is done with MRI with gadolinium. They can grow fairly large without symptoms. Early diagnosis is important to prevent loss of function. There was interest in the possible contribution of radiosurgery for cerebellar hemangioblastoma. Dr. Hsia noted that it is important to screen VHL women before childbearing because of the tendency of tumors to grow at a faster pace during pregnancy.

Dr. Dieter Schmidt of Freiburg summarized the recommendations for retinal angiomas. He screens the retina with contact glass and fluorescein angiography as needed, in an effort to find lesions when they are very small. He treats angiomas with laser, especially small ones in the periphery, treating them in multiple sessions to avoid blistering the retina. Conscientious follow-up is important, as additional lesions are not uncommon.

When lesions are close to the optic nerve or macula, treatment can be dangerous. He tends to observe these unless they are actively growing. He posed the question whether photon-beam therapy might hold promise for treatment of certain of these difficult lesions. Dr. Stephane Richard of Paris noted that since retinal angiomas are indistinguishable under a microscope from cerebellar hemangioblastomas, we should refer to them as hemangioblastomas.

Dr. Peter Choyke of the National Institutes of Health, U.S., summarized the findings on renal cell carcinoma. CT scanning is recommended with 5 mm. slice depth and contrast. One should not only identify the presence of tumors, but their size and growth rate, but re-checking twice at 6-month intervals the first year. Once this information has been gathered and the risk calculated, watch the tumors up to a size of approximately 3 cm and then perform enucleation or partial nephrectomy. Total nephrectomy should only be performed when there are no other options. Several of those present recommended the use of MRI or ultra-sound during the surgery to maximize the benefit of each surgery. Continue a conscientious follow-up program because more tumors are not uncommon. The goals are to avoid frequent surgery, and reduce metastasis to a minimum.

Dr. Atuk summarized the recommendations on pheochromocytoma. Dr. Eamonn Maher of England recommends annual urine testing. Dr. Atuk uses CT, though some felt that MRI or MIBG were preferred. He feels that of the chemical indicators, urinary catecholamines are the most useful indicators. None of those present had experienced any malignancies among pheos. Therefore the recommendation is to enucleate the tumor whenever possible. Pheos can occur outside the adrenals, so even people with bilateral adrenalectomy should continue to be screened for pheo. The presence of a pheo must be ruled out before any surgery in VHL patients, to avoid surgical complications.

Professor J.P. Grenfeld of Paris, in his concluding remarks, noted that VHL is often misdiagnosed in all countries, partially due to the risk of overly compartmentalized medicine. He noted that with the better information which is being gathered, with better training on VHL now available to physicians, better information for families, and with the participation of the families in the ongoing process of learning about VHL, progress will continue to be made.

1. J. Gnarra et al, "Mutations of the VHL tumor suppressor gene in renal carcinoma," published in Nature Genetics, May 1994, pages 85–90. This research was conducted by Drs. Barton Bar, Michael I. Legman, and Marston W. Linehan of NCI in collaboration with the Urology Departments of New York Hospital; Cornell University Medical Center, New York; University of Michigan, Ann Arbor; and Johns Hopkins Medical Institutions, Baltimore; Laboratory of Molecular Pathology, Technical University Munich; University Clinic of Surgery, Heidelberg.

2. F. Latif et al, "Identification of the Von Hipped-Landau disease tumor suppressor gene." Science, 260, 1317–1320 (1993). Reported in VHLFF, June 1993.

3. F. Chen et al, manuscript submitted.

4. Gnarra et al, p. 90.

Chapter 21

Renal Cell Cancer

What is Renal Cell Cancer?

Renal cell cancer (also called cancer of the kidney or renal adeno-carcinoma) is a disease in which cancer (malignant) cells are found in certain tissues of the kidney. Renal cell cancer is one of the less common kinds of cancer. It occurs more often in men than in women.

The kidneys are a "matched" pair of organs found on either side of your backbone. The kidneys of an adult are about 5 inches long and 3 inches wide and are shaped like a kidney bean. Inside each kidney are tiny tubules that filter and clean your blood, taking out waste products, and making urine. The urine made by the kidneys passes through a tube called a ureter into the bladder where it is held until it is passed from your body. Renal cell cancer is a cancer of the lining of the tubules in the kidney. If you have cancer in the part of the kidney that collects urine and drains it to the ureters (the renal pelvis) or if you have cancer in the ureters, refer to the PDQ patient information statement on transitional cell cancer of the renal pelvis and ureter.

Like most cancers, renal cell cancer is best treated when it is found (diagnosed) early. You should see your doctor if you have one or more of the following: blood in your urine, a lump (mass) in your abdomen, or a pain in your side that doesn't go away. If you have cancer of the kidney, you may also feel very tired or have loss of appetite, weight loss without dieting, and anemia (too few red blood cells).

The National Cancer Institute, CancerNet online information service.

If you have signs of cancer, your doctor will usually feel your abdomen for lumps. Your doctor may order a special x-ray called an intravenous pyelogram (IVP). During this test, a dye containing iodine is injected into your bloodstream. This allows your doctor to see the kidney more clearly on the x-ray. Your doctor may also do an ultrasound, which uses sound waves to find tumors, or a special x-ray called a CT scan to look for lumps in the kidney. A special scan called magnetic resonance imaging (MRI), which uses magnetic waves to find tumors, may also be done.

Your chance of recovery (prognosis) and choice of treatment depend on the stage of your cancer (whether it is just in the kidney or has spread to other places in the body) and your general state of health.

Stages of Renal Cell Cancer

Once renal cell cancer has been found, more tests will be done to find out if cancer cells have spread to other parts of the body. This is called staging. Your doctor needs to know the stage of your disease to plan treatment. The following stages are used for renal cell cancer:

Stage I

Cancer is found only in the kidney.

Stage II

Cancer has spread to the fat around the kidney, but the cancer has not spread beyond this to the capsule that contains the kidney.

Stage III

Cancer has spread to the main blood vessel that carries clean blood from the kidney (renal vein), to the blood vessel that carries blood from the lower part of the body to the heart (inferior vena cava), or to lymph nodes around the kidney. (Lymph nodes are small, bean-shaped structures that are found throughout the body; they produce and store infection-fighting cells.)

Stage IV

Cancer has spread to nearby organs such as the bowel or pancreas or has spread to other places in the body such as the lungs.

Recurrent

Recurrent disease means that the cancer has come back (recurred) after it has been treated. It may come back in the original area or in another part of the body.

How Renal Cell Cancer is Treated

There are treatments for most patients with renal cell cancer. Five kinds of treatment are used:

- surgery (taking out the cancer in an operation)
- chemotherapy (using drugs to kill cancer cells)
- radiation therapy (using high-dose x-rays or other high-energy rays to kill cancer cells)
- hormone therapy (using hormones to stop cancer cells from growing)
- biological therapy (using your body's immune system to fight cancer).

Surgery is a common treatment for renal cell cancer. Your doctor may take out the cancer using one of the following:

- Partial nephrectomy removes the cancer and part of the kidney around the cancer. This is usually done only in special cases, such as when the other kidney is damaged or has already been removed.

- Simple nephrectomy removes the whole kidney. The kidney on the other side of the body can take over filtering the blood.

- Radical nephrectomy removes the kidney with the tissues around it. Some lymph nodes in the area may also be removed.

Chemotherapy uses drugs to kill cancer cells. Chemotherapy may be taken by pill, or it may be put into the body by a needle in a vein or muscle. Chemotherapy is called a systemic treatment because the drugs enter the bloodstream, travel through the body, and can kill cancer cells throughout the body.

Radiation therapy uses x-rays or other high-energy rays to kill cancer cells and shrink tumors. Radiation may come from a machine outside the body (external radiation therapy) or from putting materials that contain radiation through thin plastic tubes (internal radiation therapy) in the area where the cancer cells are found. Radiation can be used alone or before or after surgery and/or chemotherapy.

Hormone therapy uses hormones (taken by pill or injected with a needle) to stop cancer cells from growing.

Biological therapy tries to get your own body to fight cancer. It uses materials made by your own body or made in a laboratory to boost, direct, or restore your body's natural defenses against disease. Biological therapy is sometimes called biological response modifier (BRM) therapy or immunotherapy.

Sometimes a special treatment called arterial embolization is used to treat renal cell cancer. A narrow tube (catheter) is used to inject small pieces of a special gelatin sponge into the main blood vessel that flows into the kidney to block the blood cells that feed the tumor. This prevents the cancer cells from getting oxygen or other substances they need to grow.

Treatment by Stage

Treatments for renal cell cancer depend on the type and stage of your disease, your age, and your general health.

You may receive treatment that is considered standard based on its effectiveness in a number of patients in past studies, or you may choose to go into a clinical trial. Not all patients are cured with standard therapy and some standard treatments may have more side effects than are desired. For these reasons, clinical trials are designed to find better ways to treat cancer patients and are based on the most up-to-date information. Clinical trials are going on in most parts of the country for most stages of renal cell cancer. If you want more information, call the Cancer Information Service at 1-800-4-CANCER (1-800-422-6237).

Stage I Renal Cell Cancer

Your treatment may be one of the following:

1. Surgery to remove the kidney and the tissues around it (radical nephrectomy). Lymph nodes in the area may also be removed.

2. Surgery to remove only the kidney (simple nephrectomy).
3. Surgery to remove the part of the kidney where the cancer is found partial nephrectomy).
4. External beam radiation therapy to relieve symptoms in patients who cannot have surgery.
5. Injection of small pieces of a special gelatin sponge into the main artery that flows to the kidney to block blood flow to the cancer cells (arterial embolization). This is usually done only in patients who cannot have surgery.
6. Clinical trials.

Stage II Renal Cell Cancer

Your treatment may be one of the following:

1. Surgery to remove the kidney and the tissues around it (radical nephrectomy). Lymph nodes in the area may also be removed.
2. External beam radiation therapy before or after radical nephrectomy.
3. Surgery to remove the part of the kidney where the cancer is found (partial nephrectomy).
4. External beam radiation therapy to relieve symptoms in patients who cannot have surgery.
5. Injection of small pieces of a special gelatin sponge into the main artery that flows to the kidney to block blood flow to the cancer cells (arterial embolization). This is usually done only in patients who cannot have surgery.
6. Clinical trials.

Stage III Renal Cell Cancer

Your treatment may be one of the following:

1. Surgery to remove the kidney and the tissues around it (radical nephrectomy). Lymph nodes in the area may also be removed. If the cancer has spread to the main blood vessels that carry blood to and from the kidney (the renal vein or vena cava), part of the blood vessel may also be removed.
2. Injection of small pieces of a special gelatin sponge into the main artery that flows to the kidney to block blood flow to the

cancer cells (arterial embolization) followed by radical nephrectomy.

3. External beam radiation therapy to relieve symptoms.
4. Arterial embolization to relieve symptoms.
5. Surgery to remove the kidney (simple or radical nephrectomy) to relieve symptoms.
6. External beam radiation therapy before or after radical nephrectomy.
7. Clinical trials of biological therapy in addition to other therapy.

Stage IV Renal Cell Cancer

Your treatment may be one of the following:

1. Biological therapy.
2. External radiation therapy to relieve symptoms.
3. Surgery to remove the kidney (nephrectomy) to relieve symptoms.
4. If cancer has spread only to the area around the kidney, surgery to remove the kidney and the tissue around it (radical nephrectomy). If the cancer has spread to a limited area, surgery to remove the cancer where it has spread (metastasized) in addition to radical nephrectomy.
5. Clinical trials.

Recurrent Renal Cell Cancer

Your treatment may be one of the following:

1. Biological therapy.
2. External radiation therapy to relieve symptoms.
3. Chemotherapy.

To Learn More

To learn more about renal cell cancer, call the National Cancer Institute's Cancer Information Service at 1-800-4-CANCER (1-800-422-6237). By dialing this toll-free number, you can speak with someone who can answer your questions.

The Cancer Information Service can also send you free booklets. The following booklet about renal cell cancer may be helpful to you:

— *What You Need To Know About Kidney Cancer*

The following general booklets on questions related to cancer may also be helpful:

— *What You Need To Know About Cancer*
— *Taking Time: Support for People with Cancer and the People Who Care About Them*
— *What Are Clinical Trials All About?*
— *Chemotherapy and You: A Guide to Self-Help During Treatment*
— *Radiation Therapy and You: A Guide to Self-Help During Treatment*
— *Eating Hints for Cancer Patients*
— *Advanced Cancer: Living Each Day*
— *When Cancer Recurs: Meeting the Challenge Again*

There are many other places you can get material about cancer treatment and services to help you. You can check the social service office at your hospital for local and national agencies that help with your finances, getting to and from treatment, care at home, and dealing with your problems. The American Cancer Society, for example, has many free services. Their local offices are listed in the white pages of the telephone book.

You can also write to the National Cancer Institute at this address:

National Cancer Institute
Building 31, Room 10A24
9000 Rockville Pike
Bethesda, MD 20892

What is PDQ?

PDQ is a computer system that gives up-to-date information on cancer treatment. It is a service of the National Cancer Institute (NCI) for people with cancer and their families, and for doctors, nurses, and other health care professionals.

PDQ tells about the current treatments for most cancers. The information in PDQ is reviewed each month by cancer experts. It is updated when there is new information. The patient information in PDQ also tells about warning signs and how the cancer is found. PDQ also lists information about research on new treatments (clinical trials), doctors who treat cancer, and hospitals with cancer programs. The treatment information in this summary is based on information in the PDQ treatment summary for health professionals on this cancer.

How to Use PDQ

You can use PDQ to learn more about current treatment for your kind of cancer. Bring this material from PDQ with you when you see your doctor. You can talk with your doctor, who knows you and has the facts about your disease, about which treatment would be best for you. Before you start your treatment, you might also want to seek a second opinion from a doctor who treats cancer.

Before you start treatment, you also may want to think about taking part in a clinical trial. A clinical trial is a study that uses new treatments to care for patients. Each study is based on past studies and what has been learned in the laboratory. Each trial answers certain scientific questions in order to find new and better ways to help cancer patients. During clinical trials, more and more information is collected about new treatments, their risks, and how well they do or do not work. If clinical trials show that the new treatment is better than the treatment currently being used, the new treatment may become the "standard" treatment. Listings of clinical trials are a part of PDQ. Many cancer doctors who take part in clinical trials are listed in PDQ.

If you want to know more about cancer and how it is treated, or if you wish to learn about clinical trials for your kind of cancer, you can call the National Cancer Institute's Cancer Information Service. The number is 1-800-4-CANCER (1-800-422-6237). The call is free and a trained information specialist will talk with you and answer your questions.

PDQ may change when there is new information. Check with the Cancer Information Service to be sure that you have the most up-to-date information.

Chapter 22

Transitional Cell Cancer of the Renal Pelvis and Ureter

What Is Transitional Cell Cancer of the Renal Pelvis and Ureter?

Transitional cell cancer (TCC) of the renal pelvis and ureter is a disease in which cancer (malignant) cells are found in the tissues in the kidneys that collect urine (the renal pelvis) and/or in the tube that connects the kidney to the bladder (ureter).

The kidneys are a "matched" pair of organs found on either side of your backbone. The kidneys of an adult are about 5 inches long and 3 inches wide and are shaped like a kidney bean. Inside each kidney are tiny tubules that clean your blood, taking out waste products and making urine. The urine made by the kidneys passes through the ureter into the bladder where it is held until it is passed from your body. The renal pelvis is the part of the kidney that collects urine and drains it to the ureters. The cells that line the renal pelvis and ureters are called transitional cells, and it is these cells that are affected in TCC. If you have a more common type of kidney cancer called renal cell cancer, see the patient information statement on renal cell cancer.

Like most cancers, TCC of the renal pelvis and ureter is best treated when it is found (diagnosed) early. In the early stages of TCC you may not have any symptoms. The symptoms of TCC and other types of kidney cancer are similar to other types of kidney disease.

The National Cancer Institute, CancerNet online information service.

You should see your doctor if you have blood in your urine or pain in your back.

If you have symptoms, your doctor will usually feel your abdomen for lumps. A narrow lighted tube called a ureteroscope may be inserted through the bladder into the ureter so that your doctor can look inside the ureter and renal pelvis for signs of cancer. If cancer cells are found, your doctor may take out a small piece of the tissue to look at under the microscope. This is called a biopsy. Your doctor may also do a special x-ray called a CT scan or a scan that uses magnetic waves (MRI) to look for lumps.

Your chance of recovery (prognosis) and choice of treatment depend on the stage of your cancer (whether it is just in the tissue lining the inside of the ureter or renal pelvis or has spread to other places) and your general state of health.

Stages of Transitional Cell Cancer of the Renal Pelvis and Ureter

Once transitional cell cancer is found, more tests will be done to find out if cancer cells have spread to other parts of the body (staging). Your doctor needs to know the stage to plan treatment. The following stages are used for TCC of the renal pelvis and ureter:

Localized. The cancer is only in the area where it started and has not spread outside the kidney or ureter.

Regional. The cancer has spread to the tissue around the kidney or to lymph nodes in the pelvis. (Lymph nodes are bean-shaped structures that are found throughout the body. They produce infection-fighting cells.)

Metastatic. The cancer has spread to other parts of the body.

Recurrent. Recurrent disease means that the cancer has come back (recurred) after it has been treated. It may come back in the original area or in another part of the body.

How Transitional Cell Cancer of the Renal Pelvis and Ureter Is Treated

There are treatments for all patients with transitional cell cancer of the renal pelvis and ureter. The primary treatment is surgery (taking out the cancer in an operation). Radiation therapy (using high-dose x-rays to kill cancer cells), biological therapy (using your body's immune system to fight cancer), and chemotherapy (using drugs to kill cancer cells) are being tested in clinical trials.

Surgery is the most common treatment for transitional cell cancer of the renal pelvis and ureter. Your doctor may remove the tumor using one of the following operations:

- The kidney, ureter, and top part of the bladder may be removed in an operation called a nephroureterectomy.
- Segmental resection removes only part of the ureter or kidney.
- Electrosurgery uses an electric current to remove the cancer. The tumor and the area around it are burned away and then removed with a sharp tool.
- Laser therapy uses a narrow beam of intense light to remove cancer cells.
- Electrosurgery and laser therapy are used only for cancers that are on the surface of the renal pelvis or ureter.

Chemotherapy uses drugs to kill cancer cells. Chemotherapy may be taken by pill, or it may be put into the body by a needle in the vein or muscle. Chemotherapy is called a systemic treatment because the drug enters the bloodstream, travels through the body, and can kill cancer cells throughout the body. Chemotherapy may also be put directly into the ureter or pelvis (intraureteral or intrapelvic chemotherapy).

Biological therapy tries to get your own body to fight cancer. It uses materials made by your own body or made in a laboratory to boost, direct, or restore your body's natural defenses against disease. Biological therapy is sometimes called biological response modifier (BRM) therapy or immunotherapy.

Radiation therapy uses high-energy x-rays to kill cancer cells and shrink tumors. Radiation may come from a machine outside the body (external beam radiation therapy) or from putting materials that produce radiation (radioisotopes) through thin plastic tubes (internal radiation therapy) in the area where the cancer cells are found.

Treatment by Stage

Your choice of treatment depends on how far the cancer has spread and your general health.

You may receive treatment that is considered standard based on its effectiveness in a number of patients in past studies, or you may choose to go into a clinical trial. Not all patients are cured with standard therapy and some standard treatments may have more side effects than are desired. For these reasons, clinical trials are designed to find better ways to treat cancer patients and are based on the most up-to-date information. Clinical trials are going on in most parts of the country for most stages of transitional cell cancer of the renal pelvis and ureter. If you want more information, call the Cancer Information Service at 1-800-4-CANCER (1-800-422-6237).

Localized Transitional Cell Cancer of the Renal Pelvis and Ureter

Your treatment may be one of the following:

1. Surgery to remove the kidney, ureter, and the top part of the bladder (nephroureterectomy).
2. Surgery to remove part of the ureter or kidney (segmental resection).
3. A clinical trial of electrosurgery or laser therapy.
4. A clinical trial of intrapelvic or intraureteral chemotherapy or biological therapy.

Regional Transitional Cell Cancer of the Renal Pelvis and Ureter

Your treatment will probably be a clinical trial of radiation therapy and/or chemotherapy.

Metastatic Transitional Cell Cancer of the Renal Pelvis and Ureter

Your treatment will probably be a clinical trial of chemotherapy.

Recurrent Transitional Cell Cancer of the Renal Pelvis and Ureter

Your treatment will probably be a clinical trial of new treatments.

To Learn More

To learn more about transitional cell cancer of the renal pelvis and ureter, call the National Cancer Institute's Cancer Information Service at 1-800-4-CANCER (1-800-422-6237). By dialing this toll-free number, you can speak with someone who can answer your questions.

The Cancer Information Service can also send you free booklets. The following booklets about kidney cancer may be helpful to you:

— *What You Need to Know About Kidney Cancer*
— *Research Report: Adult Kidney Cancer and Wilms' Tumor*

The following general booklets on questions related to cancer may also be helpful:

— *What You Need to Know About Cancer*
— *Taking Time: Support for People with Cancer and the People Who Care About Them*
— *What Are Clinical Trials All About?*
— *Chemotherapy and You: A Guide to Self-Help During Treatment*
— *Radiation Therapy and You: A Guide to Self-Help During Treatment*
— *Eating Hints for Cancer Patients*
— *Advanced Cancer: Living Each Day*
— *When Cancer Recurs: Meeting the Challenge Again*

There are many other places you can get information about cancer treatment and services to help you. You can check the social service office at your hospital for local and national agencies that help with your finances, getting to and from treatment, care at home, and dealing with your problems. The American Cancer Society, for example, has many free services. Their local offices are listed in the white pages of the telephone book.

You can also write to the National Cancer Institute at this address:

National Cancer Institute
Building 31, Room 10A24
9000 Rockville Pike
Bethesda, MD 20892

What is PDQ

PDQ is a computer system that gives up-to-date information on cancer treatment. It is a service of the National Cancer Institute (NCI) for people with cancer and their families, and for doctors, nurses, and other health care professionals.

PDQ tells about the current treatments for most cancers. The information in PDQ is reviewed each month by cancer experts. It is updated when there is new information. The patient information in PDQ also tells about warning signs and how the cancer is found. PDQ also lists information about research on new treatments (clinical trials), doctors who treat cancer, and hospitals with cancer programs. The treatment information in this summary is based on information in the PDQ treatment summary for health professionals on this cancer.

How to use PDQ

You can use PDQ to learn more about current treatment for your kind of cancer. Bring this material from PDQ with you when you see your doctor. You can talk with your doctor, who knows you and has the facts about your disease, about which treatment would be best for you. Before you start your treatment, you might also want to seek a second opinion from a doctor who treats cancer.

Before you start treatment, you also may want to think about taking part in a clinical trial. A clinical trial is a study that uses new treatments to care for patients. Each study is based on past studies and what has been learned in the laboratory. Each trial answers certain scientific questions in order to find new and better ways to help cancer patients. During clinical trials, more and more information is collected about new treatments, their risks, and how well they do or do not work. If clinical trials show that the new treatment is better than the treatment currently being used, the new treatment may become the "standard" treatment. Listings of clinical trials are a part of PDQ. Many cancer doctors who take part in clinical trials are listed in PDQ.

If you want to know more about cancer and how it is treated, or if you wish to learn about clinical trials for your kind of cancer, you can call the National Cancer Institute's Cancer Information Service. The number is 1-800-4-CANCER (1-800-422-6237). The call is free and a trained information specialist will talk with you and answer your questions.

PDQ may change when there is new information. Check with the Cancer Information Service to be sure that you have the most up-to-date information.

Chapter 23

Current Research Initiatives

Chapter Contents

Section 23.1

Tobacco, High Blood Pressure and Body Mass Linked to Kidney Cancer in Men

Cancer, May 15, 1994.

An article in the May 15th issue of *Cancer* reports a multicenter, hospital-based control study of the epidemiology of renal cell carcinoma. The study was conducted by Muscat etal. from 1977 to 1993 to evaluate the associations of smoking, chewing tobacco, body mass index (BMI), high blood pressure, and alcohol consumption with renal cell carcinoma in men and women. 788 patients with renal cell carcinoma were interviewed against 779 control subjects through a questionnaire. The average age of the men was 58 years and of the women was 59 years.

The odds ratio (OR) among male current smokers for renal cell carcinoma was 1.4 compared with those who never smoked, with a rising trend in the ORs with increasing pack-years, but not in the numbers of cigarettes smoked per day. For women who were current smokers compared with those who never smoked, the OR was 1.0.

There was no increased risk observed in those current smokers of filter cigarettes, but in those who exclusively smoke nonfilter cigarettes the OR in men was 2.4 and in women was 2.0. An OR of 3.2 was associated with chewing tobacco among men and no risk was found to be related to total alcohol consumption. Subjects with high BMI and a history of high blood pressure showed an OR of 1.9 in men and 3.2 in women.

The article reports that the incidence of kidney cancer in the United States has increased by 35.4% from 1973 to 1990 (2), and that many previous epidemiologic studies have shown increased risks associated with cigarette smoking. It concludes that persons with high BMI and hypertension may be at higher risk for developing the disease. There was no significant risk found between smoking and renal cell carcinoma in women, but the smoking of nonfilter cigarettes and long-term smoking were found to be risk factors for renal cell carcinoma in men.

References

Muscat JE, Hoffmann D, Wynder EL. The Epidemiology of Renal Cell Carcinoma. *Cancer* 1995; 10:2552–2557.

SEER Statistics Review 1973-1994. National Institute of Health. Bethesda (MD). *National Cancer Institute*. NIH Publication No. 94–2789.

—by Kathleen Feehary

Section 23.2

Gene for Kidney Cancer Isolated: How You Can Help

National Kidney Cancer Foundation from the OncoLink website: onco-news@oncolink.upenn.edu. Used by permission.

A research team headed by scientists at the National Cancer Institute (NCI) has identified the gene responsible for the most common type of kidney cancer. The finding is reported in the May 1994 issue of *Nature Genetics*.

The cancer, called sporadic (non-familial) clear cell carcinoma, accounts for about 23,500 newly diagnosed cases of kidney cancer each year, or about 85 percent of all cases of the disease. Currently, there are an estimated 75,000 kidney cancer patients in the U.S.

"With identification of this kidney cancer gene, it will be possible to develop new methods to improve the diagnosis and treatment of the disease and potentially to find way to prevent it," said W. Marston Linehan, M.D., of the NCI, "The finding also will make it possible to develop a blood or urine test to detect kidney cancer early when it is most treatable."

When detected in its earliest stages, the five-year relative survival rate for kidney cancer is 86 percent. If detected after it has spread to distant organs, the survival rate is 10 to 20 percent at the end of two years. In the United States, about 8,400 people will die this year of clear cell carcinoma of the kidney.

The damage or mutated gene responsible for sporadic clear cell carcinoma of the kidney is a tumor suppressor gene located on the short arm of chromosome 3. The protein produced by the gene appears to restrain normal growth. The researchers found that this gene is mutated and inactivated in 57 percent of tumors from patients with sporadic, non-familial kidney cancer.

"The disease appears to fit the two-hit model for development of cancer, where both copies of the critical gene are damaged or mutated," said co-investigator Berton Zbar, M.D., chief of NCI's Laboratory of Immunobiology. There are two copies of every gene in most cells. One normal copy of a gene is sufficient to prevent development of cancer. If both copies are damaged or mutated, (the two-hit model) cancer may develop.

The researchers also found that the kidney cancer gene is affected early in the development of the disease. This finding is important, Dr. Linehan explained, because its early presence makes it possible to consider development of treatments to halt or reverse the progression of disease in its early stages.

The gene responsible for sporadic clear cell carcinoma in the same gene that was identified last year as the cause of the inherited cancer syndrome called von Hippel-Lindau (VHL) disease. This research was conducted by Dr. Zbar and Michael Lerman, M.D., Ph.D., of NCI's Laboratory of Immunobiology, in collaboration with Dr. Linehan and colleagues. People who have VHL disease are predisposed to develop multiple tumors, including cancers of the kidney, eye, brain, spinal cord, and adrenal glands. Isolation of the VHL gene is now leading to improved identification of carriers of the gene in affected families to better manage care.

Last fall, after the VHL gene was identified, the National Kidney Cancer Association asked patients to participate in the NCI's research.

All patients and family members of patients were asked to contact the NKCA if (a) more than one person in the family had kidney cancer, including deceased family members; or (b) at least one member of the family had kidney cancer and at least one other family member had contracted or died of tumors of the eye, brain, spinal cord, ear, or adrenal gland.

Over 20 families contacted the NKCA. Each family was asked to provide some medical information which the NKCA passed on to Dr. Linehan at the NCI. Afterwards, he sent the NKCA the following note via electronic mail: "The family information you sent has been a home run. This morning we already identified one family with three affected members and another with four." Sometimes, a small amount of assistance at a critical time can lead to important progress in research. Dr. Linehan has again asked the NKCA for assistance in identifying families with kidney cancer.

Patients Wanted

Kidney cancer patients or family members of patients should call the Association at 708-332-1051. The NKCA will provide a family medical history questionnaire and information on participating in the NCI's research. The NKCA will also provide free information on kidney cancer and the genetics of kidney cancer to callers.

When the questionnaires are returned to the NKCA, they are screened and sent to the NCI in batches. This saves the NCI the effort of dealing with individual callers and NCI scientists are not tied up answering questions about kidney cancer. Once the questionnaires are received by the NCI, Dr. Linehan will call those patients and families which seem to be most relevant to the research.

If a detailed study is made of a particular family, it usually sufficient for every family member to get a simple blood test from his or her local doctor. The blood is shipped to the appropriate NCI laboratory by the doctor. (Due to AIDS and other blood transmitted diseases, it is important for all blood samples to be properly packed and handled.)

Families which have the familial kidney cancer gene should be extra vigilant so any new cases are diagnosed and treated early. Besides helping themselves, families which agree to participate in research will be helping scientists develop diagnostic tests and new treatments for all forms of kidney cancer.

Nurses, Social Workers and Doctors Can Help Too

If you know any kidney cancer patients, call them and give them the National Kidney Cancer Association phone number, 708-332-1051. Urge them to contact the NKCA. You'll be performing a valuable service, supporting research and helping patients get more information about their disease—perhaps even saving a life.

Section 23.3

Taxol May Fight Kidney Disease as Well As Cancer

University of Pennsylvania, ©1994-1996. Used by permission.

Taxol, approved by the FDA for treatment of ovarian and breast cancer, may also be an effective medication for treatment of polycystic kidney diseases, as was recently published by David D.L. Woo, et al. Polycystic kidney diseases are the most common hereditary diseases of the human kidney and account for 10% of all kidney transplant or dialysis patients. There is currently no treatment for the formation and enlargement of renal cysts. Woo, et al., developed an *in vitro* model of spontaneous cyst formation and found that taxol inhibits the process. Mice with polycystic kidney disease normally die of uremia (toxic levels of waste products in their bloodstream) by 4-5 weeks of age. Similar mice treated weekly with taxol are still alive after 200 days. This "suggests that taxol or its analogs may be useful in the treatment of human polycystic kidney diseases," the researcher said. Because taxol acts on microtubules (large cytoskeletal filaments), "our data implicate the microtubule network in the genesis of polycystic kidney disease cysts in both *in vitro* and *in vivo*."

Chapter 24

Additional Resources for Information about Kidney Cancer

Chapter Contents

265

Section 24.1

Overview of the National Kidney Cancer Association

National Kidney Cancer Association, ©1995. Used by permission.

The National Kidney Cancer Association actively works to increase the survival of kidney cancer patients and improve their care. The Association (1) provides information to patients and physicians, (2) sponsors research on kidney cancer, and (3) acts as an advocate on behalf of patients.

The NKCA publishes We Have Kidney Cancer, a 56-page booklet for patients and their families. A free copy of this booklet may be obtained by calling the NKCA at 708-332-1051 or by writing to the NKCA at 1234 Sherman Avenue, Evanston, IL 60202. The FAX number is 708-328-4425.

The Association also publishes Kidney Cancer News, a quarterly newsletter for patients and physicians. To obtain a free subscription, contact the Association. Other information is also available through the Association.

The Association also operates a free computer bulletin board for patients, physicians, and others with an interest in kidney cancer. This free BBS can be accessed at 708-332-1052 (2400 BAUD, 8 DATA BITS, 1 STOP BIT, NO PARITY, FULL DUPLEX, NO ECHO, ANSI terminal compatible). Free E-mail, information on kidney cancer and information on the NKCA are available 24 hours per day.

The Association holds regular meetings of patients, families and physicians to discuss current treatments and issues in kidney cancer. These meetings are held by local chapters in New York, Chicago, Los Angeles, and other major cities. Through these support group activities, patients can meet other patients and learn about their disease. The Association believes that patients who are well informed about their disease are more likely to make good decisions regarding treatment, and are more likely to survive their disease.

The Association operates a kidney cancer research fund which is supported by patients and their families. Income from the fund is used to sponsor research on kidney cancer. The Association's Medical Advisory Board is composed of leading physician/researchers in the field of kidney cancer and the Association's research program is directed by this board.

The Association represents patients with government and other organizations. For example, the Association has testified before the FDA on new drugs for treating kidney cancer. It also assists patients in obtaining insurance company reimbursements for new, state-of-the-art therapies. It will also help patients fight employment discrimination.

Incorporated in 1990 as a State of Illinois non-profit corporation, the Association has been recognized by the U.S. Internal Revenue Service as a tax-exempt charitable organization, 501(c)(3). Donations made to the Association qualify as tax deductible, charitable contributions.

If you have questions about kidney cancer, call the Association. Inquiries are always welcome. If you would like to participate in Association activities such as local chapter meetings, please call or write to the Association.

Section 24.2

Online Services for Kidney Cancer Patients

From a special edition of the Kidney Cancer News.
©National Kidney Cancer Association. Used by permission.

Free Online Info Services

Patients, physicians, family members, oncology social workers, nurses, drug executives, public policy makers, and others can get free information on kidney cancer and health care issues from the NKCA BBS.

Hundreds of information files are now online and free to the public. Need a copy of the Clinton Health Care Reform Plan? Want to know the latest clinical trials in renal cell carcinoma? View kidney cancer cells under a microscope? Do you need a list of doctors who specialize in urologic oncology? It's all online at the NKCA BBS—an electronic health center.

What is a BBS?

A BBS or Bulletin Board System is a computer and software system which allows users who have their own personal computers to post messages and files so other users can access the same information. Access is usually provided by dial-up telephone lines. Anyone who has a personal computer with a modem and the appropriate software can access the bulletin board.

A modem is a telecommunications device which connects to the computer and translates the digital signals of the computer into tones which can be transmitted over telephone lines. A modem at the receiving computer translates the tones back into digital signals. In this way, two computers can "talk" to each other and transmit information back and forth.

Cyberspace Support Group

When the NKCA implements multi-user chat, it will be possible for the NKCA BBS to serve as an electronic patient support group where patients and physicians can meet in "cyberspace" to exchange ideas. Patients from all over the country will be able to "talk" with each other online at the same time.

No Computer?

Visit your local public library. Many libraries have computers with modems which you can use. Take these instructions with you.

Market Research and Science

Market researchers in drug companies can "talk" directly with patients. Scientists can "mail" papers, data files, medical diagrams, and CAT scans to other scientists. Cancer organizations can exchange public policy position papers. And more.

Getting Started

To use the National Kidney Cancer Association Computer Bulletin Board System (BBS), you will need a personal computer with a modem and some telecom software. The NKCA BBS may be accessed with an IBM-compatible PC, an Apple computer such as MacIntosh, or any other computer.

Personal computer prices have dropped significantly and are now within the reach of many households. If you are about to buy one, get one with a high speed modem which will allow you faster access and file downloading. High speed modems are also "error correcting" which means that they are less troubled by static and noise on telephone lines.

Most modems come with telecom software. When the software runs on your computer, it tells your modem how to communicate. Common software packages include: *SmartCom* from Hayes Microcomputer Products, *CrossTalk* from Digital Communication Associates, *Procomm Plus* from Data Storm Technologies, *QuickLink II* from Smith Micro Software, and *QModem* from Mustang Software, and *MicroPhone* for MacIntosh.

Some of these packages, such as *QuickLink II*, will handle FAX as well as data communications if you have a combination FAX-data modem. Products such as *QModem* from Mustang Software will also handle Remote Imaging Protocol (RIP) graphics and sound as well as FAX and data communications.

The NKCA BBS supports three types of interfaces: text, ANSI, and RIP graphics. The standard interface is ANSI, which stands for the American National Standards Institute. The system will default to text if ANSI and RIP are not detected. In your telecom software, specify ANSI terminal emulation when you contact the NKCA BBS. Or, for IBMPC's, install an ANSI device driver in your CONFIG.SYS file and use VT-100 or other VT terminal emulation in your software package.

The NKCA BBS has a Graphical User Interface (GUI) using RIP but it has not yet been fully implemented. However, if you have a high speed modem and a mouse, you can give RIP graphics a try. Download the file RIPTERM.EXE from the Utilities & Software file area and install the software. Now call the NKCA BBS back and you can run in RIP mode. Be sure to set your user settings to "auto detect." The NKCA BBS will automatically determine if you are using ANSI or RIP terminal emulation.

To learn more, get a copy of *Dvorak's Guide to PC Telecommunications* published by Osborne McGraw-Hill.

Slick Technology

The NKCA BBS is a fully functional computerized system. It is available 24 hours per day, 7 days per week HELP is available throughout the system. Color is used extensively but users with monochrome systems are also supported.

The NKCA BBS has been set up on an IBM PC (a 25 MHz machine) running DOS 5.0 with one data line. More data lines will be added as the user base grows. Once the system has more than one line, it will also support on-line CHAT among users. The current data line phone number is 708-332-1052 in Illinois, or call toll free at 800-280-2032.

Baud rates up to 14.4K are supported. Set your communications software to the desired baud rate with 8 DATA BITS, 1STOP BIT, FULL DUPLEX, NO PARITY, and NO ECHO. A wide range of file transfer protocols are available for uploading and downloading files, including Ymodem, Xmodem, Kermit, and Zmodem.

How to Use the NKCA BBS

The NKCA BBS is very simple. There are only five menus:

1. Main Menu
2. Message Menu
3. Files Menu
4. Bulletins Menu
5. Questionnaires Menu

The Bulletins Menu contains news bulletins for users. The Questionnaires Menu allows you to provide information to the National Kidney Cancer Association.

Using these capabilities, you can order printed materials such as booklets and newsletters from the Association. You can also make a charitable tax deductible donation to the Association and become a member of the Association.

270

Each menu provides you with various options and functions. The following tables show a brief explanation of the three key menus.

The Online HELP system within the NKCA BBS is extensive. You can access HELP by typing "?" at the prompt.

Conferences

The NKCA BBS is organized into "conferences" which are broad topic and discussion fields. Currently, there are two:

- 0) Private E-Mail
- 1) General Public Messages

A user is automatically logged on to the BBS in one of the conferences. The default is Private E-Mail. The user may "join" any other conference, something which will be more meaningful when the NKCA BBS supports multiple concurrent users.

It is possible to link bulletins, files, and messaging to specific conferences. However, as currently configured, all bulletins and files may be accessed from all conferences. All messages posted in the Private E-Mail Conference are private. All messages posted in the other conferences are public.

Files

There are over 400 files on the NKCA BBS. Each file is in one of the designated file areas, depending upon its type or subject. The number of file areas may change as do the files in each area.

For example, each month, the NKCA posts new clinical trials to the clinical trial file areas.

File areas available:

- Private Mail
- Utilities & Software
- Clinical Trial General Info
- Kidney Cancer Expert Doctors
- Useful Text Lists
- KC News & Other NKCA Documents
- Kidney Cancer Information
- BBS User Info
- Public Policy & Pat Advocacy

- General Cancer Information
- Nutrition & Diet
- Genetics & Gene Therapy
- Basic Research
- Questions & Answers
- Legal & Patient Rights
- Insurance & Finance
- Renal Cell Carcinoma Trials
- Transitional Cell Trials
- Wilms Tumor Trials
- Other Clinical Trials
- Humor Book-Literature Reviews
- Health Care Charts & Graphs
- Advertisements & PR Releases
- Drug Package Inserts

Main Menu Functions

Message Menu. Takes you to the Message Menu where you send and read E-mail messages.

Files Menu. Takes you to the File Menu where you can Read, Search, Upload and Download files.

Bulletins. Displays list of available Bulletins like this one.

Doors. Allows you to run programs on the NKCA BBS. Currently no doors are available.

Questionnaires. Takes you to the questionnaires menu where you can make donations, order material, etc.

?. Ask the system for HELP on commands.

Join a Conference. Provides you access to one of the NKCA's conference areas.

Your Settings. Displays your settings stored in the system and allows you to make changes to them.

Initial Welcome. Displays the starting screen of NKCA BBS.

System Stats. Displays information about usage of the NKCA BBS.

Comments. Allows you to mail comments to the Sysop.

Page Sysop. Allows you to call the Sysop. If the Sysop is not available, you can leave a message.

Who's Online. Tells you who is online with you.

User Online Page. Allows you to page another online user.

Live User Chat. Allows you to chat with another user online.

Goodbye & Logoff. Goodbye and logs you out of the system.

Help. Let's you set one of three levels of HELP within the system. The default is Novice.

Newsletter. Text of the current quarterly edition of KIDNEY CANCER NEWS.

Messaging

You can send private E-mail to any user of the NKCA BBS. To send private E-Mail, join the Private E-Mail Conference and enter your message. Only the user to whom the message is addressed can read it.

Or, if you want to send a message to all users, join the General Public Messages Conference. Send a message to ALL or any user. These messages are "public" and can be read by all users. When you reply to these messages, your replies are also public.

QWK mail runs a program which creates QWK compatible downloadable mail packets. These packets usually contain a list of new files, recently updated bulletins, all your new mail, and so on. Use this feature when you prefer to do your message reading and replying offline. This option saves you online time and saves the NKCA money. To use this feature, you need a special offline message reader like *OLX* or *QModem* from Mustang Software to handle QWK mail packets.

Paging and Chatting

Paging is a special form of message that asks a user to "chat" with you immediately online. You can page either the System Operator (Sysop) or another user. If a live online chat is established, your screen will split. Your conversation will appear in half the screen and the conversation of the other person will appear in the other half.

Currently, you can only chat with the Sysop. If you page the Sysop and he is not there, you can post a message to the Sysop. Eventually, you will be able to chat with all users who are online. The target date for multi-user chat implementation is Christmas 1994. Watch the Bulletins for an announcement.

Doors

When you access Doors, you are presented with a menu which allows you to run specific programs which have been set up on the NKCA BBS computer. Currently, only test programs are available through the Doors function. The NKCA is testing and evaluating several programs which may be implemented through Doors, check the Bulletins for announcements about new Door programs.

Toll Free Access

The NKCA BBS can be dialed directly at 708-332-1052. Please use this number if you are calling locally or in the state of Illinois.

The NKCA BBS can also be reached by dialing 800-280-2032. When you use this toll free number, the National Kidney Cancer Association is paying the phone bill at $.23 per minute. Therefore, please use the highest baud rate you can, up to 14.4K baud.

Internet Access

Currently, the NKCA BBS is not accessible through Internet. It may be in the future. Watch the NKCA BBS Bulletins for all announcements about expanded access. Nevertheless, it is possible to send Internet messages to the NKCA. Our Internet address is:

nkca@merleacns.nwu.edu

and all messages are private. Do not expect these messages to be posted on the NKCA BBS but you may receive a response on Internet from the NKCA.

Each file extension specifies the graphic format which has been used to create the file. GIF is the Graphic Interexchange Format of CompuServe, Inc. JPG is the format developed by the Joint Photographic Group.

To view a graphics file, you must download the file and "view" it with a "viewing program" which will display the image on your computer screen or let you print it out. In the Utilities & Software file area, you can download several different files, such as CSHOW876.ZIP, which contain "viewing programs" for graphic files. Just download, run PKUNZIP to decompress the file, install the software, and run it to view graphic files. You may find it useful to put the CSHOW software in its own subdirectory and add it to the PATH statement in your AUTOEXEC.BAT file if you are using an IBM-PC.

Message Menu

Quit To Main. Returns you to the Main Menu

Files Menu. Takes you to the Files Menu where you can Read, Search, Upload and Download files.

Enter a New Message. Let's you send a message or E-mail to one of the other users or all users.

Read Messages. Allows you to read your messages and E-mail

Check Personal. Checks all personal mail addressed to you.

Read New Messages. Read all new public messages since you last logged onto the system or posted in "N" days.

Join a Conference. Provides you access to one of the NKCA's conference areas.

Your Settings. Displays your settings stored in the system and allows you to make changes to them.

Help. Let's you set one of three levels of HELP within the system. The default is Novice.

Goodbye & Logoff. Goodbye and logs you out of the system.

Kill a Message. Allows you to delete a message on the NKCA BBS after you have read your mail.

?. Ask the system for HELP on commands.

Update Confs. Allows you to set conferences which are searched when you read or scan for messages.

Scan Messages. Allows you to search for messages which contain specific key words.

Verify User. Allows you to determine if a specific individual is a user of the NKCA BBS.

List Users. Lists all valid users of the NKCA BBS—the people to whom you can send mail and files.

Transfer QWK Mail. Allows you to download mail so you can read it with an off line reader program

Thumbnails, Previews, Etc.

The NKCA BBS also has the ability to combine multiple GIF graphics files into a single "thumbnail" image so you can preview them. Just mark the graphics files you want to preview, download the file containing the composite "thumbnail" images and view them. Pick the ones you really want and download the full sized versions of the files.

Using this capability, you can combine two images into a new file. If you have two CT scans, such as "before" and "after" treatment, upload the two files. Download the composite thumbnail. Rename it and upload it again. The composite contains both CT scans.

You will find graphics software in the Utilities & Software file area to help you manipulate graphic images. Using this software, you can create new graphics, combine images, and do desk top publishing. AND IT'S ALL FREE!

Combining Text and Graphics

You should note that graphics files may appear as part of ZIP files in other file areas. For example, in the Public Policy & Patient Advocacy file area, there is NKCA testimony before the Joint Economic Committee of Congress on health care reform. In addition, to the text of the testimony, there are five PCX files containing graphs which were part of the testimony. Both text and graphs are part of the same ZIP file but become separate files when decompressed by PKUNZIP.

The PCX files may be viewed with CSHOW or the other graphics viewing programs. The text files may be read by any word processor or text display program.

```
[ 1] EXERCISE.TXT 1,199    11/10/93   | Exercise recommendations for kidney
     Dwnlds: 12       DL Time  00:00:10   | cancer patients in brief

[ 2] FAILURE.TXT   15,443   09/01/93   | Overview of kidney failure, dialysis,
     Dwnlds: 3        DL Time  00:02:10   | diet and other issues

[ 3] FAMILY.TXT     2,521   11/10/93   | Family considerations for care givers
     Dwnlds: 7        DL Time  00:00:21   | and patients

[ 4] FOLLOWUP.TXT 2,039    11/10/93   | Medical follow up issues for kidney
     Dwnlds: 11       DL Time  00:00:17   | cancer patients

[ 5] IL-2SUM.TXT    4,531   05/06/94   | Summary of Results of NCI High Dose
     Dwnlds: 4        DL Time  00:00:38   | IL-2 Clinical Trials

[ 6] IMMUNO.TXT    7,293   11/10/93   | Immunotherapy for metastatic disease:
     Dwnlds: 11       DL Time  00:01:01   | An introduction

[ 7] INFECTED.TXT  7,842   09/01/93   | Overview of kidney infections,
     Dwnlds: 5        DL Time  00:01:06   | symptoms, treatments, etc.

[C]ont, [H]elp, [N]stp, [P]rev, [M]ark, [D]nld, [I]nfo, [V]iew, [S]top?
```

**Figure 24.2.1.** Sample files screen—type "H" for help.

Your Files

Users are welcome to send files to the NKCA for posting on the system. Read any good books lately? The NKCA wants you to submit files such as book reviews.

We want doctors to submit CT scans, bones scans, slide presentations, and scientific papers. Companies can submit "electronic advertisements" for clinical trials, products, and services. Drug companies can upload package inserts for cancer drugs. Cancer centers can submit profiles of their treatment programs. If it can be typed on a computer, digitized or scanned into a standard format, it can be put on the NKCA BBS.

If you type something in WordPerfect or other word processor, output the file as an ASCII text file with a TXT file extension. Then upload it into the system using a telecom protocol such as Zmodem.

If you want to include graphs or charts or photographs, create a PCX or GIF image file with a GIF or PCX or other graphic file extension. Use PKZIP to combine the text file and the graphics file together into a single ZIP file. Then upload the ZIP file to the NKCA BBS. It may be obvious, but check your files before you send them. If you create an ASCII text file, be sure that you can read the file as an ASCII text file. (HINT: Be sure there are no more than 78 characters on a line.) If you create a ZIP file, "unzip" it to make sure it contains what you intend. If you make a graphic image file, be sure it can be read with standard software such as CSHOW. If you upload a program, be sure that it runs properly and that it is accompanied by appropriate documentation. NOTE: all programs submitted by users are scanned for viruses and are tested by the Sysop.

All uploads should be sent to file area 99, New Uploads from Users. The Sysop will put your file into the appropriate file area. If you want to suggest placement in a specific file area, send the Sysop a message.

The NKCA BBS is your BBS. You can make it great by contributing new material and uploading great stuff.

Files on the NKCA BBS come from a variety of sources: the NKCA itself, the National Cancer Institute, other bulletin board systems, users of the NKCA BBS, drug companies, publishers of software, etc. Every file on the NKCA BBS has a file name from one to eight characters, followed by a "." and a file extension from one to three characters. For example: gnomist.

To see the files on the NKCA BBS, list the files in a specific file area. AU files listed on your screen will be numbered starting at 1. Some files will be "flagged" *INFO* to indicate that a long description is available for these files. Simply type "I" followed by a space and the number of the file to display the long description.

File Transfers

Some files may be read online. Some must be "downloaded" and decompressed to be read or used. To download a file, you simply type "D" and enter the file name. You can also mark several files and download them all at one time.

The NKCA BBS supports a variety of communication protocols for downloading and uploading files. Zmodem is recommended, particularly if you do not have an error correcting modem. Kermit may also be used. (Yes, it really is named after the late Jim Henson's green frog.) Protocols such as Xmodem and Ymodem should only be used if you are using an error correcting modem.

File Extensions

A file extension indicates a file's "type." For example, files that have a TXT extension are ASCII text files and may be read online or downloaded. To read a TXT file, simply "View" it or "Read" it.

Files with a ZIP extension have been compressed with a program called PKZIP and are in "ZIP" format. More than one file may be compressed into a single ZIP file. Compression is useful for large files, particularly to save storage space and online transmission time. You may read a list of the files which may make up a ZIP file, but the contents of the files in a ZIP fib may not be read online. Simply "View" the ZIP file to read the names of the compressed files it contains.

If you download a ZIP file, you should also download PKZ204G.EXE from the Utilities and Software file area.

PKZ204G.EXE should be copied to a subdirectory such as PKWARE and then executed. It will decompress itself and create a series of programs including PKUNZIP.EXE and PKZIP.EXE. You can use PKUNZIP to decompress any ZIP file which you download from the NKCA BBS or other bulletin boards. You can use PKZIP to compress files for uploading or storage on your own system. For sake of convenience, you may wish to add the subdirectory PKWARE to the PATH statement in your AUTOEXEC.BAT file, if you are using MS-DOS.

MacIntosh users should download UNZIP20.SIT or ZIPIT1.CPT which allow Mac users to decompress ZIP files.

Graphics

The NKCA BBS has a fib area with Health Care Charts & Graphs. The files in this fib area have extensions such as GIF, PCX, and JPG. These extensions indicate that the fib contains graphic information such as a picture, a graph, a chest X-ray, a CAT scan, an MRI scan, a microscopic slide image, a diagram, or other visual information.

Files Menu

Quit To Main. Returns you to the Main Menu.

Message Menu. Takes you to the Message Menu where you send and read E-mail messages.

Personal Statistics. Displays your personal download and upload statistics.

Info on a File. Allows you to read any long description on a fib put there by the user who uploaded it.

View a ZIP File. Shows you all files contained in a M file.

Read a Text File. Allows you to read the contents of a text fib, those with TXT fib extensions.

Join a Conference. Provides you access to one of the NKCA's conference areas.

Help. Let's you set one of three levels of HELP within the system. The default is Novice.

?. Ask the system for HELP an commands.

Goodbye & Logoff. Goodbye and logs you out of the system.

Search for Files. Allows you to search for fibs by keywords such as "diet," "IL-2," "Wilms."

List Files. Displays a list of files on the system by fib area.

New Files Since. Displays only new files since you last logged onto the system or within "N" number of days.

Download Files. Allows you to download one or more files.

Upload Files. Allows you to upload files to a file area.

Edit a Marked List. Allows you to edit a list of files which you want to download.

File Transfer Info. Allows you to select a file transfer Protocol such as Kermit, Ymodem, etc.

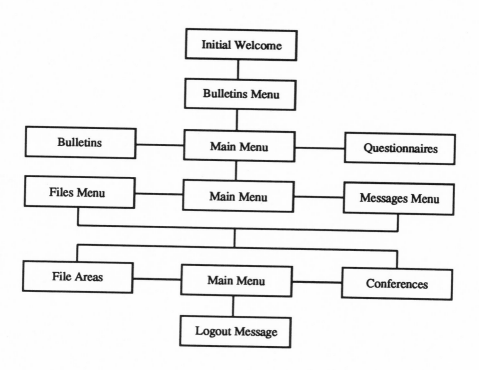

Figure 24.3.2. Structure of the NKCA BBS.

Overall Structure of the NKCA BBS

The NKCA BBS has a very simple structure. When a user signs onto the system with his name and password, he proceeds through the Initial Welcome message to the Bulletins Menu which alerts him or her to any new Bulletins since the last sign-on. Then, the Main Menu appears.

From the Main Menu, the user can proceed to any other menu or part of the system, including the Questionnaires Menu, Bulletins Menu, Message Menu, or Files Menu.

The overall structure of the NKCA BBS is simple. However, using the system is the best way to learn it.

Do not be afraid to make mistakes. All important parts of the NKCA BBS are protected from accidental erasure. If you see something which doesn't seem right, please feel free to call the Association or send the Sysop a message.

Part Six

End-Stage Renal Disease, Dialysis, and Amyloidosis

Chapter 25

End-Stage Renal Disease: Choosing a Treatment That's Right for You

Introduction

This text is for people whose kidneys fail to work. This condition is called end-stage renal disease (ESRD).

Today, there are new and better treatments for ESRD that replace the work of healthy kidneys. By learning about your treatment choices, you can work with your doctor to pick the one that's best for you. No matter which type of treatment you choose, there will be some changes in your life. But with the help of your health care team, family, and friends, you may be able to lead a full, active life.

This text describes the choices for treatment: hemodialysis, peritoneal dialysis, and kidney transplantation. It gives the pros and cons of each. It also discusses diet and paying for treatment. It gives tips for working with your doctor, nurses, and others who make up your health care team. It provides a list of groups that offer information and services to kidney patients. It also lists magazines, books, and brochures that you can read for more information about treatment.

You and your doctor will work together to choose a treatment that's best for you. This text can help you make that choice.

When Your Kidneys Fail

Healthy kidneys clean the blood by filtering out extra water and wastes. They also make hormones that keep your bones strong and

NIH Publication 94–2412, June 1994.

blood healthy. When both of your kidneys fail, your body holds fluid. Your blood pressure rises. Harmful wastes build up in your body. Your body doesn't make enough red blood cells. When this happens, you need treatment to replace the work of your failed kidneys.

Hemodialysis

Hemodialysis is a procedure that cleans and filters your blood. It rids your body of harmful wastes and extra salt and fluids. It also controls blood pressure and helps your body keep the proper balance of chemicals such as potassium, sodium, and chloride.

Hemodialysis uses a dialyzer, or special filter, to clean your blood. The dialyzer connects to a machine. During treatment, your blood travels through tubes into the dialyzer. The dialyzer filters out wastes and extra fluids. Then the newly cleaned blood flows through another set of tubes and back into your body.

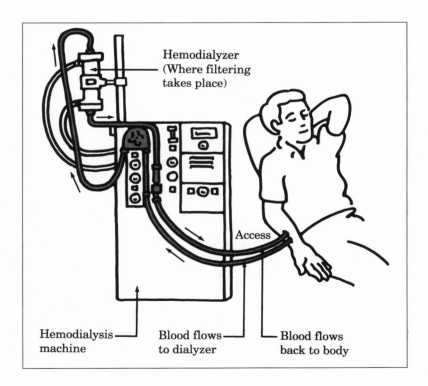

Figure 25.1.

286

Before your first treatment, an access to your bloodstream must be made. The access provides a way for blood to be carried from your body to the dialysis machine and then back into your body. The access can be internal (inside the body—usually under your skin) or external (outside the body).

Hemodialysis can be done at home or at a center. At a center, nurses or trained technicians perform the treatment. At home, you perform hemodialysis with the help of a family member or friend. If you decide to do home dialysis, you and your partner will receive special training.

Hemodialysis usually is done three times a week. Each treatment lasts from 2 to 4 hours. During treatment, you can read, write, sleep, talk, or watch TV.

Side effects can be caused by rapid changes in your body's fluid and chemical balance during treatment. Muscle cramps and hypotension are two common side effects. Hypotension, a sudden drop in blood pressure, can make you feel weak, dizzy, or sick to your stomach.

It usually takes a few months to adjust to hemodialysis. You can avoid many of the side effects if you follow the proper diet and take your medicines as directed. You should always report side effects to your doctor. They often can be treated quickly and easily.

Hemodialysis and a proper diet help reduce the wastes that build up in your blood. A dietitian can help you plan meals according to your doctor's orders. When choosing foods, you should remember to:

- Eat balanced amounts of foods high in protein such as meat and chicken. Animal protein is better used by your body than the protein found in vegetables and grains.

- Watch the amount of potassium you eat. Potassium is a mineral found in salt substitutes, some fruits, vegetables, milk, chocolate, and nuts. Too much or too little potassium can be harmful to your heart.

- Limit how much you drink. Fluids build up quickly in your body when your kidneys aren't working. Too much fluid makes your tissues swell. It also can cause high blood pressure and heart trouble.

- Avoid salt. Salty foods make you thirsty and cause your body to hold water.

• Limit foods such as milk, cheese, nuts, dried beans, and soft drinks. These foods contain the mineral phosphorus. Too much phosphorus in your blood causes calcium to be pulled from your bones. Calcium helps keep bones strong and healthy. To prevent bone problems, your doctor may give you special medicines. You must take these medicines everyday as directed.

Each person responds differently to similar situations. What may be a negative factor for one person may be positive for another. However, in general, the following are pros and cons for each type of hemodialysis.

In-Center Hemodialysis

Pros

• You have trained professionals with you at all times.
• You can get to know other patients.

Cons

• Treatments are scheduled by the center.
• You must travel to the center for treatment.

Home Hemodialysis

Pros

• You can do it at the hours you choose. (But you still must do it as often as your doctor orders.)
• You don't have to travel to a center.
• You gain a sense of independence and control over your treatment.

Cons

• Helping with treatments may be stressful to your family.
• You need training.
• You need space for storing the machine and supplies at home.

Questions You May Want To Ask

- Is hemodialysis the best treatment choice for me? Why or why not?
- If I am treated at a center, can I go to the center of my choice?
- What does hemodialysis feel like? Does it hurt?
- What is self-care dialysis?
- How long does it take to learn home hemodialysis? Who will train my partner and me?
- What kind of blood access is best for me?
- As a hemodialysis patient, will I be able to keep working? Can I have treatments at night if I plan to keep working?
- How much should I exercise?
- Who will be on my health care team? How can they help me?
- Who can I talk with about sexuality, family problems, or money concerns?
- How/where can I talk to other people who have faced this decision?

Peritoneal Dialysis

Peritoneal dialysis is another procedure that replaces the work of your kidneys. It removes extra water, wastes, and chemicals from your body. This type of dialysis uses the lining of your abdomen to filter your blood. This lining is called the peritoneal membrane.

A cleansing solution, called dialysate, travels through a special tube into your abdomen. Fluid, wastes, and chemicals pass from tiny blood vessels in the peritoneal membrane into the dialysate. After several hours, the dialysate gets drained from your abdomen, taking the wastes from your blood with it. Then you fill your abdomen with fresh dialysate and the cleaning process begins again.

Before your first treatment, a surgeon places a small, soft tube called a catheter into your abdomen. This catheter always stays there. It helps transport the dialysate to and from your peritoneal membrane.

There are three types of peritoneal dialysis.

Continuous Ambulatory Peritoneal Dialysis (CAPD). CAPD is the most common type of peritoneal dialysis. It needs no machine. It can be done in any clean, well-lit place. With CAPD, your blood is always being cleaned. The dialysate passes from a plastic bag through the catheter and into your abdomen. The dialysate stays in your abdomen with the catheter sealed. After several hours, you drain the solution back into the bag. Then you refill your abdomen with fresh solution through the same catheter. Now the cleaning process begins again. While the solution is in your body, you may fold the empty plastic bag and hide it under your clothes, around your waist, or in a pocket.

Continuous Cyclic Peritoneal Dialysis (CCPD). CCPD is like CAPD except that a machine, which connects to your catheter, automatically fills and drains the dialysate from your abdomen. The machine does this at night while you sleep.

Intermittent Peritoneal Dialysis (IPD). IPD uses the same type of machine as CCPD to add and drain the dialysate. IPD can be done at home, but it's usually done in the hospital. IPD treatments take longer than CCPD.

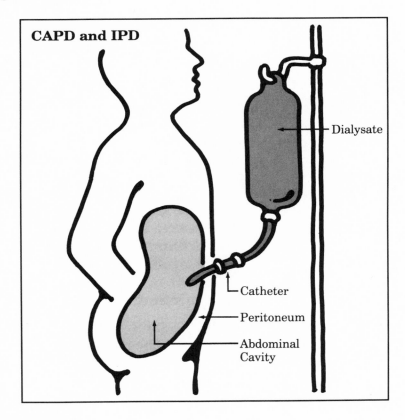

Figure 25.2.

CAPD is a form of self-treatment. It needs no machine and no partner. However, with IPD and CCPD, you need a machine and the help of a partner (family member, friend, or health professional).

With CAPD, the dialysate stays in your abdomen for about 4 to 6 hours. The process of draining the dialysate and replacing fresh solution takes 30 to 40 minutes. Most people change the solution four times a day.

With CCPD, treatments last from 10 to 12 hours every night.

With IPD, treatments are done several times a week, for a total of 36 to 42 hours per week. Sessions may last up to 24 hours.

Peritonitis, or infection of the peritoneum, can occur if the opening where the catheter enters your body gets infected. You can also get it if there is a problem connecting or disconnecting the catheter from the bags. Peritonitis can make you feel sick. It can cause a fever and stomach pain.

To avoid peritonitis, you must be careful to follow the procedure exactly. You must know the early signs of peritonitis. Look for reddening or swelling around the catheter. You should also note if your dialysate looks cloudy. It is important to report these signs to your doctor so that the peritonitis can be treated quickly to avoid serious problems.

Diet for peritoneal dialysis is slightly different than diet for hemodialysis.

- You may be able to have more salt and fluids.
- You may eat more protein.
- You may have different potassium restrictions.
- You may need to cut back on the number of calories you eat. This limitation is because the sugar in the dialysate may cause you to gain weight.

CAPD

Pros

- You can perform treatment alone.
- You can do it at times you choose.
- You can do it in many locations.
- You don't need a machine.

Cons

- It disrupts your daily schedule.

CCPD

Pros

- You can do it at night, mainly while you sleep.

Cons

- You need a machine and help from a partner.

IPD

Pros

- Health professionals usually perform treatments.

Cons

- You may need to go to a hospital.
- It takes a lot of time.
- You need a machine.

Questions You May Want To Ask

- Is peritoneal dialysis the best treatment choice for me? Why or why not? Which type?
- How long will it take me to learn peritoneal dialysis?
- What does peritoneal dialysis feel like? Does it hurt?
- How will peritoneal dialysis affect my blood pressure?
- How do I know if I have peritonitis? How is peritonitis treated?
- As a peritoneal dialysis patient, will I be able to continue working?
- How much should I exercise?
- Who will be on my health care team? How can they help me?
- Who can I talk with about sexuality, finances, or family concerns?
- How/where can I talk to other people who have faced this decision?

Dialysis Is Not a Cure

Hemodialysis and peritoneal dialysis are treatments that try to replace your failed kidneys. These treatments help you feel better and live longer, but they are not cures for ESRD. While patients with ESRD are now living longer than ever, ESRD can cause problems over the years. Some problems are bone disease, high blood pressure, nerve damage, and anemia (having too few red blood cells). Although these problems won't go away with dialysis, doctors now have new and better ways to treat or prevent them. You should discuss these treatments with your doctor.

Kidney Transplantation

Kidney transplantation is a procedure that places a healthy kidney from another person into your body. This one new kidney does all the work that your two failed kidneys cannot do.

A surgeon places the new kidney inside your body between your upper thigh and abdomen. The surgeon connects the artery and vein of the new kidney to your artery and vein. Your blood flows through the new kidney and makes urine, just like your own kidneys did when they were healthy. The new kidney may start working right away or may take up to a few weeks to make urine. Your own kidneys are left where they are, unless they are causing infection or high blood pressure.

You may receive a kidney from a member of your family. This kind of donor is called a living-related donor. You may receive a kidney from a person who has recently died. This type of donor is called a cadaver donor. Sometimes a spouse or very close friend may donate a kidney. This kind of donor is called a living-unrelated donor.

It is very important for the donor's blood and tissues to closely match yours. This match will help prevent your body's immune system from fighting off, or rejecting, the new kidney. A lab will do special tests on blood cells to find out if your body will accept the new kidney.

The time it takes to get a kidney varies. There are not enough cadaver donors for every person who needs a transplant. Because of this, you must be placed on a waiting list to receive a cadaver donor kidney. However, if a relative gives you a kidney, the transplant operation can be done sooner.

The surgery takes from 3 to 6 hours. The usual hospital stay may last from 10 to 14 days. After you leave the hospital, you will go to the clinic for regular followup visits.

If a relative or close friend gives you a kidney, he or she will probably stay in the hospital for one week or less.

Transplantation is not a cure. There is always a chance that your body will reject your new kidney, no matter how good the match. The chance of your body accepting the new kidney depends on your age, race, and medical condition.

Normally, 75 to 80 percent of transplants from cadaver donors are working one year after surgery. However, transplants from living relatives often work better than transplants from cadaver donors. This fact is because they are usually a closer match.

Your doctor will give you special drugs to help prevent rejection. These are called immunosuppressants. You will need to take these drugs every day for the rest of your life. Sometimes these drugs cannot stop your body from rejecting the new kidney. If this happens, you will go back to some form of dialysis and possibly wait for another transplant.

Treatment with these drugs may cause side effects. The most serious is that they weaken your immune system, making it easier for you get infections. Some drugs also cause changes in how you look. Your face may get fuller. You may gain weight or develop acne or facial hair. Not all patients have these problems, and makeup and diet can help.

Some of these drugs may cause problems such as cataracts, extra stomach acid, and hip disease. In a smaller number of patients, these drugs also may cause liver or kidney damage when used for a long period of time.

Diet for transplant patients is less limiting than it is for dialysis patients. You may still have to cut back on some foods, though. Your diet probably will change as your medicines, blood values, weight, and blood pressure change.

- You may need to count calories. Your medicine may give you a bigger appetite and cause you to gain weight.
- You may have to limit eating salty foods. Your medications may cause salt to be held in your body, leading to high blood pressure.
- You may need to eat less protein. Some medications cause a higher level of wastes to build up in your bloodstream.

Pros

- It works like a normal kidney.
- It helps you feel healthier.
- You have fewer diet restrictions.
- There's no need for dialysis.

Cons

- It requires major surgery.
- You may need to wait for a donor.
- One transplant may not last a lifetime. Your body may reject the new kidney.
- You will have to take drugs for the rest of your life.

Questions You May Want To Ask

- Is transplantation the best treatment choice for me? Why or why not?
- What are my chances of having a successful transplant?
- How do I find out if a family member or friend can donate?
- What are the risks to a family member or friend if he or she donates?
- If a family member or friend doesn't donate, how do I get placed on a waiting list for a kidney? How long will I have to wait?
- What are the symptoms of rejection?
- Who will be on my health care team? How can they help me?
- Who can I talk to about sexuality, finances, or family concerns?
- How/where can I talk to other people who have faced this decision?

Conclusion

It's not always easy to decide which type of treatment is best for you. Your decision depends on your medical condition, lifestyle, and personal likes and dislikes. Discuss the pros and cons of each with your health care team. If you start one form of treatment and decide you'd like to try another, talk it over with your doctor. The key is to learn as much as you can about your choices. With that knowledge, you and your doctor will choose a treatment that suits you best.

Paying for Treatment

Treatment for ESRD is expensive, but the Federal Government helps pay for much of the cost. Often, private insurance or state programs pay the rest.

Medicare

Medicare pays for 80 percent of the cost of your dialysis treatments or transplant, no matter how old you are. To qualify, you must have worked long enough to be insured under Social Security (or be the child of someone who has) or you already must be receiving Social Security benefits.

You should apply for Medicare as soon as possible after beginning dialysis. Often, a social worker at your hospital or dialysis center will help you apply.

Private Insurance

Private insurance often pays for the entire cost of treatment. Or it may pay for the 20 percent that Medicare does not cover. Private insurance also may pay for your prescription drugs.

Medicaid

Medicaid is a state program. Your income must be below a certain level to receive Medicaid funds. Medicaid may pay for your treatments if you cannot receive Medicare. In some states, it also pays the 20 percent that Medicare does not cover. It also may pay for some of your medicines. To apply for Medicaid, talk with your social worker or contact your local health department.

Veterans Administration (VA) Benefits

If you are a veteran, the VA can help pay for treatment. Contact your local VA office for more information.

Social Security Income (SSI) and Social Security Disability Income (SSDI)

These benefits are available from the Social Security Administration. They assist you with the costs of daily living. To find out if you qualify, talk to your social worker or call your local Social Security office.

Organizations That Can Help

There are several groups that offer information and services to kidney patients. You may wish to contact the following:

American Kidney Fund
Suite 1010
6110 Executive Boulevard
Rockville, MD 20852
(800) 638-8299

American Association of Kidney Patients
1 Davis Boulevard, Suite LL1
Tampa, FL 33606
(813) 251-0725

National Kidney Foundation, Inc.
30 East 33rd Street
New York, NY 10016
(800) 622-9010

National Kidney and Urologic Diseases Information Clearinghouse
Box NKUDIC
9000 Rockville Pike
Bethesda, MD 20892
(301) 654-4415

Additional Reading

If you would like to learn more about ESRD and its treatment, you may be interested in reading:

Your New Life With Dialysis—A Patient Guide for Physical and Psychological Adjustment. Edith T. Oberley, M.A., and Terry D. Oberley, M.D., Ph.D. Fourth edition, 1991. Charles C. Thomas Publishers, 2600 South First Street, Springfield, IL 62794-9265

Understanding Kidney Transplantation. Edith T. Oberley, M.A., and Neal R. Glass, M.D., F.A.C.S., 1987. Charles C. Thomas Publishers, 2600 South First Street, Springfield, IL 62794-9265

Kidney Disease: A Guide for Patients and Their Families. American Kidney Fund, Suite 1010, 6110 Executive Boulevard, Rockville, MD 20852. (800) 638-8299

National Kidney Foundation Patient Education Brochures. Includes information on treatment, diet, work, and exercise. National Kidney Foundation, Inc., 30 East 33rd Street, New York, NY 10016. (800) 622-9010

Medicare Coverage of Kidney Dialysis and Kidney Transplant Services: A Supplement to Your Medicare Handbook. Publication Number HCFA-02183. U.S. Department of Health and Human Services Health Care Financing Administration, Suite 500, 1331 H Street, NW, Washington, DC 20005. (301) 966-7843

Renalife magazine. Published Quarterly. American Association of Kidney Patients (AAKP), 1 Davis Boulevard, Suite LL1, Tampa, FL 33606. (813) 251-0725

Family Focus Newsletter. National Kidney Foundation, Inc., 30 East 33rd Street, New York, NY 10016. (800) 622-9010

For Patients Only magazine, Suite 400, 20335 Ventura Boulevard, Woodland Hills, CA 91364. (818) 704-5555. Published six times per year.

Chapter 26

Nutrition and Dialysis

Chapter Contents

299

Section 26.1

Intradialytic Parenteral Nutrition for Hemodialysis Patients

Health Technology Review, No. 6, August 1993, AHCPR Pub. No. 93-0068.

Most patients with end-stage renal disease (ESRD) who are undergoing hemodialysis (HD) have intact and fully functional gastrointestinal systems. However, many of these patients become malnourished from inadequate intake of nutrients as the result of anorexia, frequent acute intercurrent illness, dietary restrictions, or nutrient losses into the dialysate.[1] Evidence such as the finding that serum albumin levels appear to inversely correlate with mortality in a large population of dialysis patients[2] suggests that poor nutrition may contribute to increasing the morbidity and mortality of HD patients.[3] In view of these indications, nutritional supplements, referred to as intradialytic parenteral nutrition (IDPN), have been administered intravenously during hemodialysis treatment in attempts to improve the nutritional status of these patients. The amount and composition of solutions administered during dialysis are adjusted according to the patient's estimated needs.

Background

Whether parenteral administration of nutrients during the course of dialysis improves nutritional status and is beneficial to ESRD patients has been debated for more than 20 years. Most studies described in the literature have failed to demonstrate consistent positive effects of IDPN or have lacked the information necessary for interpretation of the reported results.

Foulks et al[4] reviewed the data from eight studies[5-12] published from 1975 to 1987 that purported to evaluate the effects of providing either parenteral or oral nutritional supplements during the dialysis

300

period as a treatment for malnutrition. Since the studies had many shortcomings, Foulks et al[4] were unable to conclude whether IDPN served any role in the nutritional management of HD patients. Most of the studies were of short duration, and patients were given both oral feedings and parenteral solutions of varying compositions. The number of subjects in each study ranged from 4 to 21, with half of the studies having fewer than 10 patients. The beneficial effects of IDPN as a treatment for malnourished HD patients were not clearly evident, especially since the investigators failed to indicate the means by which they assessed the nutritional status of their subjects and whether their patients were malnourished. In two of the studies[8,9] in which the patients had documented malnourishment, the number of patients with positive responses to IDPN was equal to the number who had no response or whose nutritional status continued to decline.

Discussion

Since the publication of Foulks and colleagues' review, additional studies of the effects of IDPN in HD patients have been reported.

Equivocal results were observed in two studies. Madigan et al[13] treated nine dialyzed diabetic patients with IDPN. After 2 months, three patients had gained weight, four had lost weight, and two had no change in weight. Four patients had increased appetites and five had decreased appetites. In the second study, data available from five of nine patients[14] demonstrated no significant effect of IDPN on the serum chemistry values of these patients, but IDPN appeared to stimulate their appetites.

Two case reports related beneficial effects of IDPN. The first described a diabetic woman with ESRD who had lost weight and strength as a result of persistent nausea and vomiting and frequent episodes of diarrhea.[15] After 6 months of IDPN administration, the patient regained weight and strength to the extent that she was able to ambulate for short distances without assistance and resume many daily activities. The second report described the administration of IDPN to a malnourished man undergoing HD who was losing weight and was unable to maintain nutritional adequacy by oral feeding.[16] Three months after IDPN therapy was started, the patient's nutritional parameters showed significant improvement and his nausea, vomiting, and anorexia were resolved.

Bilbrey and Cohen[3] ascertained the incidence and severity of protein-calorie malnutrition and mortality in 204 long-term HD patients with various degrees of malnutrition. Twenty of these patients, who had moderate to severe malnutrition, were treated with IDPN three times per week for 90 days. Although all malnutrition parameters were not improved, the baseline malnutrition index of these 20 patients improved significantly with the IDPN therapy. Significant increases were noted in protein-calorie malnourishment parameters such as body weight, mid-arm circumference, transferrin, blood urea nitrogen, and protein catabolic rate, but no change in other parameters such as serum albumin, triceps skinfold thickness, total lymphocyte count, and midarm muscle circumference (mid-arm circumference: 3.14 x triceps skinfold thickness) was reported.

In a controlled study, Cano et al[17] showed that administration of IDPN had positive effects on the nutritional status of HD patients. Twenty-six patients were included in this study: 12 were randomly assigned to receive IDPN and the remaining 14 served as controls. IDPN solutions containing amino acids and lipids were administered three times a week during hemodialysis for 3 months. Significant improvements in the nutritional status of HD patients were noted in those who received IDPN, while a general decline was noted in the control subjects. Specifically, serum albumin levels, skintest scores, transthyretin levels (formerly termed thyroxine-binding prealbumin), creatinine levels, weight, and appetite responded positively.

The American Society for Parenteral and Enteral Nutrition (ASPEN), a voluntary, professional society composed primarily of physicians, nurses, dietitians, and pharmacists involved in nutrition-support services, provided information indicating that the effects of IDPN in the care of patients with renal failure have varied. Although malnourished HD patients with significant gastrointestinal dysfunction appear to have benefitted from IDPN, data from studies of IDPN therapy have not given clear evidence of benefit because of the lack of uniform patient selection criteria, failure to randomize, small sample size, and other problems that arise in clinical trials. Even though IDPN may be of benefit to some malnourished HD patients, there are no data on which to base criteria for selection of patients who might benefit, the volume and composition of the solution to use, or the length of time IDPN should be administered. ASPEN stated that there is a small subset of HD patients with significant gastrointestinal symptoms who might be selected for and benefit from IDPN on a case-by-case basis.

Summary

Results such as those observed by Cano et al,[17] and the accepted intravenous administration of nutrients to support the nutritional status of patients with totally dysfunctional gastrointestinal systems, would indicate that IDPN may be beneficial for HD patients with significant gastrointestinal dysfunction who become severely malnourished. However, with the exception of the study by Cano et al,[17] the effects of IDPN have been equivocal. Although Bilbrey and Cohen[3] suggest measurable parameters that may identify malnutrition in HD patients, the characteristics of those patients who appeared to have benefitted from IDPN treatment were not evident from the published literature. Other important issues that have not been addressed are:

- Is IDPN of benefit to HD patients?
- What are the criteria for selection of patients who might benefit from intravenous supplemental nutrients?
- How long should IDPN therapy be applied?
- How much volume should be administered?
- What is the composition of an effective IDPN solution?

Well-controlled studies to answer these questions are needed before the role of IDPN therapy in the treatment of HD patients can be defined. The possibility remains that improving the nutritional status may improve the morbidity and mortality outcomes of some HD patients. These conclusions are in agreement with those expressed in comments and statements received from ASPEN.

References

1. Wolfson M. Use of nutritional supplements in dialysis patients. Semin Dial 1992;5:285–290.
2. Lowrie E.G., Lew N.L. Death risk in hemodialysis patients: The predictive value of commonly measured variables and an evaluation of death rate differences between facilities. Am J Kidney Dis 1990;15:458–482.
3. Bilbrey G.L., Cohen T.L. Identification and treatment of protein calorie malnutrition in chronic hemodialysis patients. Dial Transplant 1989;18:669–700.
4. Foulks C.J., Goldstein J., Kelly M.P., Hunt J.M. Indications for the use of intradialytic parenteral nutrition in the malnourished hemodialysis patient. J Renal Nutr 1991;1:23–33.

5. Heidland A., Kult J. Long-term effects of essential amino acids supplementation in patients on regular dialysis treatment. Clin Nephrol 1975;3:234–239.

6. Hecking E., Port F., Brehm R., et al. A controlled study on the value of amino acid supplementation with essential amino acids and keto analogues in chronic hemodialysis. Proc Clin Dial Transplant Forum 1977:7:157–161.

7. Guarnieri G., Faccini L., Lipartiti T., et al. Simple methods for nutritional assessment in hemodialyzed patients. Am J Clin Nutr 19R033 1598–1607.

8. Thunberg B., Jain V.K., Patterson P.G., et al. Nutritional measurements and urea kinetics to guide intradialytic hyperalimentation. Proc Clin Dial Transplant Forum 1980;10:22–28.

9. Piraino A.J., Firpo J.J., Powers D.V. Prolonged hyperalimentation in catabolic chronic dialysis therapy patients. JPEN J Parenter Enteral Nutr 1981;5:463–477.

10. Wolfson M, Jones MR, Kopple JD. Amino acid losses during hemodialysis with infusion of arnino acids and glucose. Kidney Int 1982;21:500–506.

11. Olshan A., Bruce J., Schwartz A.B. Intradialytic parenteral nutrition administration during outpatient hemodialysis. Dial Transplant 1987;16:495–496.

12. Moore L., Acchiardo S. Aggressive nutritional supplementation in chronic hemodialysis patients. CRN Q 1987; 11:14.

13. Madigan K.M., Olshan A., Yingling D.J. Effectiveness of intradialytic parenteral nutrition in diabetic patients with end-stage renal disease. J Am Diet Assoc 1990;90:861–863.

14. Snyder S., Bergen C., Sigler M.H., Teehan B.P. Intradialytic parenteral nutrition in chronic hemodialysis patients. ASAIO Trans 1991; 37:M373–M375.

15. Fausz C., Sostaric B. Diabetic ESRD patient supported with intradialytic parenteral nutrition. ANNA J 1992; 19:485–486.

16. Baltz P.S., Shuster M. Intradialytic parenteral nutrition as a therapy for malnourished hemodialysis patients. ANNA J 1992;19:72–73.

17. Cano N., Labastie-Coeyrehourq J., Lacombe P., et al. Perdialytic parenteral nutrition with lipids and amino acids in malnourished hemodialysis patients. Am J Clin Nutr 1990;52:726–730.

—by S. Steven Hotta, M.D., Ph.D.

Section 26.2

Diet Guide for the Hemodialysis Patient

American Kidney Fund ©1995. Used by permission.

By the time you need dialysis treatments, approximately 90% of your kidneys is no longer functioning. This means that only 10% (or less) of your kidneys is left to do the job of eliminating excess water and waste products from your bodies. It becomes necessary to rely on some type of dialysis treatment to restore a more normal balance in the body since your kidneys can no longer remove sufficient amounts of certain waste products. By controlling your diet these harmful waste products can be reduced. Your feeling of well being will be dependent not only on regular hemodialysis treatments and your medications, but also on how well you follow your renal diet.

Persons who are well dialyzed should feel well, should have good appetites and should have normal blood pressure. If you are a dialysis patient, then these goals should be yours. The doctor has ways to check what is called "adequacy of dialysis." The words used to describe adequacy of dialysis are either **the URR or the KtV**. Without adequate dialysis, there is poor appetite and weight loss, which may lead to hospitalization and decreased lifespan. So it is very important to be aware of your URR or your KtV. That way you have an idea of what is being done to enable you to reach your goals.

Calories

Calories provide the energy we need. It is important to obtain adequate calories from your diet for this energy. Calories are present in carbohydrates, fats and proteins. If the level of calories taken daily is below what you need, your body will burn its own tissues and muscles to get the necessary energy.

Good sources of **carbohydrates** are sugars, honey, jellies, syrup, mints and hard candies. These concentrated sweets are not recommended for the diabetic.

Fats are important in the diet because they add interest and flavor and provide us with a feeling of satisfaction. We emphasize the use of polyunsaturated (vegetable) fats like corn oil instead of lard. It is suggested that you trim the visible fat from meat and remove the skin of poultry to avoid unnecessary animal saturated fats.

Proteins are responsible for growth, building muscles and repairing tissues. They are broken down in the body upon digestion into waste products. It is necessary to limit protein in the diet to minimize these waste products. The waste product we most often talk about is *urea*. When the kidneys are not filtering as they should, urea remains in the blood and can build up to very high levels, which may never cause nausea, vomiting, hiccups, or general malaise. Though dialysis will lower the level of urea, protein restriction is still necessary to limit the buildup of urea between hemodialysis treatments.

Animal proteins such as milk, eggs, fish, poultry, cheese and meat are called "high quality" proteins because they contain all the essential building blocks of protein (called "essential amino acids"). These leave the least amount of waste products after digestion. Vegetable proteins such as cereals, starches and vegetables are called "low quality" proteins because they do not contain all the essential amino acids. These low quality proteins produce more waste products when digested. Consequently the majority of protein in your diet will be invested in the high quality ones in order to maintain muscles, make new tissues and prevent wasting.

Your protein allowance is prescribed according to your size. For example a man weighing 70 kilograms [154 pounds] will be allowed about 1.2 grams of protein per kilogram of desirable body weight. He will have a protein prescription of 84 grams of protein per day (1.2 x 70 kilos). Your dietitian will help plan a meal pattern suitable to you.

Sodium

Sodium is a mineral. Your body operates in an intricate balance with this mineral. Normal kidneys eliminate excess sodium in the urine to maintain the necessary balance. Sodium is found naturally in almost all foods. Salt is sodium chloride. One teaspoon of salt has 2000 milligrams of sodium. It is the total sodium intake for the day that may need to be limited, so beware of hidden sodium in food. Your dietitian will teach you how much (if any) salt you may add to your food. Too much sodium will cause high blood pressure, thirst and fluid retention. It can lead to heart failure. If your blood pressure remains high, you are at risk for a stroke or heart damage.

Some foods high in sodium are salt, seasoning salts, soy sauce, canned soups, pickles, olives, bacon, ham and some cheeses. It is wise to avoid these unless the dietitian can advise you how these can be included in the diet.

Potassium

Potassium is also a mineral. Healthy kidneys excrete any excess intake of potassium. If your kidneys are damaged, they may not be able to excrete potassium adequately. The principal danger of potassium overload is that it may cause an irregularity of the heart beat. This can occur without warning. HIGH LEVELS OF POTASSIUM IN YOUR BLOOD CAN CAUSE YOUR HEART TO STOP. Too little potassium in the diet may also be harmful.

Major sources of potassium are milk, potatoes (especially potato chips!), bananas, oranges, dried fruit, legumes, nuts, salt substitute and chocolate. The dietitian can help you plan your diet accordingly.

Since high potassium in the blood (hyperkalemia) can be life threatening, it should be treated as a medical emergency. Some patients, for whatever reason, are simply unable to maintain a safe level of potassium in the blood. In severe cases the physician can prescribe a combination of medicines called Kayexalate and Sorbitol. Kayexalate binds potassium in the intestines and Sorbitol is not absorbed by the intestines, thus it helps propel the Kayexalate through the intestines. This combination of medicines is not always recommended because it can cause an excess of sodium to accumulate.

Phosphorus

Phosphorus is another mineral found in all foods, but it is particularly high in milk, cheese, liver, legumes, nuts, fish and milk products. It is normally eliminated in the urine, but tends to accumulate in the blood of the person with diseased kidneys. A high phosphate level in the blood causes a lowering (like a see saw) of the calcium in your blood which results in an increased activity of the small glands in the neck called parathyroid glands. Ultimately this can lead to bone disease. A side effect of high phosphorus may be itching.

307

Since it is impossible to eliminate phosphorus entirely from the diet, phosphorus-binding antacids like Phoslo, Oscal or Tums are usually prescribed. This medication binds the phosphorus in food into the intestines, so that it may be excreted in the stool and therefore not be absorbed into the bloodstream. Dialysis removes very little phosphorus, so it is important to take your antacid as it is prescribed, which is usually WITH MEALS. Years ago the doctor prescribed antacids with aluminum. But research has shown that these aluminum containing antacids can cause bone disease. Learn to read the labels. [Magnesium-containing antacids such as Maalox or Mylanta, should be avoided.] Again, ask your physician for help.

Fluids

Usually a dialysis patient requires a fluid restriction with the diet. The less urine you excrete, the less fluid you can drink. Fluid overload may be very dangerous, causing high blood pressure, tissue swelling and heart failure. Fluid can build up in the lungs, causing difficulty in breathing and shortness of breath. It can overwork the heart, causing the heart to become enlarged and weak.

True weight gains do not occur overnight. Fluid weight builds up quickly. A rapid weight gain may mean you are drinking too much and/or eating too much sodium or salt in the diet. To reduce thirst, avoid salty foods.

There are other types of fluids besides water. Anything that melts at room temperature is fluid. This includes ice, ice cream, sherbet and jello. Fruits and vegetables are 90% water. Don't forget soups contain water.

Your daily fluid allowance will be individualized. It is usually equal to the amount of urine you produce in 24 hours plus a pint (16 ounces).

Vitamins and Minerals

A water soluble vitamin with folic acid is prescribed, as these are unfortunately removed during a hemodialysis exchange. Vitamin A is not recommended.

In addition to the water soluble vitamins, a very special type of Vitamin D may be ordered. If it is given orally as an orange capsule, it is called "Rocaltrol". If it is given as an injection, it is called "IV Calcijex." This particular vitamin may be referred to as a hormone and it is not part of your usual vitamin pill. It has a most important function in promoting the absorption of calcium and preventing the bones from becoming brittle. It may improve muscle weakness, aches and pains which often accompany kidney disease.

Dairy products, milk and cheese are excellent sources of calcium but they are also high in phosphorus. Consequently these are usually limited. A calcium supplement, such as Titralac or Tums, is usually prescribed to be taken between meals to promote its absorption. This calcium will be used to keep the bones strong. It should be discontinued if the blood calcium levels rise excessively. Your physician/nurse/dietitian will keep you informed.

Often patients are anemic, because diseased kidneys no longer make another special hormone. Fortunately now there is a medication called "EPO" that helps to reverse the anemia. Iron supplements are prescribed along with the EPO, so that red blood cells can be made. The iron is either given orally as a pill or as an injection. Don't forget the iron, because EPO does not work alone.

Some researchers have reported that zinc supplements may improve appetite and loss of taste. It may improve libido in males. It is suggested that dialysis patients avoid taking laxatives or enemas with magnesium.

Fiber

Decreased fluid intake, lack of exercise, lack of dietary fiber, iron supplementation and the daily use of antacid phosphate binders may result in constipation. Fiber from wheat bran is a highly concentrated form of fiber and therefore it is fairly effective in reducing constipation. Frequently the use of bran cereals is suggested for this problem. Though bran is high in potassium, it does not appear to be absorbed. Laxatives that contain magnesium, such as Ex Lax, Milk of Magnesia, or Citrate of Magnesia should be avoided. Instead, ask your physician for an appropriate laxative.

There is no established Recommended Dietary Allowance (RDA) for dietary fiber. Current recommendations vary, suggesting that individuals should consume between 20 and 25 grams per day. Larger individuals would consume more fiber than smaller individuals.

Diabetics on Dialysis

Since high blood sugar produces thirst, perhaps the most important part of the diet is to control the blood sugar. The insulin dependent diabetic may need supplementary doses of insulin to control blood sugar.

The new diet management of the diabetic emphasizes complex carbohydrates like whole grain bread, and fresh vegetables in an effort to reduce the coronary artery disease that particularly effects the diabetic patient. Now more than half of the total daily calories should be taken from complex carbohydrates. Polyunsaturated fats are also important. These include margarine (with liquid oil as the first ingredient) and oils, such as safflower, sunflower or corn oil.

If you are a diabetic that experiences low blood sugar attacks, never use orange juice because it is high in potassium. Instead use regular coca cola or regular lemonade or cranberry juice. These are low in potassium but high in sugar.

Ask your physician about using a glucometer if you are not already using one to monitor your blood sugar.

— by Peggy Harum

Section 26.3

Diet Guide for the CAPD Patient

American Kidney Fund ©1995. Used by permission.

By the time you need dialysis treatments, approximately 90% of your kidneys is no longer functioning. This means that only 10% (or less) of your kidneys is left to do the job of eliminating excess water and waste products from your bodies. It becomes necessary to rely on some type of dialysis treatment to restore a more normal balance in the body.

Continuous Ambulatory Peritoneal Dialysis (CAPD) is a type of dialysis that allows the patient a fairly liberal diet. CAPD does not cause large fluctuations in the amount of fluid retained by the body, as hemodialysis does. This may mean reduced stress on the heart and blood vessels as well as fewer dietary restrictions. With CAPD waste products and water may be removed each time you do an exchange. We will concentrate on emphasizing the need to replace valuable proteins that are lost each time an exchange is done. And we will discuss each nutrient involved in maintaining your nutritional status at the best possible level.

Persons that are well dialyzed should feel well, should have good appetites and should have normal blood pressure. If you are a CAPD patient, then these goals should be yours. Without adequate dialysis, there is poor appetite and weight loss, which may lead to hospitalization and decreased lifespan. Be sure to tell your doctor if you lose your appetite because it is one indication that your peritoneum may not be working well.

Calories

Calories provide the energy we need. It is important to obtain adequate calories from your diet for this energy. Calories are present in carbohydrates, fats and proteins. If the level of calories taken daily is below what you need, your body will burn its own tissues and muscles to get the necessary energy.

Carbohydrate is one source of energy. In addition to the carbohydrate available in the diet, the dialysate used in doing a CAPD exchange contains carbohydrate in the form of dextrose.

There are various concentrations of dextrose in the dialysate solution. For example, a 2000 milliliter bag of 1.5% dextrose has 105 calories, while a 2000 milliliter bag of 2.5% dextrose has 170 calories. And the 2000 milliliter bag of 4.25% dextrose has 289 calories. Of this, 70% of the calories is absorbed. The trick then is to avoid needing the bag with the most calories. The way to do that is to avoid drinking excessively and limiting the use of salt and salty foods which will cause the body to retain excess water. Retaining excess water may also cause the blood pressure to rise.

Fats are the most concentrated source of energy. They add interest and flavor to the diet, providing us with a feeling of satisfaction. We emphasize the use of polyunsaturated (vegetable) fats like corn oil instead of butter or sour cream. It is suggested that you trim the visible fat from meat and remove the skin of poultry to avoid unnecessary animal saturated fats.

Proteins are responsible for growth, building muscles and repairing tissues. They are broken down in the body upon digestion into waste products. We encourage you to eat more protein with CAPD than with hemodialysis because each time you do an exchange, protein is removed. After a period of time or years, this causes your muscles to waste. Your dietitian may measure your arm to determine the muscles present at the time of the initiation of CAPD. By doing this, we can follow your progress in maintaining your muscle mass.

In addition to measuring your muscle proteins, the physician does a blood test to measure your blood proteins. This blood protein is called albumin. It should be maintained between 3.5 to 5.5 grams %. Your dietitian or nurse will keep you informed on the progress of this as well as other blood tests.

Animal proteins such as milk, meat, eggs, poultry and fish are called "high quality" proteins because they contain all the essential building blocks of protein (called essential amino acids). These leave the least amount of waste products after digestion. Vegetable proteins such as cereal, starches, and vegetables are called "low quality" proteins because they do not contain all the essential amino acids. These low quality proteins produce more waste products when digested. Consequently the majority of protein in your diet will be invested in the high quality ones in order to maintain muscles, make new tissues, prevent wasting and replace the proteins lost when you do an exchange.

Your protein allowance is prescribed according to your size. For example a man weighing 70 kilograms or 154 pounds will be allowed about 1.2 grams of protein per kilogram desired body weight or 84 grams of protein per day. If the man experiences peritonitis, the protein needs will increase to about 1.5 grams per kilogram per day or 105 grams per day. Your renal dietitian will help plan a diet suitable to you and your needs.

Often CAPD patients describe an inability to take the protein allowance that is prescribed for them. We suggest taking 6 small meals instead of 3 large ones. And we recommend the use of protein supplements like Casec, Propac, Promod or Electrodialyzed Whey to raise the amount taken daily when the patient is unable to eat adequate protein in the diet. Your dietitian will teach you how to use these supplements if necessary.

Sodium

Sodium is a mineral. Your body operates in an intricate balance with this mineral. Normal kidneys eliminate excess sodium in the urine to maintain the necessary balance. Sodium is found naturally in almost all foods. Salt is sodium chloride. One teaspoon of salt has 2000 milligrams of sodium. It is the total sodium intake for the day that may need to be limited, so beware of hidden sodium in food. Your dietitian will teach you how much (if any) salt you may add to your food. Too much sodium will cause high blood pressure, thirst and fluid retention. It can lead to heart failure. If your blood pressure remains high, you are at risk for a stroke or heart damage.

Some foods high in sodium are salt, seasoning salts, soy sauce, Chinese food, canned soups, pickles, olives, potato chips, bacon, ham, some cheeses and "Fast Foods." It is wise to avoid these unless the dietitian can advise you how these can be included in the diet.

Remember the CAPD patient must use the high concentration dextrose like 4.25% to help "pull off" the excess fluids that accumulate from salty foods. The 4.25% has the most calories—the patient gains weight from too many calories—and it becomes a vicious cycle. The trick then is to avoid the salty foods in the beginning if your dietitian advises you to do so.

Potassium

Potassium is also a mineral. Healthy kidneys excrete any excess intake of potassium. If your kidneys are damaged, they may not be able to excrete potassium adequately. The principal danger of potassium overload is that it may cause an irregularity of the heart beat. This can occur without warning. HIGH LEVELS OF POTASSIUM IN YOUR BLOOD CAN CAUSE YOUR HEART TO STOP. Too little potassium in the diet may also be harmful. Fortunately, the majority of CAPD patients do not experience problems with control of potassium. It is relatively easy to control, as it is removed to some degree each time an exchange is done. Normally we do not restrict potassium in the diet for the CAPD patient. We monitor the levels carefully and advise you on a regular basis of the results. It may be necessary for some CAPD patients to eat more potassium in the diet. Some patients need to take a potassium supplement such as K-Lyte, Kay Ciel or Micro K if the potassium level is too low. The range we expect is about 3.5 to 5.5 milliequivalents per liter of blood.

Major sources of potassium are milk, potatoes, bananas, oranges, orange juice, dried fruit, legumes, nuts, salt substitute and chocolate. The dietitian can help you plan your diet accordingly.

Phosphorus

Phosphorus is another mineral found in all foods, but it is particularly high in milk, cheese, liver, legumes, nuts, fish and milk products. It is normally eliminated in the urine, but tends to accumulate in the blood of the person with diseased kidneys. A high phosphate level in the blood causes a lowering (like a see saw) of the calcium in your blood. This results in an increased activity of the small glands in the neck called parathyroid glands. Ultimately this can lead to bone disease.

Since it is impossible to eliminate phosphorus entirely from the diet, phosphorus-binding antacids like Phoslo, Oscal or Tums are usually prescribed. This medication binds the phosphorus in food into the intestines, so that it may be excreted in the stool and therefore not be absorbed into the bloodstream. Dialysis removes very little phosphorus, so it is important to take your antacid as it is prescribed, which is usually WITH MEALS. Years ago the doctor prescribed antacids with aluminum. But research has shown that these aluminum containing antacids can cause bone disease. Learn to read the labels. Antacids containing magnesium, such as Maalox or Mylanta, should also be avoided. Again, ask your physician for help.

Fluids

The CAPD patient may require a fluid restriction in the diet. The less urine you excrete, the less fluid is usually allowed in the diet. Fluid overload may be very dangerous, causing high blood pressure, tissue swelling and heart failure. Fluid can build up in the lungs, causing difficulty in breathing and shortness of breath. It can overwork the heart, causing the heart to become enlarged and weak. The CAPD patient normally has a more lenient fluid allowance because this type of dialysis allows a more steady state with fluid being removed each time an exchange is done.

Generally speaking, if a patient puts 4 exchanges of 2000 milliliters each into the peritoneum per day, this equals a total of 8000 milliliters (about 2 gallons). Then it is necessary to remove this plus any other fluids that accumulate in the body. If the patient uses excess sodium in the diet, and retains more fluids, particular attention must be paid to the fluid gains each day.

True weight gains do not occur overnight. Fluid weight builds up quickly. A rapid weight gain may mean you are drinking too much and/or eating too much sodium or salt in the diet. To reduce thirst, avoid salty foods.

There are other types of fluids besides water. Anything that melts at room temperature is fluid. This includes ice, ice cream, sherbet, soup and jello. Fruits and vegetables are 90% water.

Normally patients on CAPD are allowed about 2 quarts (liters) fluids per day. The physician prescribes this on an individual basis.

Vitamins and Minerals

A water soluble vitamin with folic acid is prescribed as these are unfortunately removed during a CAPD exchange. Vitamin A is not recommended.

In addition to the water soluble vitamins, a very special type of Vitamin D may be ordered. If it is given orally as an orange capsule, it is called "Rocaltrol". If it is given as an injection, it is called "IV Calcijex." This particular vitamin may be referred to as a hormone and it is not part of your usual vitamin pill. It has a most important function in promoting the absorption of calcium and preventing the bones from becoming brittle. It may improve muscle weakness, aches and pains which often accompany kidney disease.

Dairy products, milk and cheese are excellent sources of calcium but they are also high in phosphorus. Consequently these are usually limited. A calcium supplement, such as Titralac or Tums, is usually prescribed to be taken between meals to promote its absorption. This calcium will be used to keep the bones strong. It should be discontinued if the blood calcium levels rise excessively. Your physician/nurse/dietitian will keep you informed.

Often patients are anemic, because disease kidneys no longer make another special hormone. Fortunately now there is a medication called "EPO" that helps to reverse the anemia. Iron supplements are prescribed along with the EPO, so that red blood cells can be made. The iron is either given orally as a pill or as an injection. Don't forget the iron, because EPO does not work alone.

Some researchers have reported that zinc supplements may improve appetite and loss of taste. It may improve libido in males. It is suggested that dialysis patients avoid taking laxatives or enemas with magnesium.

Fiber

We must not overlook the importance of including adequate fiber in the diet of the CAPD patient. If constipation occurs, then the peritoneum does not function efficiently to remove waste products. Maintenance of good daily bowel habits are necessary. The use of high fiber foods like bran, bran cereals, fresh fruits (with skins), fresh vegetables must be included in the diet. Laxatives that contain magnesium, such as Ex Lax, Milk of Magnesia or Citrate of Magnesia should be avoided. Instead, ask your physician for an appropriate laxative.

Since the CAPD patient has less of a problem with control of potassium, the inclusion of fresh fruits and fresh vegetables into the diet is much simpler than including them into the diet of the hemodialysis patient. Ask your renal dietitian to help you establish a plan to include high fiber foods into your diet.

There is no established Recommended Dietary Allowance (RDA) for dietary fiber. Current recommendations vary, suggesting that individuals should consume between 20 and 25 grams per day. Larger individuals would consume more fiber than smaller individuals.

Children

When figuring diets for children on CAPD the calories in the dialysate are not subtracted from the daily allowance.

Diabetics on Dialysis

Since high blood sugar produces thirst, perhaps the most important part of the diet is to control the blood sugar. The insulin dependent diabetic may need supplementary doses of insulin to control blood sugar.

The new diet management of the diabetic emphasizes complex carbohydrates like whole grain bread, and fresh vegetables in an effort to reduce the coronary artery disease that particularly effects the diabetic patient. Now more than 55% of the total daily calories should be taken from complex carbohydrates. Polyunsaturated fats are also important. These include margarine (with liquid oil as the first ingredient) and oils, such as safflower, sunflower or corn oil.

Ask your physician about using a blood sugar monitoring device like Glucometer, Accucheck or One Touch 2 to monitor your blood sugar. It is very important in the control of your diabetes.

—by Peggy Harum

For Additional Information

The American Kidney Fund is a non-profit, national, voluntary health organization providing direct financial assistance to thousands of Americans who suffer from kidney disease. Since its inception in 1971, the AKF has served as the primary non-governmental funding source for kidney patients in need of assistance. In addition to the direct financial aid program, the Fund provides services through its community services, public and professional education, kidney donor development and research programs. These activities are made possible through the generosity and continued support of the general public.

American Kidney Fund
6110 Executive Boulevard, Suite 1010
Rockville, MD 20852
National Toll Free Number: 1-800-638-8299

Chapter 27

AIDS Information for the Dialysis Patient

How do I protect myself against getting AIDS? Can AIDS spread in the dialysis unit? The answers to these and other questions are in this chapter. This chapter will help you understand how HIV is spread and how you and the dialysis staff can prevent the spread of HIV in the dialysis unit. AIDS can be frightening when we don't know what it is or how it is spread. When we have the facts, we are able to control the disease better. This chapter will answer some of your questions about AIDS, but don't stop here. If you want more facts, talk to your doctor, nurse, or social worker, or contact one of the organizations listed at the end of the brochure.

What is AIDS? What is HIV?

AIDS stands for acquired immunodeficiency syndrome. It is a disease caused by a virus that enters the blood. Human immunodeficiency virus (HIV) is the virus that causes AIDS. HIV destroys a person's ability to fight infections.

How Is HIV Generally Spread?

HIV is spread through blood and certain body fluids, such as semen and vaginal fluids, from infected individuals. You cannot "catch" it like a cold or the flu. HIV is usually spread by having oral, anal, or vaginal sex with someone who is infected with HIV or by using drug

DHHS Publication FDA 90–4240.

319

needles previously used by a person infected with HIV. HIV can also be spread to babies from their infected mothers before or during birth.

How Can HIV Spread in a Dialysis Unit?

HIV can spread in a dialysis unit through direct exposure to infected blood or body fluids on broken skin and mucous membranes (for example, mouth, nose, anus, and vagina). HIV cannot be spread through contact with equipment or other surfaces in the dialysis unit. The spread of HIV in the dialysis unit can be prevented by following routine infection control procedures that have been used for many years. Dialysis staff members take precautions to keep you and themselves safe from the spread of all infection. Staff members are well trained to prevent the spread of any infection in the dialysis unit. This includes preventing the spread of HIV infection.

What Do Dialysis Staff Members Do to Prevent and Control the Spread of Infection?

Staff members follow infection control measures to prevent the spread of infection. Examples of the precautions they take are:

- Wearing gloves, scrub suits, lab coats or aprons
- Wearing gowns and protective eyewear and masks when blood splashes are likely
- Washing hands and putting on a fresh pair of gloves for each patient
- Cleaning and disinfecting equipment and other surfaces in the dialysis unit
- Disposing of needles or other sharp instruments in puncture-resistant containers located close to dialysis areas
- Never recapping needles

Staff members take these steps to prevent the spread of all infective agents to patients and staff.

Why Are Hepatitis B Patients Treated Differently than HIV Patients?

Staff members take extra steps to protect themselves and patients from the spread of hepatitis B virus (HBV). This virus is more easily spread than HIV. Patients infected with HBV are separated from the rest of the patients in the unit. This is because, unlike HIV, HBV can be spread through contact with equipment or with other surfaces in the dialysis area. HIV is not spread this way, so it is not necessary to isolate patients with HIV.

Could I Get HIV from a Health Care Worker in My Unit?

There is very little chance that you will get HIV from a health care worker. Staff members take proper steps to prevent the spread of infection. In fact, among the more than 100,000 dialysis patients in the United States, there is no known case of a dialysis patient getting HIV from a health care worker.

My Center Reuses Dialyzers. Does this Increase the Chance for HIV to Spread?

No. Specific dialyzers are assigned to specific patients. Each patient reuses his or her own dialyzer after it has been properly disinfected by staff members. This prevents the chance for HIV and other blood-borne infections to spread to other patients. Check your dialyzer to be sure it has your name on it before your treatment begins.

How Will I Know If There Are Patients with HIV Dialyzing in My Center?

You probably won't. Staff members probably won't know either. This is confidential patient information

Staff members do not need to know if a patient is infected with HIV because they always take special care with every patient to prevent the spread of any infective agent. The steps they take will keep you safe from all types of blood-borne infections in the dialysis unit.

Are Blood Transfusions Safe?

There is a very low risk of getting HIV through blood transfusions. All blood is tested and screened for HIV before it is accepted for donation. This lessens the chance for HIV to spread through blood transfusions.

Can I Get HIV from a Kidney Transplant?

The blood for all potential organ donors must be tested for HIV. Organs from donors who are HIV positive are not used for transplantation.

If you are a transplant candidate and are worried about the risk of being infected, discuss your concerns with your transplant surgeon. The two of you can review the pros and cons of transplantation.

What Should I Do If I Think I Have HIV or AIDS?

If you think you may have been exposed to HIV, get tested for the virus. Ask your doctor to arrange for a blood test. If the test results show you are HIV positive, see a doctor for treatment. The staff working where you are tested must keep this information confidential. They are responsible for answering your questions and giving you support before and after the test—no matter what the results are.

If My Center Wants to Test Me for HIV Can I Refuse?

Yes. You can refuse to be tested for HIV. The center may not test patients without their permission. If the question of testing comes up in your dialysis unit, you may want to discuss it with your doctor.

If I Test Positive for HIV, Will My Care in the Dialysis Unit Change?

You have a right to receive complete and appropriate care whether you have HIV or not. You should not be treated differently because you have HIV. Some centers, however, may take extra steps to prevent the spread of HIV.

Some dialysis units may separate patients who have HIV from the other patients in the unit. Although this is not necessary, local practices may vary.

When you plan to travel, check the policies of the dialysis centers where you may need treatment. Although there is no infection control reason to do so, some centers may refuse treatment to transient patients who are HIV positive. Be sure to call ahead.

Where Can I Get More Information about AIDS and HIV Infection?

Many local and national organizations have the information about AIDS, including the following:

National AIDS Information Clearinghouse: (301) 762-5111

National AIDS Hotline: (800) 342-AIDS

American Association of Kidney Patients: (813) 251-0725

National Kidney Foundation: (800) 622-9010

Chapter 28

Dialysis-Related Amyloidosis

Chapter Contents

Section 28.1

What Is Dialysis-Related Amyloidosis?

NKF Family Focus, Volume 4, No. 1, Winter 1993,
©National Kidney Foundation. Used by permission.

Twenty or thirty years ago dialysis was not very available. It was not until 1972, through the efforts of the National Kidney Foundation and others that Congress passed the law that provided Medicare coverage for dialysis and transplant treatments. Since that landmark law was passed, dialysis has become available for almost everyone who needs it, regardless of age, employment status, or other disability or illness. Now, it is not unusual to meet patients who have been on dialysis for ten or fifteen years or even longer.

Long-term (more than eight or ten years) dialysis may be associated with new problems or medical conditions that were not noticed before. In other words, patients were not dialyzed long enough to develop these problems. One of these medical conditions that has only been recognized by most renal doctors in the last three or four years is dialysis-related amyloidosis. Here, let's answer some of the most common questions about this condition.

What is dialysis-related amyloidosis?

Dialysis-related amyloidosis (DRA) refers to a condition in which an abnormal protein, Beta$_2$-microglobulin or Beta$_2$-M, is deposited in the tissues around joints and tendons. In addition, tests that measure this protein show that dialysis patients have very high levels of Beta$_2$-M in their bloodstream. Patients with DRA may develop pain or stiffness or collection of fluid in their joints, cysts or hollow cavities in some of their bones, or they may develop a condition called Carpal Tunnel Syndrome. Carpal Tunnel Syndrome occurs when abnormal protein or tissue is deposited in the wrist. Patients notice numbness or tingling in their fingers and hand, sometimes associated with muscle weakness. Some patients with DRA even have unexpected bone fractures or tears in the tendons or ligaments that connect their muscles to bone.

What is the chance that I will have DRA?

DRA is probably fairly common in patients who have dialyzed for a long time, that is, more than eight or ten years. A study of dialysis patients in Europe showed that 20 percent of patients had Carpal Tunnel Syndrome after ten years on dialysis, and 30 to 50 percent of dialysis patients had it after 15 years on dialysis. In Japan, however, less than ten percent of patients had Carpal Tunnel Syndrome after ten years on dialysis. There are a lot of things we don't understand yet about DRA, including who gets it, why they get it, why more patients in Europe are affected than patients in Japan, and so forth. There is a lot of research going on now all over the world to answer some of these questions.

Do CAPD patients get DRA?

The answer is yes. Originally it was thought that CAPD patients were less likely to get dialysis-related amyloidosis because $Beta_2$-M protein is a protein that is removed from the body more easily by CAPD than by the hemodialysis. We now know, however, that CAPD patients can develop DRA also.

How will I know if I have DRA?

If you have DRA, symptoms might include pain, stiffness or swelling of joints such as the knee, shoulder, hip or wrist, numbness or tingling in your fingers, weakness of one or both hands, or pain or stiffness in your neck. You might have a spontaneous fracture, that is unexpectedly break a bone, without falling or injuring your arm or leg, although this is fairly unusual. A few patients have an unexpected tear in a tendon or ligament in their leg, arm or heel (Achilles tendon), but this seems to be pretty rare. It is possible that you might not have symptoms. Your doctor might have noticed cysts in your bones on a routine X-ray. If you think you may have DRA talk to your renal doctor about it. He or she will evaluate your symptoms, physical exam and tests and help decide if you have DRA.

Is there a treatment for DRA?

Symptoms of arthritis can be treated and relieved with medication. Carpal Tunnel Syndrome can be treated medically, at least in the beginning but may require surgery for complete relief of symptoms or if muscle weakness develops. Spontaneous fractures are treated just like any other fractures, with a cast and rest. If a tendon tears it usually is fixed with surgery.

Certain types of artificial kidneys remove the abnormal $Beta_2$-M protein from the body better than others, but removing the protein from the bloodstream does not seem to treat the disease. Different types of artificial kidneys are now being developed that may help in the future.

None of these things stop DRA, however. The only treatment that stops DRA from getting worse is a successful kidney transplant. Patients with DRA have almost immediate relief of symptoms following kidney transplant (probably because of the steroid medicines that are used to help the body accept the kidney). In addition, most transplant patients who have been followed for as long as six years after transplant do not seem to develop new symptoms or new signs of DRA. Many kidney doctors feel that transplant is the best treatment for patients with DRA.

—by Wendy Weinstock Brown, MD

Section 28.2

Additional Resources on Amyloidosis and Kidney Disease

Searches on File from the NKUDIC.

Legend

TI   Title
AU   Author
CN   Corporation Author
SO   Source
AV   Producer/Availability

TI   *Amyloid and Amyloidosis* **1990.**
AU   Natvig, J.B., et al, eds.
SO   Hingham, MA: Kluwer Academic Publishing. 1991. 965 p.
AV   Available from Kluwer Academic Publishers. P.O. Box 358, Accord Station, Hingham, MA 02018. (617) 871-6600. Price: $270.00 plus shipping and handling. ISBN: 0792310896.

TI   *Amyloidosis.*
SO   New Fairfield, CT: National Organization for Rare Disorders. 1987. 5 p.
CN   National Organization for Rare Disorders.
AV   Available from National Organization for Rare Disorders. NORD Literature Department. P.O. Box 8923, New Fairfield, CT 06812. (203) 746-6518. Price: $2.50 plus $0.50 postage and handling. Also available from CompuServe 76703, 4, or 'Go NORD'.

TI   *Amyloidosis.*
AU   Skinner, M.; Cohen, A.S.
SO   Boston, MA: Arthritis Center. 1988. 6 p.
AV   Available from Arthritis Center. Amyloid Treatment and Re-source Center, Conte Building, 80 East Concord Street, Boston, MA 02118-2394. (617) 638-4310. Single copy free for reprint.

TI   *An Informational Guide for Patients with Amyloidosis.*
AU   Lyons, S.; Stolz, K.; Skinner, M.
SO   Boston, MA: Arthritis Center, Amyloid Treatment and Re-source Center. 199x. 9 p.
AV   Available from Arthritis Center. Amyloid Treatment and Re-source Center, Conte Building, 80 East Concord Street, Boston, MA 02118-2394. (617) 638-4310. Single copy free.

TI   **Hereditary Amyloidosis Disease Entity and Clinical Model.**
AU   Benson, M.
SO   *Hospital Practice.* 23(3):125–141. March 15, 1988.

Chapter 29

Dialysis Statistics

Abstract

The National Institutes of Health Consensus Development Conference on Morbidity and Mortality of Dialysis brought together experts in general medicine, nephrology, pediatrics, biostatistics, and nutrition as well as the public to address the following questions: (1) How does early medical intervention in predialysis patients influence morbidity and mortality? (2) What is the relationship between delivered dialysis dose and morbidity/mortality? (3) Can co-morbid conditions be altered by nondialytic interventions to improve morbidity/mortality in dialysis patients? (4) How can dialysis-related complications be reduced? and (5) What are the future directions for research in dialysis? Following 1-1/2 days of presentations by experts and discussion by the audience, a consensus panel weighed the evidence and prepared their consensus statement.

Among their findings, the consensus panel concluded that (1) patients including children in the predialysis phase should be referred to a renal team in an effort to reduce the morbidity and mortality incurred during both the predialysis period and when receiving subsequent dialysis therapy; (2) the social and psychological welfare and the quality of life of the dialysis patient are favorably influenced by the early predialytic and continued involvement of a multidisciplinary

Morbidity and Mortality of Dialysis, NIH Consensus Statement Vol.11, No.2, November 1-3,1993.

renal team; (3) attempts should be made by instituting predialytic intervention and the appropriate initiation of dialysis access to avoid a catastrophic onset of dialysis; (4) quantitative methods now available to objectively evaluate the relationship between delivered dose of dialysis and patient morbidity and mortality suggest that the dose of hemodialysis and peritoneal dialysis has been suboptimal for many patients in the United States; (5) factors contributing to underdialysis of some patients include problems with vascular and peritoneal access, nonadherence to dialysis prescription, and underprescription of the dialysis dose; (6) cardiovascular mortality accounts for approximately 50 percent of deaths in dialysis patients, and relative risk factors such as hypertension, smoking, and chronic anemia should be treated as soon as possible after diagnosis of chronic renal failure; (7) early detection and treatment of malnutrition contribute to improved survival of patients on dialysis; and (8) until prospective, randomized, controlled trials have been completed, a delivered hemodialysis dose at least equal to a measured $K_{dr}t/V$ of 1.2 (single pool) and a delivered peritoneal dialysis dose at least equal to a measured $K_{pr}t/V$ of 1.7 (weekly) are recommended.

The full text of the consensus panel's statement follows.

Introduction

Prior to 1960 end-stage renal disease (ESRD) was uniformly fatal. However, with the development by Wayne Quinton and Belding Scribner of an external shunt to provide repeated vascular access coupled with the use of dialysis technology that had evolved some years earlier for the treatment of acute renal failure, chronic intermittent hemodialysis for the management of ESRD was launched in March 1960 at the University of Washington. The application of peritoneal dialysis for the management of ESRD soon followed. A little over a decade elapsed before Congress legislative the provision of Medicare coverage, regardless of the patient's age, for the treatment of ESRD. These as well as subsequent events have made it possible for hundreds of thousands of patients with ESRD to receive life-sustaining renal replacement therapy.

The incidence of treated ESRD in the United States is 180 per million population and continues to rise at a rate of 7.8 percent per year. In 1990, over 45,000 new patients were enrolled in the Medicare ESRD program of which 66 percent were white, 28 percent were African Americans, 2 percent represented Asian/Pacific Islanders, and

1 percent were Native Americans. Forty-three percent were at least 64 years of age and fewer than 2 percent were under 20 years of age. On average, African Americans and Native Americans are younger at the onset of treated ESRD and show dramatically higher incidence rates than whites or Asian/Pacific Islanders. Although clinical experience suggests that the incidence of ESRD in Hispanics is also greater than in whites, data from the United States Renal Data System are not available to confirm this clinical impression. Hypertension and diabetes accounted for 63 percent of the new cases in 1990. The incidence of diabetic ESRD in Native Americans was almost twice that of African-Americans and 6 times that of whites.

Of the more than 195,000 ESRD patients receiving renal replacement therapy during 1990, 70 percent were being treated with either hemodialysis or peritoneal dialysis. Although kidney transplantation is the treatment of choice for many patients with ESRD, the increase in waiting time for cadaveric organs, the presence of disqualifying comorbid conditions, and the low transplantation rates in an aging ESRD population will likely ensure that dialysis remains the primary method of renal replacement therapy in the foreseeable future.

The cost for care of patients with ESRD from all sources including Federal, State, and private funding was approximately $7.26 billion in 1990, an increase of 21 percent over a similar estimate for the preceding year. Not reflected in this figure are additional expenditures for outpatient drugs and supplies, the cost of disability, and Social Security payments. As the U.S. population continues to grow and a larger proportion of the population at risk attains the age of 65 and beyond, the cost of kidney disease including this end-stage component is projected to increase. According to an analysis conducted by the Health Care Financing Administration, by the turn of the century it is estimated that more than 300,000 patients will be enrolled in the ESRD Program. Furthermore, 85,000 new patients will enter the program in the year 2000 alone. Most of the increase will come from the aged and the diabetic population.

Despite improvements in dialysis technology over the past decade, mortality in the ESRD population remains high. For instance, at age 49 the expected duration of life of an ESRD patient is 7 years compared with approximately 30 years for an individual of the same age from the general population. In addition to increased mortality, patients with ESRD also experience significantly greater morbidity, including a substantial loss in quality of life. In 1986, for example, for all Medicare patients over 65 years of age, hospitalization averaged

2.8 days per year, whereas for those after 1 year on dialysis the median number was 15.0 days per year. The relevant information available to prescribe the appropriate dialysis dose is limited and subject to gross errors. As a consequence, "what is an adequate dialysis dose" remains a controversial question among professionals caring for patients on dialysis.

To resolve questions concerning delivered dialysis dose, as well as co-morbid conditions and dialysis-related complications, all of which appear to cause an increased morbidity and mortality in the United States dialysis population when compared to certain European countries and Japan, the National Institute of Diabetes and Digestive and Kidney Diseases and the Office of Medical Applications of Research of the NIH convened a consensus development conference November 1-3, 1993. Following 1-1/2 days of testimony by experts in the field, a consensus panel representing the professional fields of general medicine, nephrology, pediatrics, biostatistics, nutrition, and nursing, and a representative of the public considered evidence and agreed on answers to the questions that follow.

- How does early medical intervention in predialysis patients influence morbidity and mortality?
- What is the relationship between delivered dialysis dose and morbidity/mortality?
- Can co-morbid conditions be altered by nondialytic interventions to improve morbidity/mortality in dialysis patients?
- How can dialysis-related complications be reduced?
- What are the future directions for research in dialysis?

How Does Early Medical Intervention in Predialysis Patients Influence Morbidity and Mortality?

It is clear that factors influencing the morbidity and mortality in dialysis patients are operative for an extended period before ESRD is present and the need for dialysis is imminent. Unfortunately, only a minority of patients (20 to 25 percent) are referred to a renal physician prior to the initiation of dialysis. Managed care programs must recognize the importance of the continued involvement of the renal team in the care of these patients. A number of conditions related to renal failure are present prior to the onset of dialysis including anemia, hypertension, malnutrition, renal osteodystrophy, lipid abnormalities, and metabolic acidosis. In addition, smoking and poor glycemic control in diabetics will influence subsequent morbidity and mortality. The costs of delayed referral include both emergency dialysis, with its higher morbidity and mortality, and excessive utilization of health care dollars. Emergency dialysis jeopardizes the choice for modality of dialysis, endangers the ability to maintain prolonged vascular access, precludes psychological preparation of the patient for ESRD care and necessitates hospitalization for a catastrophic complex illness. The mortality in this crisis situation can be as high as 25 percent.

In the patient with progressing renal insufficiency, early intervention should be aimed at reversal of hypertension and correction of identified nutritional deficiencies and acidosis. While data are limited, the use of erythropoietin will prevent severe anemia and may reverse its associated complications. There is no consensus on the ultimate role of dietary protein restriction in slowing the progression of renal failure. However, an intake level of 0.7 to 0.8 g/kg/day can maintain nutritional status in noncatabolic patients with ESRD without placing an undue burden on the capacity to eliminate potentially toxic metabolites including acid, potassium, sulfate, phosphorus, magnesium, and unidentified uremic toxins. Because of deleterious effects of parathyroid hormone, therapies aimed at prevention or reversal of secondary hyperparathyroidism should be initiated in the predialysis phase.

Referral of a patient to a renal team should occur when the serum creatinine has increased to 1.5 mg/dL in women and 2.0 mg/dL in men. Predialysis referral to a renal team, consisting of a nephrologist, dietitian, nurse, social worker, and mental health professional, allows time to establish a working relationship, to acquaint the patient with the various modes of renal replacement therapy, and to provide information on dialysis access, nutritional modification, avoidance of potentially nephrotoxic drugs, and potential financial support for services. It is essential to initiate the medical interventions, discussed below, to reduce mortality and morbidity as soon as possible.

Hypertension

Increasing evidence suggests that aggressive therapy of hypertension in the predialysis period delays progression of renal disease and is the most potent intervention to decrease subsequent cardiovascular mortality in dialysis patients. As in patients without renal disease, hypertension is the most important etiologic factor in the development of left ventricular hypertrophy (LVH) and diastolic dysfunction. It has been proposed that delay of adequate therapy or failure to lower blood pressure to normal over several years results in changes that become irreversible or only slowly reversible on dialysis. Hypertension is the highest risk factor for coronary artery disease and cerebral vascular disease. The goal of therapy is a normal systolic and diastolic pressure.

Anemia

Studies now suggest that aggressive treatment of anemia in the predialysis period is as important as during dialysis. In fact, to reduce cardiovascular morbidity and mortality, predialysis therapy may be critical, since longstanding LVH associated with anemia may be poorly reversible or irreversible if therapy is delayed until the commencement of dialysis. In addition, predialysis correction of anemia appears to improve or maintain functional capacity, nutritional adequacy, sexual function, and psychological health. It also reduces the risk of hepatitis and sensitization to transplant antigens associated with transfusion. As in the dialysis patient, the predialysis patient should be evaluated for other causes of anemia besides the renal failure, and any nutritional deficiencies should be corrected. As the anemia worsens, the physician should initiate therapy with subcutaneous erythropoietin. The target hematocrit has not yet been determined. At present, it is recommended that the hematocrit be maintained above 30 percent, but studies are now being conducted to determine if higher hematocrit levels produce better results.

Renal Osteodystrophy

It is known that the factors mediating renal osteodystrophy are present early in the course of progressive renal disease. These factors need to be managed throughout the entire predialysis course to prevent the ravages of severe, potentially irreversible hyperparathyroidism. Patients should be instructed early in dietary phosphate restriction, probably before the serum phosphate is elevated. Calcium-containing phosphate binders should be initiated when minimal elevations of phosphate are evident. Metabolic acidosis should be rigorously treated to maintain bicarbonate near or at the normal range because of the effect of acidosis in increasing bone dissolution and inhibiting osteoblastic activity, especially in children and women. Treatment of acidosis may also improve protein metabolism.

Nutritional Therapy

At an early meeting with the renal team, a nutritional assessment by a trained dietitian should be accomplished and should include as a minimum weight, height, recent weight loss, upper arm anthropometry, and serum proteins (albumin, transferrin, and/or prealbumin). In the absence of obvious malnutrition a modest protein-restricted diet of 0.7 to 0.8 g of protein/kg/day will provide good nutrition. When malnutrition is present, emphasis on adequate caloric intake, greater amounts of dietary protein of up to 1 to 1.2 g/kg are called for in order to allow nutritional repletion or to counter the catabolic effects of stress. Measurement of urinary urea nitrogen to assess net protein catabolic rate (PER) can be useful for monitoring protein intake. In certain patients in the predialysis period, fluid retentive states will make nutritional assessment more difficult. Newer techniques such as multifrequency bioimpedance analysis and dual-emission x-ray absorptiometry offer promise for ease, reproducibility, and accuracy for assessing states of fluid overload and bone mineral status, respectively.

The dietitian should also design dietary prescriptions for energy, fat and carbohydrate, fluid, sodium, and phosphate, as well as other micronutrients, recognizing that the adequacy of energy intake will be largely monitored by weight change in outpatients. Although modification of the diet to minimize lipid abnormalities is reasonable, such modifications should not be so rigid that they limit energy intake below daily requirements. Lipid abnormalities, particularly hypertriglyceridemia and reduced high-density lipoprotein (HDL) cholesterol along with elevations in lipoprotein(a), are common in ESRD, but there are limited data supporting the efficacy of diet or drug therapy, and there is some evidence that the drugs usually employed have more serious side effects.

Quality of Life

Quality of life is very important in the predialysis period and should be given strong consideration in the decision to initiate dialysis. Maintenance of physical strength, appetite, and sense of well-being, as well as optimal physiologic functioning promotes interpersonal relationships with family and friends as well as rehabilitation and job retention in the working patient. As the likely need for dialysis approaches, preparation of the patient by introduction to various aspects of the therapy, to members of the renal team, and to the physical site of the therapy as well as to other patients undergoing dialysis will generally facilitate acceptance and compliance. Another potential benefit is the opportunity to discuss the characteristics of the various modes of the therapy in order to involve the patient in this selection and to allow early placement of vascular access if hemodialysis is the method chosen.

Dialysis Access

The benefits of early establishment of vascular access should be emphasized. Arteriovenous (A-V) fistula surgery must occur weeks to months before the initiation of dialysis to permit maturation of the fistula. Likewise, a peritoneal dialysis catheter should be placed at least 1 month prior to its anticipated use. There may exist advantages to newer catheters in which the external segment is initially buried subcutaneously and exteriorized when needed at a later date. Late referral is clearly associated with increased complications, the need for emergency hemodialysis, and possible long-term access problems.

Interventions in Renal Failure in Childhood

Chronic renal failure is different in childhood than in adults in that its incidence is low (11 per 10^6 per year) and its causes are obstructive uropathy, renal dysplasia, and congenital or inherited diseases in a majority of cases. Morbidities associated with childhood chronic renal failure are growth failure, osteodystrophy with bone deformity, salt and water losses due to urologic abnormalities, and neurologic abnormalities, including seizures, deafness, retardation, and learning disabilities. Because of growth requirements, dietary protein intake should be higher than for adults, perhaps as high as 1.3 to 1.5 g/kg/day or even higher for children receiving peritoneal dialysis. The production of erythropoietin and calcitriol and the functions of the growth-hormone-IGF-I axis may be impaired from birth onward. Because of these features, predialysis therapy should be aimed at correcting malnutrition, hormone deficiencies, salt depletion, and neurologic dysfunction.

What is the Relationship between Delivered Dialysis Dose and Morbidity/Mortality?

Hemodialysis

Indices of hemodialysis adequacy have historically included measurements of serum creatinine and urea, estimates of dialysis delivery (square meter-hour), and assessment of patient well-being. Recently, an estimate of fractional urea clearance during dialysis has been suggested as a more quantifiable measurement of dialysis efficacy. This estimate uses urea as a marker for uremic toxins cleared during the dialysis procedure. The fractional urea clearance model for hemodialysis is expressed as $K_{dr}t/V$, where K_d is dialyzer clearance (ml/min), r is residual renal urea clearance (ml/min), t is treatment time (min), and V is total-body urea distribution volume in a single pool (ml). A simpler and more common measurement of fractional urea clearance during a single dialysis treatment is the urea reduction ratio (URR). This ratio is expressed as a percentage and is calculated as [(predialysis BUN minus postdialysis BUN)/predialysis BUN] x 100. An approximate relationship between these two means of expressing dialysis dose can be made: $K_{dr}t/V$ of 1.2 is approximately equal to URR 60 percent. Although urea may be distributed in multiple body pools most current measurements use a single-pool model to calculate urea clearance.

Recent reports demonstrated a direct correlation between dialysis mortality and $K_{dr}t/V$ (or URR). Several studies have also suggested that the dialysis dose delivered to many hemodialysis patients in the United States was less than that recommended by the National Cooperative Dialysis Study. Although data from controlled, prospective studies are not available, retrospective data presented and opinions expressed at the consensus conference favor a recommendation for a minimum delivered hemodialysis (conventional dialyzer, single urea pool analysis) $K_{dr}t/V$ of 1.2 in patients with protein intake of approximately 1.0 to 1.2 g/kg/day. It is suggested that assessment of dialysis dose, by formal $K_{dr}t/V$ modeling, be performed on a regular basis. Opinions were expressed that dialysis time may be an independent predictor of mortality irrespective of the dialyzer urea clearance. It is obvious that a prospective, randomized, controlled study relating the dose of delivered dialysis to morbidity and mortality is of great importance.

339

In the metabolically stable patient, net protein catabolic rate reflects protein intake. As changes in $K_{dr}t/V$ may be paralleled by corresponding changes in net protein catabolic rate, dietary protein intake may decrease if the dialysis prescription fails to achieve the desired goal and the patient becomes symptomatic.

Morbidity

Attainment of the recommended $K_{dr}t/V$ is influenced by a number of factors, modifiable and unmodifiable, which may alter the delivered dose. These include, but are not limited to, the following:

- Vascular access: Obstruction to blood flow in the vascular access may occur and result in recirculation of blood through the dialysis circuit, thereby contributing to decreased dialysis.

- Equipment: Blood flow rate and dialyzer surface area and mass-transfer coefficient must be considered to give optimal delivery to achieve the calculated dialysis dose. Effective dialyzer surface area must be carefully monitored because excessive reuse of dialysis membranes results in loss of dialyzer efficiency and reduction of the delivered dialysis dose.

- Patient factors: Adherence to salt and water intake limitations must be met to avoid unnecessary fluctuations in blood volume during hemodialysis and the associated loss of effective dialysis. Other patient compliance issues include adherence to appointment schedules and time on dialysis. Patients with certain underlying diseases (e.g., diabetes, amyloidosis, drug dependence) have special problems that may interfere with dialysis.

Dialysis Biocompatibility

The composition of the hemodialyzer membrane may be a factor in establishing urea clearance goals, i.e., biocompatible polymer membranes such as polysulfones, polyacrylonitrile, and polymethylmethacrylate have permeability characteristics different from cellulosic membranes. In addition, the composition of the membrane may be a factor in the nature and intensity of the interaction between the membrane and blood. Generally, cellulosic-based membranes, in contrast to the more biocompatible membranes, have a greater capacity to activate complement and to attenuate the granulocyte response. It has also been suggested that the use of biocompatible membranes may result in lower mortality rates.

Peritoneal Dialysis

Peritoneal dialysis utilizes a natural membrane to remove nitrogenous products from the body fluids of individuals with impaired renal function. The use of relatively long dwell-time peritoneal exchanges [continuous ambulatory peritoneal dialysis (CAPD)] has enabled individuals to carry on normal daily activities without the use of machines or other appliances. The dose of peritoneal dialysis has been established empirically and depends to some extent on patient acceptance of frequent interruptions for the exchange of peritoneal fluid. Recently, an effort has been made to prescribe for each individual patient the dose of peritoneal dialysis needed to attain target levels of urea clearance. In general, four exchanges of 2 liters each may generate as much as 10 liters of dialysate (allowing for the removal of ultrafiltrate). Assuming nearly complete equilibration of urea between plasma and peritoneal fluid, this equates to a weekly urea clearance of approximately 70 liters. For a 70kg man with a urea "space" of 42 liters, the calculated $K_{pr}t/V$ is 1.7. The weight of current evidence indicates that this value of $K_{pr}t/V$ is a reasonable minimal delivered dose for most functionally anephric CAPD patients who daily eat approximately 0.9 to 1.0 g/kg of protein. The dose of nighttime peritoneal dialysis is usually increased above that of CAPD.

The prescription of dialysis will depend on the volume of urea distribution, the efficiency of peritoneal exchange, and the residual renal urea clearance.

Peritoneal dialysis is a demanding and time-consuming therapy. Omission of exchanges or shortening exchange times by the patient will reduce urea clearance and lead to increased morbidity and mortality. The use of urea as an index of peritoneal dialysis efficiency is complicated because the peritoneal membrane is more permeable to large molecules than are dialyzer membranes.

Peritoneal dialysis efficiency can be increased by more frequent exchange (5/day), increased volume per exchange (2.5 to 3.0 liters), and the coupling of CAPD with nighttime cycler dialysis in large individuals or those with relatively low peritoneal clearances.

Children

Children undergoing chronic dialysis therapy are more likely to receive peritoneal dialysis than adults. This preference is based on technical factors including problems maintaining chronic hemodialysis access. Because of the serious problems of growth failure and neurologic dysfunction, children require appropriate hormone therapy (erythropoietin, calcitriol, and growth hormone), nutrition support services, and neurologic evaluation. A qualified pediatric nephrologist is an essential member of the renal team. Data exist that intervention with specified nutrition, growth hormone, erythropoietin and calcitriol therapy, and avoidance of aluminum can clearly improve growth velocity. Because of the serious problems of growth failure and neurologic dysfunction, children with renal insufficiency should be referred to centers with specialized pediatric nephrologic care. Children also require educational and play facilities at the dialysis center.

Children of all ages with ESRD benefit from treatment with peritoneal and hemodialysis. The principles of dialysis outlined for adults generally hold for children, although no retrospective or prospective studies have been performed that indicate reasonable targets of $K_{pr}t/V$ or $K_{dr}t/V$ to maximally allay morbidity and mortality.

Children with chronic renal failure suffer from a cycle of depression, anxiety and loss of self-esteem. The difficulties encountered often result in family stress with a high divorce rate among the parents of a child undergoing dialysis. For these reasons, a mental health professional is an essential component of the pediatric renal disease center.

Finally, dialysis should be a temporary therapy, since renal transplantation is considered the treatment of choice for children.

Can Co-Morbid Conditions Be Altered By Nondialytic Interventions To Improve Morbidity/Mortality in Dialysis Patients?

Cardiovascular Abnormalities

Cardiovascular events (principally systolic and diastolic dysfunction, myocardial infarction, and stroke) account for 50 percent of the mortality in dialysis patients, and also contribute importantly to mortality after renal transplantation.

Studies of patients entering dialysis treatment demonstrate a high prevalence of established cardiovascular abnormalities including hypertension, LVH, coronary artery disease, and cardiac failure. For example, two-dimensional echocardiograms are abnormal in 70 percent of such patients. The rising mean age of dialysis patients likely will further increase this cardiovascular pathology.

We believe that optimum reduction of dialysis morbidity and mortality begins with predialysis intervention. The patient with chronic renal failure is at high risk for cardiovascular events. It is likely, but not yet proven, that prevention of severe anemia by erythropoietin will also prevent, diminish, or partially reverse left ventricular overload.

Cessation of smoking, correction of obesity, and regular aerobic exercise may also contribute to reducing mortality from cardiovascular disease. Normotension and non-smoking have been two characteristics of 20-year-plus survivors on chronic dialysis.

It is not yet known whether modifications of the common lipid abnormalities in chronic renal failure and ESRD patients can be safely achieved in the long term by currently available lipid-lowering agents or whether this would be beneficial.

Because myocardial calcification and fibrosis may contribute especially to diastolic dysfunction (which accounts for 50 percent of cardiac failure in dialysis patients) control of calcium, phosphorus, and parathyroid hormone levels may help to prevent cardiovascular disease as well as bone disease.

Two-thirds of ESRD is due to two primary diseases—diabetes mellitus and essential hypertension—that themselves contribute importantly to cardiovascular disease. Not infrequently such patients have had erratic treatment and followup programs prior to the onset of chronic renal disease. The identification of a diabetic patient has not routinely led to inclusion of that patient in a program of strict glycemic control and followup of potential microvascular and renal complications, such as micro or gross albuminuria. We also now understand that careful control of blood pressure upon diagnosis of diabetes mellitus is crucial.

Current studies suggest that blood pressure is not being adequately controlled in many dialysis patients. Blood pressure at the initiation of each dialysis treatment should be in the normal range or as near as possible to it. Adequate ultrafiltration and restriction of interdialytic intake of sodium chloride should establish normotension in up to 80 percent of dialysis patients. Mechanisms of hypertension in the remainder include an inappropriately hyperactive renin-angiotensin system, nephrogenic activation of the sympathetic nervous system and, possibly, an altered balance of endothelial factors (nitric oxide and endothelin) influencing arteriolar smooth muscle tone.

Nutritional Deficiency

The nutritional status of the patient is a major factor in the outcome of hemodialysis treatment and may be maintained in the predialysis period by the use of low-protein diets, in the range of 0.7 to 0.8 g/kg/day together with adequate calorie intake of 35 kcal/kg/day. It is essential that during this period, malnutrition, as evidenced by a decrease in albumin and body weight, is not allowed to develop in renal patients. Serum albumin levels above 3.5 g/dL are associated with little mortality, while mortality rises dramatically with lower values for serum albumin.

Once the patient is on hemodialysis, dietary protein should be liberalized to equal 1.0 g/kg/day, with appropriate calorie supplementation, to sustain nutrition at a normal level. The complexity of nutritional intervention for the renal patient is of such degree and, at the same time, of such importance as to require the expert guidance of a well-trained renal dietitian. High cholesterol is indicative of increased risk of morbidity and mortality, but values below 100 mg/dL are also associated with increased mortality. The reasons why hypoalbuminemia and hypocholesterolemia are indexes of high mortality are not known.

Educational programs instituted by the renal center and by organizations concerned with the welfare of all kidney patients should explain the need for adequate dialysis time and correction of malnutrition, because these factors contribute to longer life of higher quality and correction of many co-morbid conditions. Patient participation, as an integral part of the renal team, is of the essence if success in improving quality of life is to be achieved.

Current concerns about morbidity and mortality raise issues regarding the present uniform reimbursement system for dialysis, especially in the area of nutritional and psychosocial support systems. Linking direct reimbursement for such care to important outcomes such as levels of serum albumin, mean blood pressure, and measurements of fractional urea clearance during dialysis should be explored.

How Can Dialysis-Related Complications Be Reduced?

Although dialysis allows effective and productive lives for many patients with ESRD, a variety of complications can occur. Problems with dialysis access, infections, atherosclerosis and cardiovascular disease, malnutrition, and metabolic abnormalities, as well as persisting uremic symptoms and acute symptoms related to the dialysis procedure itself, may limit a patient's health and quality of life. Disorders of calcium, phosphorus, vitamin D, and parathyroid hormone are common and may be disabling.

Hemodialysis

Perhaps the major complication limiting continued effective hemodialysis involves vascular access a satisfactory fistula cannot be established in many patients, because of inadequate vessels (especially in diabetic patients). The chances of a successful fistula are enhanced by early planning and placement well before dialysis becomes necessary. When early planning is not possible, the use of a tunneled subcutaneous catheter may make dialysis possible while an A-V fistula is maturing, but repeated use of temporary subclavian catheters is often accompanied by infection or thrombosis with ultimate impairment of subclavian flow and loss of the whole arm for dialysis access purposes. Use of temporary catheters should be avoided when possible.

When a fistula is unsuccessful or not feasible, a synthetic graft is ordinarily placed. Current experience indicates that 60 percent of these grafts fail each year due to thrombosis. Anatomic stenosis is responsible for four-fifths of these clots (almost all are on the venous side of the anastomosis) while the rest result from other causes such as excessive post-venepuncture pressure by manual compression or clamp or sleeping on the graft. Medical thrombolysis may remove the clot and restore flow, but often surgical thrombectomy is required. The stenosis, usually formed by endothelial proliferation, sometimes responds to percutaneous angioplasty but may require surgical intervention. The present life of a synthetic graft is about 2 years with loss due to thrombosis in 80 percent and infection in 20 percent of patients.

Consistently elevated venous dialysis pressure may provide a warning of developing stenosis and hence of impending thrombosis and may indicate the need for a fistulogram. An increase in recirculation may also indicate an incipient problem. Attention to these signs may allow for intervention prior to clotting of the graft and prevent its loss.

The need for meticulous, experienced surgical skill in establishing satisfactory fistulas and shunts must be emphasized. Although the procedure may not be dramatic, a dialysis patient's life often depends on the presence of a reliable access. Nursing skill in access use has a major influence on dialysis success.

Infection

Infection remains the major cause of death in 15 to 30 percent of all dialysis patients; a figure that has not changed significantly over the years. Infections are usually due to common organisms and often appear to be access-related. About 60 percent of bacteremic infections are Gram-positive, especially *Staphylococcus aureus*. Perhaps 50 to 60 percent of dialysis patients are carriers of this organism (compared to 10 to 30 percent of the general population), and the carrier rate among diabetic patients is still higher. It is possible to reduce the carrier rate with prophylactic antibiotic treatment, but this may encourage the emergence of resistant organisms.

Uremia itself causes an impairment in cell-mediated immunity that is not totally corrected by dialysis. In addition, granulocyte phagocytosis and killing functions appear to be impaired by cellulosic dialysis membranes. Biocompatible membranes may have less deleterious effects on white cell function and other defense mechanisms. Some studies suggest a 50 percent fall in incidence of infection accompanying a switch to more biocompatible dialyzers.

Peritoneal Dialysis

The overwhelming cause of unsuccessful peritoneal dialysis is peritonitis. Although improvement has followed recent changes in tubing and connection systems, recurrent peritonitis is a continuing problem for many patients. Catheter tunnel infection often underlies this peritonitis, and changes in catheter design (e.g., U shape), placement (with both peritoneal and skin ends directed caudad and a cuff placed in the rectus muscle), and the use of prophylactic antibiotics at the time of placement or thereafter have been proposed as deterrents to infection. The use of vaccine against Staphylococcus organisms and of bacteriostatics such as silver-coated catheters are under investigation.

Calcium, Phosphorus, and Parathyroid Hormone

The disturbances in body calcium, phosphorus, vitamin D, parathyroid hormone, and bone disease that usually start prior to the initiation of dialysis continue to demand consistent attention so long as dialysis is required. Mainstays in therapy include control of dietary phosphorus, minimization of its absorption by use of phosphate-binders, and the use of calcitriol. Control of dietary intake of phosphorus requires patient education by the renal team and adherence by the patient to the recommended diet. Previous reliance on aluminum hydroxide to prevent absorption of phosphorus has been largely discontinued because of accumulation of aluminum in the brain and bone, leading to severe neurological disorders and osteomalacia. Ingestion of calcium carbonate or calcium acetate with meals is currently recommended for most patients to prevent absorption of phosphorus. Use of these calcium salts may require adjustments in the concentration of calcium in the dialysate fluid to prevent hypercalcemia and consequent deposition of calcium phosphate salts with damage to the heart, blood vessels, and other tissues. Careful titration of the calcitriol dosage is required to obtain its benefits without causing hyperphosphatemia or hypercalcemia. Careful attention to dietary phosphorus, calcium salts, and calcitriol often enable parathyroid hormone concentrations to be maintained at or near normal. Of serious concern is the emergence of "adynamic bone disease," a condition diagnosed by bone biopsy in which the normal correction of bone wear and tear by "remodeling" fails to occur. The exact cause(s) and consequences of adynamic bone disease are not yet known.

Amyloid

Amyloidosis in dialysis patients is associated with long-term (greater than 6 years) dialysis, and is increased in frequency in older patients. The deposition of beta-2-microglobulin protein as amyloid causes carpal tunnel syndrome, destructive arthropathy in medium- and large-sized joints, and cystic bone disease. The disorder may be due both to increased release of beta-2-microglobulin from macrophages and, significantly, to reduction in the destruction of beta-2-microglobulin that normally occurs in functioning kidneys. Some evidence indicates that amyloidosis is a lesser problem in patients dialyzed with high-flux membranes than in those with cellulosic membranes, perhaps because of both decreased release of the protein from macrophages and from partial removal of the protein during dialysis by filtration or binding with some synthetic polymer membranes. Serious consideration should be given to the use of these membranes for dialysis of patients in whom amyloidosis is a problem or may become a clinical concern.

Anemia

Attention to the management of anemia, begun in the predialysis phase of care, must be continued into dialysis.

Intradialytic Complications

Acute complications related to the dialysis procedure itself may severely compromise the quality of life in chronic dialysis patients. A mild degree of hypotension is "normal" in dialysis, but severe degrees may be disabling. Muscle cramps, chest or back pain, hypoxemia, fever, nausea, seizures, or cardiac arrhythmias may occur. In addition, mechanical problems related to dialysis machines, cartridges, and water purifiers may occur.

Some of these problems have been lessened by the use of bicarbonate rather than acetate dialysis solutions, by longer dialysis periods with lower rates of ultrafiltration, with the use of synthetic polymer dialysis membranes that are more biocompatible, and perhaps by reuse of these membranes. Reuse brings the potential for problems as well as benefits; however, additional research will be necessary to define the optimum mix of membranes, reuse, solutions, and time and intensity of dialysis to ensure maximum safety and minimum complications of dialysis.

Psychosocial Concerns

Early predialysis assessment and continuous, active intervention by the renal team, including mental health professionals, in the care of a patient beginning dialysis are more likely to be effective than efforts initiated later in treatment. This assessment should include measures of quality of life and social role function in addition to lack of mental acuity and depression. Ensuring patients' understanding and positive participation in their care is a primary goal of this intervention in addition to optimizing the relationship between patient and physician and patient with staff. The earlier this assessment is accomplished the greater will be the potential for a positive impact on physical and social rehabilitation. Exercise and physical training can add to physical well-being and should also be initiated at the beginning of dialysis, or in the predialysis period.

What Are the Future Directions For Research in Dialysis?

- Studies should be conducted to evaluate the effect of aggressive nutritional support in malnourished predialysis patients, and to determine the mechanisms by which malnutrition increases mortality and morbidity rates, and to develop sensitive and specific methodology to detect the early stages of malnutrition.

- Studies should be instituted to determine the benefits and risks of early control of renal osteodystrophy on morbidity and to explore the causes and therapy of disturbances in calcium, phosphorus, and vitamin D, both at the basic level on regulation of bone metabolism and at the clinical level on the importance of soft tissue calcium deposition. Studies should include development of new phosphate-binding agents and noncalcemic analogues of vitamin D, and determination of the optimal degree of suppression of parathyroid hormone.

- Basic and clinical studies should be initiated to evaluate the effect of chronic uremia on neurologic function.

- Basic and clinical studies should be conducted to evaluate the effect of uremia on growth in children.

- Studies should be initiated to determine the impact of early treatment of anemia on mortality, morbidity, and rehabilitation. Studies to determine when to initiate treatment of anemia and what the target hematocrit should be are needed in both the predialysis and dialysis patient.

- A prospective, randomized, controlled clinical trial should be initiated to examine the differences in patient morbidity and mortality at to examine the differences in patient morbidity and mortality at $K_{dr}t/V$ levels of 1.2 (single pool) and 1.6 for hemodialysis patients.

- A prospective, randomized, controlled clinical trial should be initiated to examine the differences in patient morbidity and mortality at delivered weekly $K_{pr}t/V$ levels of 1.47 and 2.10 in peritoneal dialysis patients.

- A prospective, randomized, controlled clinical trial should be initiated to determine the differences in the effects of biocompatible, high-flux versus cellulosic membranes in studies which include, but are not limited to, patient survival, incidence of infection, and incidence and course of beta-2-microglobulin amyloidosis.

- Additional studies to establish the effect of reuse of dialysis membranes on hemodialysis effectiveness and morbidity and mortality are recommended.

- A prospective study of the feasibility and effectiveness of modification of cardiovascular risk factors in chronic renal failure patients both before and after initiation of dialysis should be undertaken. Risk factors to be evaluated would include hypertension (mechanism of development and regression of left ventricular hypertrophy and characterization of the best pharmacological approaches to antihypertensive treatment), smoking, obesity, and uremic dyslipidemia. The role of metabolic factors such as hyperinsulinemia and parathyroid hormone and calcium phosphorous relationships including tissue calcium burden in the myocardium and methods of its detection should be examined. Finally, development of noninvasive testing for coronary artery disease in this patient population should be explored.

- Studies to determine the mechanisms of interdialytic hypertension should be initiated and should include the respective roles of abnormal renin-angiotensin responses, abnormal thirst and salt craving, vascular endothelial factors (endothelin, nitric oxide production, and inhibitors), the renal-sympathetic axis, the relationship to erythropoietin administration, and the role for continuous blood pressure monitoring.

- Studies of the mechanisms by which malnutrition increases mortality and morbidity rates due to infections, anorexia, hypogusia, and related problems in the dialysis patient should be undertaken.

- Improved methods for detecting stenosis and thrombosis of access grafts and understanding the mechanism of endothelial proliferation leading to vascular graft stenosis are needed. Improved material and techniques should be developed to diminish access clotting and infection and new methods identified for cost-effective thrombolysis in clotted grafts.

- Study of the immunodeficiency of uremia and evaluation of antibacterial vaccines, antibiotic prophylaxis, and dialyzer membrane characteristics in the prevention of infection in dialysis patients should be initiated.

- Evaluating and standardizing methods for measurement of psychological well-being and quality of life in dialysis patients, and applying these instruments in studies on the effectiveness of interventions should be undertaken.

Conclusions

- Patients, including children, in the predialysis phase should be referred to a renal team consisting of a nephrologist, dietitian, nurse, social worker, and mental health professional in an effort to reduce the morbidity and mortality incurred during both the predialysis period and when receiving the subsequent dialysis therapy.

- The social and psychological welfare and the quality of life of the dialysis patient are favorably influenced by early predialytic and continued involvement of a multidisciplinary renal team.

- Attempts should be made through predialytic intervention and the appropriate initiation of dialysis access to avoid a catastrophic onset of dialysis.

- Quantitative methods to measure the delivered dose of hemodialysis and peritoneal dialysis have now been developed. These methods permit an objective evaluation of the relationship between the delivered dose of dialysis and patient morbidity and mortality. These methods suggest that the dose of hemodialysis and peritoneal dialysis has been suboptimal for many patients in the United States.

- Factors contributing to underdialysis of some patients include problems with vascular and peritoneal access, nonadherence to the dialysis prescription, and underprescription of the dialysis dose.

- Until prospective, randomized, controlled trials have been completed, a delivered hemodialysis dose at least equal to a measured $K_{dr}t/V$ of 1.2 (single pool) and a delivered peritoneal dialysis dose at least equal to a measured $K_{pr}t/V$ of 1.7 (weekly) are recommended.

- Cardiovascular mortality accounts for approximately 50 percent of deaths in dialysis patients. Relevant risk factors should be treated as soon as possible after diagnosis of chronic renal failure. These factors include hypertension, smoking, and chronic anemia.

- Patients with diabetes mellitus face especially severe cardiovascular risk, which contributes to reduced survival on dialysis.

- Malnutrition is another important co-morbid condition contributing to mortality. A serum albumin of less than 3.5 g/dL is clearly associated with increased relative risk. Early detection and treatment of malnutrition should substantially improve survival.

- Control of renal osteodystrophy requires patient adherence to the prescribed regimen and careful attention by the renal team to calcium and phosphorus intake and to the use of phosphate binders and calcitriol.

- Early creation of an A-V fistula is preferable to placement of a synthetic graft for vascular access. Both require an experienced, meticulous surgeon.

- Skilled management by nursing and other clinical personnel will help prolong the life of the vascular access.

- Attention to catheter design, placement, and care, and to exchange procedures can minimize infection in patients on peritoneal dialysis.

- Biocompatible dialysis membranes may reduce infection and amyloid deposition in hemodialysis patients, but evidence is inconclusive at present.

- Financial support to conduct clinical investigation, including outcomes and health services delivery research, should be incorporated into the budgets of the Medicare End-Stage Renal Disease program, Health Care Financing Administration, Agency for Health Care Policy Research, and the Food and Drug Administration. This support will enable the conduct of studies that promise to improve morbidity and mortality, enhance cost-effective care, and create long-term financial savings in the Medicare ESRD program.

Part Seven

General Information on Urinary Tract Disorders

Chapter 30

Twelve Facts You Should Know about Urologic Diseases

Kidney and urologic diseases are among the most widespread health problems in the United States. Kidney stones affect more than 1 million Americans annually, and urinary tract infections are one of the most frequent causes of work loss among women. Each year, hundreds of thousands of men undergo surgery for relief of benign prostatic enlargement. One of the major goals of The National Kidney Foundation's public education program is to increase public awareness about these diseases and how to prevent them. Here are some facts everyone should know.

1. Benign prostatic hyperplasia is a noncancerous enlargement of the prostate that occurs in almost all men as they age. An estimated 350,000 to 400,000 operations will be performed this year. for the relief of the symptoms of this disorder.

2. Benign prostatic hyperplasia is most often treated by surgical removal of the enlarged portion of the prostate gland. However, some newer, more limited procedures are being developed to treat benign prostatic hyperplasia. Certain drugs that may be capable of relieving the symptoms of this disorder also are being studied.

Excerpts from "Fifteen Facts You Should Know about Urologic Diseases," an Unnumbered pamphlet from the National Kidney Foundation. Used by permission.

357

3. More than 1 million cases of kidney stones occur annually in the United States. This disorder occurs primarily in young and middle-aged adults and is more common in men (four of five cases).

4. New, less invasive methods of treatment involving the use of shock waves and laser beams have reduced the days of hospitalization and home recuperation associated with kidney stones.

5. Treatment for prevention of kidney stone recurrences has also advanced. Laboratory tests are available to detect metabolic abnormalities in people who have recurrent stones, and, in many cases, treatments are available to correct the abnormal patterns.

6. Urinary tract infections are among the most common infections in the human body, second only to respiratory infections. They are responsible for about 8 million physician office visits annually at a cost of more than $4 billion.

7. Urinary tract infections often can be cleared up with antibiotics. However, many people, particularly women, seem to be susceptible to recurrent urinary tract infections.

8. Research into ways of preventing recurrent urinary tract infections has focused on both the characteristics of the bacteria that cause these infections and on abnormalities in the urinary tract of susceptible people. This new information may lead to the development of more effective treatments.

9. Another common urologic problem is urinary incontinence, which is the involuntary loss of urine. An estimated 10 million adult Americans have urinary incontinence.

10. Urinary incontinence is a symptom rather than a disease. It is frequently associated with obstructive diseases such as benign prostatic hyperplasia, with neurologic diseases such as multiple sclerosis, and with diabetes.

11. The use of absorbent pads to treat urinary incontinence is frequently not the only method of treatment available, and in many cases, may not be the most appropriate treatment.

12. Treatment for incontinence should be based on careful diagnosis of the underlying causes. It can sometimes be corrected with surgery or drugs. Techniques such as biofeedback, electrical stimulation, and exercises to strengthen the muscles involved also have proven helpful in some cases.

Knowledge about the normal and abnormal function of the urinary tract has increased significantly during the past decade. This knowledge will enable more effective methods of prevention and treatment to be developed for many urologic diseases. However, these answers can be found only through research. Each year the National Kidney Foundation provides more than $2 million for research into the causes, cure, and prevention of kidney and urologic diseases. In addition to research, other Foundation programs include: patient services, professional education, organ donation, and public information.

Chapter 31

Urinalysis:
Looking into the Void

One of the most familiar (if undignified) experiences during a visit to the doctor is that trip to the bathroom, cup in hand. Indeed, more than 36.7 million urinalyses were carried out in U.S. hospitals in 1988, making the urinalysis second only to the complete blood count as the most frequently performed group of tests.

The idea of examining urine for signs of disease is centuries old. When diabetes was suspected in a patient in ancient China, for instance, the physician would simply spill the urine sample on the ground, wait a while, and then check to see whether ants had gathered. Father of medicine Hippocrates also saw diagnostic value in watching bodily waters. He correctly observed that frothy urine is associated with kidney disease.

Today, urinalysis is more precise and systematic, thanks to increased knowledge of the body and such advances as the high-power microscope and chemical dipsticks. A single dipstick can be used to check for pH, sugar, protein, bilirubin (bile), ketones (waste products of the body's breakdown of fatty acids), and blood. The results are rapidly expressed as a color change. These tests and a visual inspection of the urine sample are easily done in the physician's office. A complete urinalysis, though, includes a weight comparison called urine specific gravity and a microscopic examination of small particles called urinary sediment. If the physician's office isn't set up to do these

FDA Consumer, October 1989.

tests, the sample can be sent to an outside laboratory. Ranges of normal vary with such factors as patient age and sex and the equipment used, so it should be kept in mind that the following "normals" are only examples.

Visual Inspection

Measurement: Evaluation of the appearance and odor of urine.
Normal range: Pale to dark yellow color, clear to slightly cloudy transparency, and a mild, faintly pungent odor.
Significance of results: Urine appearance and odor can vary for reasons as serious as kidney failure or as harmless as last night's dinner. Numerous medications, such as sulfa drugs, can affect urine color. Examples of other changes and their possible causes are:

- colorless—increased fluid intake or inability of the kidneys to concentrate minerals, salts, and other substances in urine (as occurs in diabetes insipidus);
- cloudy—alkalinity, pus or bacteria;
- opalescent—bacteria; fat due to kidney disease or a crushing injury, especially to the long bones;
- yellow-orange—excess urine concentration due to fever or to bilirubin buildup caused by liver or gallbladder disease;
- red—from eating foods such as beets or from blood in the urine due, for instance, to urinary tract injury or bladder cancer;
- pungent, grass-like odor—asparagus consumption;
- asparagus odor—kidney failure;
- sharp, medicine-like odor—multivitamins in the diet;
- pleasant, fruity odor—infection with *Pseudomonas* bacteria (also turns the urine blue-green), responsible for such diseases as meningitis, pneumonia, and a type of ear malady known as hotweather ear.

Urine Specific Gravity

Measurement: Concentration of urine.
Normal range: 1.003 to 1.030 specific gravity.
Comments: Urine specific gravity is a comparison of urine weight with the weight of an equal volume of distilled water. Specific gravity increases in proportion to increases in the concentration of minerals, salts, and other substances in urine. The resulting measurement reflects how well the kidneys concentrate and dilute urine.

Method: In one method, the operator sets afloat in the sample a small tubular device called a urinometer. Urine density determines the depth to which the device sinks, and a graduated measurement on the tube is read. The operator makes corrections for variables such as temperature and the presence of sugar or excess protein and then records the results. The devices can be inaccurate, however, so before their first use they must be checked using a solution with a known specific gravity.

The refractometer, another hand instrument, gives a more dependable test. Instead of measuring specific gravity, it measures what is known as the urine refractive index, a comparison of the velocity of light in urine to that in a vacuum. Like specific gravity, the refractive index increases in proportion to increases in the amount of dissolved substances in urine. For easy use by people unfamiliar with this measurement, the device is calibrated in terms of specific gravity. It requires only a few drops of urine, has a built-in temperature control, and provides a convenient, accurate and rapid test.

There also are automated specific gravity tests, including a dipstick test. These and the other dipstick tests can be performed on equipment connected to a computer to get a printout of the findings. Significance of results: High values can accompany reduced fluid intake, dehydrating conditions (such as fever and profuse sweating), ingestion of preservatives or X-ray contrast media, diabetes mellitus, shock, congestive heart failure, and certain tumors. Low values may be seen following use of diuretics and in exaggerated fluid intake, abnormally low body temperature, kidney disease, diabetes insipidus, and sickle cell anemia. Severe kidney damage causes urine specific gravity to remain fixed at 1.0010 to 1.0012.

Urinary pH

Measurement: Degree of acidity or alkalinity in urine.
Normal range: 5 to 7 pH units.
Comments: Kidney secretion of acidic or alkaline urine helps the body maintain its acid/alkaline balance. This status is measured as pH units, or "hydrogen ion" concentration. On a scale of 1 to 14, concentration values less than 7 indicate acidity, 7 is neutral, and higher values reflect alkalinity. The urinary pH is used to monitor the adequacy of certain treatments. The pH should be kept alkaline, for instance, during treatment of transfusion reactions and in streptomycin therapy.
Method: Dipstick.

Significance of results: Acid urine can be caused by starvation, a high-protein diet, metabolism of fat, drugs (such as ammonium chloride, sometimes used as an expectorant or diuretic), acid-producing bacteria, or an abnormal condition of decreased alkalinity in the blood and tissues (acidosis). Even sleep may cause acid urine. Alkaline urine may be due to factors such as a vegetarian diet, an abnormal condition of increased alkalinity in the blood and tissues (alkalosis), potassium deficiency, kidney disease, some bacterial infections, and certain drugs (such as antacids or chlorothiazide, a diuretic).

Substances Abnormal in Urine

Measurement: Detection of glucose (a type of sugar), protein, bilirubin, ketones, or blood in urine.

Normal range: Normal urine usually does not contain measurable levels of these substances.

Comments: Substances can appear in the urine for a number of reasons. Glucose, for instance, begins to spill into the urine when its level in blood exceeds the amount the kidneys can reabsorb (about 180 milligrams per deciliter of blood). Protein that escapes filtration by the kidneys will appear in urine, and urinary bilirubin occurs when the liver IS unable to excrete it into the small intestine. Ketones will show up in urine when excessive fatty acids increase ketones beyond what the liver can process (metabolize). Pink urine is an obvious sign of blood, but blood in urine cannot always be seen, because there must be at least 66,000 red blood cells per milliliter (RBC/mL) of urine before blood is visible to the human eye, even under a microscope. Fortunately, a dipstick test for blood in urine reacts to hemoglobin (the main component of red cells) at levels equal to as little as 10,000 RBC/mL of urine.

Method: Dipstick.

Significance of results: Urine tests for sugar may not detect the substance in older diabetics who have hardening of the arteries (arteriosclerosis) or in patients taking large amounts of ascorbic acid (vitamin C). Urine glucose is most commonly due to diabetes mellitus but can also occur with fever, severe emotional stress, kidney problems, during pregnancy, or after eating large amounts of carbohydrates.

Measurable amounts of protein found persistently in urine nearly always indicate kidney problems. Still, urine protein isn't always a sign of disease, not all disease-causing urine protein is persistent, and such problems as severe emotional stress or dehydration can cause protein to be in the urine. It's important therefore to have confirmative testing after a positive result.

Bilirubin in urine may be due to gallstones or other bile duct obstruction or to such liver conditions as hepatitis or cirrhosis. When a great amount of bilirubin is present, the urine changes color to dark amber or deep yellow orange and produces yellow foam when agitated.

Urinary ketones can be due to a high-fat diet, weight loss as the body taps its fat stores for energy, or inability of the body to properly process carbohydrates—as in diabetes mellitus. They also are seen in starvation, after anesthesia when nutritional intake is low but demands are high, and infrequently during pregnancy when the mother may go through a starvation of sorts due to a combination of vomiting, decreased food intake due to nausea, and stress of the baby's growth.

A number of conditions can cause hemolysis, red blood cell destruction with release of hemoglobin into surrounding fluid. When this is significant, blood may be present in the urine. Blood in urine has been associated with extreme exercise, ingestion of certain drugs (such as sulfonamides and phenacetin), urinary tract cancer or infection, kidney stones and other kidney disease, reaction to an incompatible blood transfusion, and pervasive infection (such as blackwater fever, which can occur after repeated bouts of malaria). Excessive ascorbic acid in urine, resulting from ingestion of large amounts of vitamin C, can cause a false negative test result.

Microscopic Examination

Measurement: Evaluation of urinary sediment substances that are visible within the field of a high-power microscope.

Normal range: 0 to 2 or 3 red blood cells, 4 to 5 white blood cells, and an occasional glassy-looking cast (described under "Significance of results").

Comments: This procedure can indicate or confirm kidney problems.

Method: A urine sample is spun in an instrument called a centrifuge, causing the sediment to fall to the bottom by centrifugal force. The liquid (called the supernatant) is poured off, and a drop of the sediment is viewed under a microscope.

Significance of results: Increased red blood cells reflect much the same conditions mentioned for blood under "Abnormal Substances in Urine." Conditions in which red cells can be seen with the microscope but may only occasionally be visible to the naked eye include: therapy with anticoagulant drugs, bleeding and clotting disorders such as purpura, blood component disorders such as sickle cell anemia, and collagen tissue disorders such as lupus erythematosus.

An increase in white blood cells—particularly ones called neutrophils—occurs with nearly any disease of the kidneys and urinary tract, but primarily with infection. Clumps of epithelial cells, which line the various tubes and organs of the body, are seen with deterioration of the kidney tubules, structures that participate in forming urine. In some kidney disease, other disorders (such as lupus), or poisoning (from such toxins as mercury), the epithelial cells may degrade to fatty droplets called "oval fat bodies."

Urinary casts are formed in a kidney tubule called a nephron by the gelling of protein from concentrated tubular fluid or by the clumping of cells in a matrix of protein. The gelled substance is "cast" in the shape of the tubule and excreted from the body.

Because urinary casts are formed in the kidney tubules, their presence in urine sediment can indicate kidney problems. Red blood cell casts identify the kidney as the source of bleeding, and white blood cell casts show the kidney is the source of infection. "Fatty" casts are a sign of damage to the kidney tubules. "Broad" casts, formed in the larger tubules where large ducts drain several small ones, can indicate potential kidney failure. "Hyaline" casts are translucent. If they persist and increase despite treatment, they also can suggest serious problems.

An unusually large number of crystals in the sediment may signal the actual or potential formation of kidney stones or (urinary) amino acid loss due to inherited metabolic disease.

Bacteria can indicate either urinary tract infection or specimen contamination.

Specimen Collection

In urinalysis, the specimen can be collected at random (any time of day), from the more concentrated first voiding of the morning, or from a "second-voided" (double-voided) specimen. For the latter, the patient empties the bladder 30 to 60 minutes before the test specimen is due. This method is preferred in glucose testing of diabetics. Specimens taken at timed intervals (2, 12, or 24 hours) are considered most accurate and are therefore used to confirm a finding of glucose.

Regardless of collection time, a "clean-catch midstream" may be requested. To do this, the patient first swabs around the genital area antiseptic towelettes and dries with toilet tissue. Then urination is begun into the toilet bowl, a few ounces are "caught" midstream into the specimen cup, and urination is completed into the toilet bowl.

To help prevent skewed results, patients should:

- Report any medication being taken.
- Follow carefully any special directions about timing the sample collection.
- Don't allow the rim or lid of the specimen container to touch the genital area.
- Store the sample covered in a clean, dry, glass or plastic container. Refrigerate the sample if it will be stored for an hour or more, though it should be allowed to come to room temperature for testing.

— by Dixie Farley

Chapter 32

A Practical Workup for Hematuria

Whether gross or microscopic, hematuria must always be taken seriously. It may signal cancer, but not all discoloration is blood. This concise workup plan focuses on what the findings mean.

Any patient who has hematuria, gross or microscopic, deserves immediate and careful evaluation. Whether or not pain is involved, any degree of hematuria requires attention until you have completely ruled out disease. With a few patients, you may be able to stop the workup after basic screening tests, but for patients older than 40, who may well have a bladder tumor or other malignancy of the urinary tract, consider more sophisticated tests or consultation with a urologist.

If pain accompanies gross hematuria, examine the stained urine sediment for signs of infection. In a young woman, rule out acute hemorrhagic cystitis; in a young man, acute prostatitis or cystitis.

If a young person comes in with gross hematuria after extremely vigorous exercise, do basic screening and wait 24 hours after onset. If the urine is clear, grossly and microscopically, and nothing suspicious turns up in the screening, it is probably safe to do no further workup.

When a patient reports gross hematuria, you may want to take a freshly voided urine sample for cytologic testing. The result will probably not be positive for cancer too often, but it may identify the occasional young athlete whose overexertion or trauma disrupts the

Patient Care, Vol. 24, No. 3, February 1990. Copyright Medical Economics. Reprinted with permission of Patient Care.

integrity of a tumor. Many physicians feel that cytology at this stage is not cost effective in general. Those who favor cytologic testing under this circumstance, however, believe that the benefit of finding even one tumor that is causing bleeding far exceeds the cumulative costs of this type of testing.

Advise the patient that a second occurrence will be cause for a full investigation. A child who plays hard may have this kind of hematuria without serious consequences. But if hematuria recurs or persists beyond 24 hours, a thorough urologic workup is virtually mandatory to rule out malignancy or congenital abnormalities. Most younger patients will require only basic tests including an intravenous pyelogram (IVP) or cytoscopy, while patients older than 40 may require more extensive tests including urine for cytology or renal computed tomography scans to rule out possible bladder tumor or other malignancy.

The patient older than 40 who reports painless hematuria but passes no blood in the urine during the office visit should undergo IVP. If the patient passes cloudy or smoky urine, he may have a large stone in the renal pelvis.

It may be helpful to learn just where blood enters the urine. To determine whether hematuria is initial, total, or terminal—that is, whether it occurs at the start of urination, throughout, or only at the end—do the simple three-glass test, with a sample taken at the start, middle, and end of urination. The findings of the three-glass test are not diagnostic in themselves, but they may give you a head start toward pinning down the cause of hematuria.

Initial hematuria suggests a lesion in the penis or urethra. Inflammation, a foreign body, or carcinoma in the urethra is a possible cause. If all three samples show blood, all the urine in the bladder is affected so the lesion is probably in the bladder or higher. Possible causes run the gamut from bleeding in the bladder to bleeding in the kidneys. Carcinoma, urinary stones, and infection are likely culprits, depending on patient age. If only the final sample contains blood, consider bladder carcinoma and acute inflammation of the posterior urethra; in men consider as well bleeding in the prostatic urethra.

Occasionally you will discover hematuria in a patient who is being examined following trauma. Make sure the workup for hematuria remains independent of the trauma investigation because there may be no correlation with the accident.

Likewise, if you stop at infection when you are trying to find the cause of hematuria, you may miss a more serious condition. Resolving the question of etiology, however slight or microscopic the uria may be, is necessary for determining the correct treatment.

Infection may be only one of the causes of hematuria, so a thorough workup to determine the exact cause is essential.

Often, patients referred to urologists after months of failed anti-microbial treatments for urinary tract infection (UTI) turn out to have a cancer that appropriate attention could have detected earlier. There is a tendency to prescribe antibiotics for a woman with symptoms of cystitis and hematuria without performing a culture. The omission may be a costly one. Although bacterial cystitis may cause hematuria, do not rule out one of the irritative forms of bladder cancer, such as an in situ or squamous cell carcinoma, until the culture confirms the cause as infection.

Cultures, which are inexpensive and can be done in any physician's office, can save a lot of time and prevent delay in recognizing cancer. If you choose not to do your own cultures, another option is to examine the spun sediment of the urine under a microscope, noting the presence or absence of any bacteria. Dipstick kits are also available; simply dip the commercially prepared slide in the urine sample, incubate it overnight, and read it the next day (see "Dipstick assessment of hematuria").

The causes of hematuria vary somewhat in frequency according to age, so take the history and conduct the physical examination with the patient's age in mind. In children and adolescents, acute glomerulonephritis is the most likely cause of hematuria, followed by acute UTI, congenital abnormalities overexertion, and sports injuries or other trauma. In your physical examination, make a thorough check for hypertension and edema. Check the urine for RBCs, red cell casts and proteinuria, and evaluate serum creatinine and BUN. If the bleeding is coming from the kidneys and is glomerular in origin (as with one of the forms of glomerulonephritis) the patient's RBCs will usually be dysmorphic.

If your patient is in the 20–40 age range, the most likely cause of hematuria is acute UTI regardless of gender. Urinary stones are the second most likely cause, followed by trauma—not just severe injury, but also minor accidents at work or play that may go unnoticed. A less likely cause, but one you must rule out, is cancer of the bladder or, more unlikely still, cancer of the kidney. After age 40, gender seems to alter the frequency pattern of hematuria. In 40–60 year-old women, acute UTI remains the most likely cause, with uxinary stones and cancer of the bladder or kidney following. In men of this age group, bladder cancer is first, urinary stones second, UTI third, and renal carcinoma a distant fourth. At about age 60, benign prostatic hypertrophy becomes the leading cause of hematuria in men, with cancer of the bladder and acute UTI following. In women after age 60, bladder cancer becomes the leading cause, ahead of acute UTI.

For the patient of any age, consider less common causes such as anticoagulant therapy, diseases particular to ethnic groups (sickle cell disease in blacks, for example), and lesions or inflammation in the lower urinary tract. What the patient reports as blood in the urine may not be blood at all, but false hematuria. Certain foods and drugs—beets and laxatives containing phenolphthalein, for example—color the urine enough to frighten patients not familiar with this phenomenon. A high level of urates in the urine may give it a decidedly pink tinge that many patients will mistake for blood.

Remember, however, that urine stained by food or other agents may also contain blood; the patient may be coming to see you because the urine has a redder tinge than usual, for example. Other unusual causes for hematuria include Goodpasture's syndrome and Schonlein-Henoch purpura. Goodpasture's syndrome occurs mainly in young men recovering from upper respiratory infection; there is evidence of hemoptysis and anemia, with progressive renal disease and worsening azotemia, hematuria, proteinuria, and hypertension. Schonlein-Henoch purpura is a rare pediatric condition and is manifested by arthropathy, erythema, GI upset, and urticaria. Schistosomiasis is a common parasitic cause of hematuria in immigrants from areas where the parasite is endemic. Travelers to these areas are also likely candidates for this type of hematuria.

When either unexplained gross or microscopic hematuria persists or recurs, go directly to the IVP; if no cause is found, do cytologic testing if you have not already done it. Cytology, a noninvasive, simple, and cost-effective approach, when coupled with an IVP provides a very effective screening tool. And whereas cystoscopy only lends itself to evaluation of the bladder, bleeding frequently occurs in the upper urinary tract. Many urologists feel that a patient with frequent microscopic hematuria would benefit more from an initial evaluation by cytology than by cystoscopy. Then if cytology results are normal but you still suspect something serious, consider cystoscopy, which many urologists consider a necessary immediate step. Urine flow cytometry may be helpful when you suspect urothelial cancers.

If hematuria persists, you can be virtually certain that the underlying cause is significant. When hematuria warrants IVP, the procedure is a little different from the standard IVP for calculi. Tomograms ᶜthe kidney are necessary to make sure the entire collecting system ⁿᵉd out; otherwise, a patient's small cortical lesions might not be ⁿ. An area with such lesions may look perfectly normal on a five-minute film, yet the lesions are easily demonstrated with tomography. Oblique films help define the upper collecting systems and ureters. Renal ultrasonography is indicated when the renal outlines and collecting systems are not clearly seen on the IVP. For the patient who is allergic to contrast media (iodine sensitivity), order a plain kidney-ureter-bladder study and a sonogram.

A continuing trace of blood in the urine may be due to a low-grade glomerular disease or, in certain women, to urethrotrigonitis. The former may need a kidney biopsy, and the latter cystoscopy, if not already done. Although this is largely a matter of clinical judgment, a reasonable recommendation is that certain patients with hematuria of known origin, such as sickle cell disease or thalassemia, do not require extensive evaluation every time they experience gross hematuria.

Hemospermia is frightening enough to bring most men to a physician's office. There may be no significant underlying cause, although it is sometimes associated with acute prostatitis or inflammation in the prostatic urethra.

In addition, hemospermia may be associated with irritation or, rarely, with seminal vesiculitis, in which case chlamydial infection is a possible cause. Doxycycline hyclate (Doryx, Vibramycin, Vibra-Tabs, etc.), 100 mg bid, is appropriate empiric therapy.

Many patients with hemospermia report having had a recent vasectomy. The cause of hemospermia is less likely to be related to vasectomy itself than to increased sexual activity following the procedure. The first step in evaluation is to ensure that there is no hematuria accompanying the hemospermia. Then do a prostate massage and examine the fluid. If the patient does not have prostatitis, reassure him that occasional bloody ejaculate is no cause for concern and that it may simply reflect rigorous sexual activity.

Nor is it unusual for an elderly man to report bloody ejaculate after weeks or months of abstinence. In the absence of infection or hematuria, reassurance is probably all the patient needs. Many older men, too, may need your frank advice on preventing recurrence, by masturbation if necessary.

Chapter Highlights

Investigating hematuria, first steps: Any degree of hematuria requires attention until serious disease can be ruled out. If the patient has pain as well, examine the stained urine sediment for signs of infection. Hematuria lasting 24 hours or less in an athlete is probably not serious, but if it persists or recurs in a patient of any age, do a thorough workup. Order an intravenous pyelogram (IVP) in the patient older than 40 who has had painless hematuria but no longer has obviously bloody urine.

Investigating hematuria, advanced steps: Unusual causes of hematuria include Goodpasture's syndrome, endemic hematuria, and Schonlein-Henoch purpura. False hematuria is possible but uncommon. When hematuria persists or recurs and the cause remains unknown after IVP and cytologic testing, cystoscopy is indicated. Insist on tomography and oblique films when IVP is ordered; tomography may reveal lesions not apparent on IVP films. Low-grade glomerular disease or urethrotrigonitis may cause a continuing trace of hematuria.

Hemospermia: Often there is no significant underlying cause of hemospermia, but think of seminal vesiculitis or other infection. Harmless hemospermia may follow rigorous sexual activity. Hemospermia after vasectomy is more apt to be due to sudden increased sexual activity than to the procedure. Long abstinence may cause hemospermia in elderly men; masturbation or increased sexual activity may prevent recurrence.

Dipstick Assessment of Hematuria

Bladder cancer is the fifth in cancer in males and tenth most common in women. Acting on evidence that a patient has microscopic hematuria increases the likelihood of detecting and effectively treating urologic malignancy at an early stage. Urine dipsticks, commonly used in health screening clinics, occupational health departments, and in office practice, provide an accurate method of detecting red cells in urine. The results of a recent British study support the view that the urine dipstick is a convenient and cost-effective way to detect microscopic hematuria when screening a large population. In fact, the British investigators support the clinical impression that dipstick hematuria is a common incidental finding in men older than 60 and emphasize that it is associated with appreciable urologic disease.

In a study undertaken at St. James University Hospital in Leeds, 855 elderly men, aged 60–85, were invited to attend a health center for urine screening as part of a health-check. Of the 855 men, 578 agreed to have their urine tested with a dipstick (Multistix) for the presence of blood initially and then once a week for the next ten weeks. over 10% of the men had dipstick hematuria initially and subdipstick monitoring was positive in another 9% at some time during the follow-up period. Evaluation of hematuria, which in many patients was done by flexible cystoscopy and ultrasonography, revealed no correlation between the degree of hematuria and the severity of the underlying cause. Of the men with positive screening results, 45 had significant urologic disease (including four who had bladder tumor, seven with epithelial dysplasia, and one with a prostate tumor), but no urologic malignancies were discovered in those men found to have hematuria only after the initial test.

When examining urine slides for hematuria, how many RBCs per field are cause for concern? There is no set answer to this question. Most physicians designate a range between 0-4 RBCs per high power field as an acceptable standard, regardless of the patient's sex. Evidence of microscopic hematuria requires an initial workup, but the vast majority of patients will have no major problem. And although the likelihood of malignancy is slightly higher for an elderly patient, chances are still good that there is nothing seriously wrong.

— by Harold A. Fuselier, Jr.,
Stephen N. Rous, MD,
Jerry W. Sullivan, MD.

Part Eight

Children and Urinary Tract Disorders

Chapter 33

Enuresis

Chapter Contents

Section 33.1

Childhood Bed-wetting: Cause for Concern?

FDA Consumer, May 1989.

During grade school, Patsy (not her real name) never asked friends to spend the night. When invited to birthday party "sleep-overs," she declined. She worried about the possible lingering odor in her room. And she hated the plastic sheet that accompanied family vacations. Then, shortly after entering middle school, Patsy no longer had her "problem" bed-wetting.

Fourteen percent of 5- to 13-year-olds wet the bed, according to a recent population study. For many such children, like Patsy, the consequences are humiliation and damaged self-esteem. Fortunately, this common childhood affliction, known medically as "primary enuresis" usually disappears on its own, and proper treatment can often hurry it on its way.

Bed-wetting is considered normal up to age 5. When the problem persists, however, a visit to the doctor is in order. Bed-wetting rarely signals a health problem, but daytime wetting—which often occurs with bed-wetting yet may be overlooked if it's only a dribble—can represent serious illness. Indeed, if the wetting disorders known as dysfunctional voiding go untreated, kidney failure—even death—can result.

Delayed Development and Other Causes

The precise cause of bed-wetting is unknown. Most cases appear to be due to delayed physical development. Bladder capacity may be less than half what is considered normal for the child's age. Bed-wetting is up to three times more common in boys than girls—linked, perhaps, to boys' slower rate of maturation. Some researchers, in fact, argued that boys aren't normally dry at night until age 8.

al studies point to a genetic link in enuresis. When both par- problem as youngsters, 77 percent of the children in these studies developed it. But the figure dropped to 44 percent when only one parent had wet the bed in childhood. By contrast, when neither parent had enuresis, only 15 percent of the children did.

✗ A frequent cause of bed-wetting is constipation. In fact, treatment of constipation in enuretic children often resolves the wetting, report Sean O'Regan, M.D., and others of the Pediatric Research Center, University of Montreal. In the March 1986 *American Journal of Diseases of Children*, they explained that, in chronically constipated children, the rectum is probably never empty so the rectal sphincter muscle remains contracted to hold back stool. This, in turn, can dilate the rectum, which then presses on the small, immature bladder to cause the enuresis.

Attempts to hurry toilet training may backfire and actually contribute to bed-wetting; experts advise letting a child develop bladder control at his or her own pace. Other contributing factors include hospitalization (especially between ages 2 and 4), arrival of a baby, loss of a parent, and entering school.

In rare cases, emotionally disturbed children may respond to their illness with loss of bladder and bowel control according to Gordon McLorie, M.D., and D.A. Husmann, M.D., of Toronto's Hospital for Sick Children, in the October 1987 *Pediatric Clinics of North America*. But in other cases, they wrote, "emotional disturbances may be primarily a result of the enuresis."

Diaries and Other Diagnostic Tools

Diagnosis at the Center to Assist the Regulation of Enuresis (C.A.R.E.) in Chicago involves use of a diary. Before the first appointment, parents complete a psychological questionnaire and keep a three-day record on their child's diet and wetting pattern (times, duration and volume of daytime urination and times of bed-wetting. The record may suggest a wetting pattern abnormality, recurring urinary tract infection, or unrecognized constipation.

"I do not believe that all children with these complaints merit a full scale urodynamic evaluation," wrote C.A.R.E. director Max Maizels in the April 1982 *Journal of Urology*. (Urodynamic tests use electrodes and flexible thin tubes called catheters to gain information about urinary tract flows, muscle movement and pressure changes.) A "hands off" approach is how Maizels describes C.A.R.E.'s diagnosis and treatment. "I have been content with eliciting a detailed history, performing a physical examination of the genitalia, and observing the voided stream to guide the need for . . . urodynamic evaluation."

What can a patient's history reveal? Compared with youngsters with normal bladder control, bed-wetting children are more likely to have experienced problems while still in the womb, such as maternal illness or bleeding or, after birth, colic or jaundice (skin yellowing from bile pigment buildup in the blood), according to Maizels. "Perhaps these . . . are stresses that later lead to the 'maturational delay' believed responsible for primary enuresis," Maizels and Diane Rosenbaum wrote in the December 1985 *Primary Care*.

A thorough physical examination includes inspecting the rectum for impacted stool, checking the gait and reflexes of the legs and feet for nerve defects, and gently feeling the abdomen, genitals, buttocks, anus and spine for abnormalities. Observing the child's urination is important because different problems may be reflected by the nature of the stream, which may be weak, unusually forceful, intermittent, continuous, spraying, or painful. Intermittent flow, for instance, suggests obstruction.

Flow-rate measurements show how many ounces or milliliters of urine are passed in how many seconds. Ultrasound examination (a painless procedure, made by applying sound waves to the skin) may be needed to check the size and shape of the kidneys and to see how well the bladder empties. Laboratory analysis of urine screens for diabetes, kidney disease, or other disorders.

Among the candidates for further examination with more complicated tests are patients for whom conventional treatment has failed and those with recurrent urinary infection, wetting day and night without an obvious cause, coexisting loss of bowel control, and suspected dysfunctional voiding. Parents should ask questions to be sure the understand why a particular test is recommended and what is involved.

To Treat or Not

But if the diagnosis is that the nighttime wetting is simply due to an immature bladder, the examination will probably end there. Physician and parent can move on to discussions about treatment. It's reasonable to consider doing no more than being patient and supportive until the child is older. Still, for families facing great stress over the problem and for children feeling shame and low self-worth, there are potentially effective therapies. The choice of therapy and effectiveness of individual treatment depend on the severity of the problem, the child's age and emotional maturity, and the level of commitment of the child and parent. Certainly, scolding and punishment are ineffective and inappropriate.

Behavior Modification

For behavior modification to be effective, child and parents must be highly motivated to follow the physician's instructions exactly and to persist long enough, which may mean several months. It's very easy to become lax or give up. Rewards alone—no punishments—are used. Among the techniques:

Responsibility reinforcement training. The child takes charge of making one last trip to the bathroom, changing and laundering soiled bed linens, and charting progress (dry nights earn rewards). These responsibilities should help improve the child's feelings of self-worth and prevent parental anger over a wet bed. Hints from the Mayo Clinic: Use a plastic mattress pad and pillowcases, and buy lots of inexpensive sheets and blankets for storage in a tightly sealed plastic bag for weekly washing.

Urinary alarm. Wetting sets off the battery-powered alarm: the child wakens, turns off the switch, and finishes urinating in the bathroom. Eventually, the child is supposed to learn to wake before wetting. Lightweight pajamas are best because thick ones slow down the time between the first drops of urine and the sounding of the alarm. It's a good idea to replace batteries at set intervals because weakened ones may not trigger the alarm and may damage the device. The success rate with the alarm is as high as 75 percent, but the relapse rate can be as high as 30 percent. Maizels says that, by combining the alarm with other therapies, he and his colleagues can correct about 80 percent of wetting within the first month or two, with a relapse rate of only around 13 percent.

Another treatment often reported involves retaining urine to enlarge bladder capacity. But Terry Allen, M.D., urology professor at Southwestern Medical School in Dallas, says "this is bad policy because it puts undue pressure on the urinary tract."

Drugs Have Drawbacks

The Food and Drug Administration has approved one drug as safe and effective for bed-wetting: imipramine (Tofranil), an antidepressant. It can immediately produce dry nights, but there are drawbacks.

It can cause a number of side effects, including blood pressure changes, irregular heartbeat, anxiety, insomnia, dry mouth, blurred vision, nausea, vomiting, diarrhea, dizziness, drowsiness, and headache. Bed-wetting often resumes when treatment stops. And, while the drug is safe at recommended dosages, an overdose can cause convulsions, coma and death. "One third of the physicians who use the drug do not recognize its toxic potential," wrote Betsy Foxman of the University of Michigan School of Public Health, Ann Arbor, and others in the April 1986 *Pediatrics*. The researchers were commenting on the results of the Rand Health Insurance Experiment, a population study. "We suggest that physicians explore less hazardous alternatives before relying on pharmacologic (drug) treatment for this generally benign condition," they concluded. The April 1987 *Mayo Clinic Health Letter* advised: "We rarely recommend this drug for children with enuresis."

If the decision is nevertheless made to use imipramine, parents should take extreme care to give it exactly as prescribed, to keep it in a locked cabinet out of reach of children, and to seek immediate medical help in case of overdose. Any substance potentially poisonous to a child should be labeled with warning stickers, such as "Mr. Yuk." These are available from regional poison control centers (not emergency rooms), listed with emergency numbers at the front of the telephone directory.

Physicians are investigating enuresis treatment with oxybutynin chloride (Ditropan). The drug is approved by FDA for certain nerve-related bladder disorders, but its safety and effectiveness for bed-wetting remain unproven.

Counseling and Other Treatments

Some physicians may recommend psychological counseling or hypnosis. In the C.A.R.E. program, fluids are not restricted at bedtime, but patients are advised to drink nectars, apple juice, cranberry juice, and water rather than carbonated drinks. "As these beverages may be less interesting," says Maizels, "children tend to drink more for thirst than for recreation."

Dealing with bed-wetting can be frustrating, even traumatic. It might help to keep in mind that nearly every child will outgrow the problem.

— by Dixie Farley

Section 33.2

Approaching Enuresis in an Uncomplicated Way

Contemporary Urology, Vol. 3, No. 2, February 1991.
Copyright Medical Economics.
Reprinted with permission of Contemporary Urology.

Because enuresis is self-correcting and, in general, harmless, some physicians try to ignore it. They reassure parents that the child will outgrow the bedwetting problem. On the other hand, some physicians, concerned that they might miss a significant urologic problem, subject every enuretic child to an extensive urologic evaluation.

Neither of these approaches is appropriate. The facts are that the term enuresis does not define a homogeneous condition and that it may be the only symptom of a significant urologic abnormality.

At our hospital, we find we can determine the need for additional testing and identify treatment that will work in a particular patient by using a simple office evaluation strategy.[1] That plan is described here.

How Big a Problem?

Most children achieve bladder control and are free of diapers by the time they reach the age of 3 or 4 years. After that age, children who repeatedly and involuntarily pass urine are said to have enuresis. In primary enuresis, the child has never been dry since birth; in secondary enuresis, the child has been continuously dry for at least 6 to 12 months. Overall, enuresis is more common in boys than in girls. The spontaneous annual cure rate for primary enuresis is approximately 15% to 20%.[2] So while as many as 20% of 5-year-old children wet their bed, fewer than 1% of youths are still enuretic at the age of 18 years.[3,4]

Evaluation in the Office

The workup comprises the history, physical examination, and imaging study. The pattern of enuresis determined by the initial office evaluation divides enuretic children into three subgroups and guides therapy.

History. This is the most important aspect of office evaluation. Carefully delineate the pattern of micturition (frequency, presence of urgent urination, adequacy of the urinary stream, and so forth). Characterize the enuresis: day only, night only, both; frequency; and duration of the dry interval.

Ask if the child has had any other urologic problems, such as painful urination, straining to void, urinary tract infection, hematuria, or if the family history includes enuresis. Likewise, look for other significant medical problems, such as constipation, fecal soiling, behavioral disturbance, neurologic or orthopedic abnormality, and diabetes.

Physical examination. The purpose of the exam is to detect a physical abnormality that might explain the enuresis. This includes distended bladder; hydronephrotic kidney; bifid clitoris; muscular atrophy of the trunk, buttocks, or lower extremities; club foot; and spinal abnormality. The history often signals the potential for such deformities.

When a child has a disturbance of his urinary stream or strains to void, it may help to watch him void. When he is incontinent day and night, evaluate perineal sensation, peripheral reflexes, buttock musculature, and sacral region. Observe his gait. Perform a complete urinalysis and culture the urine, including a colony count.

Imaging. Ultrasonography (US) has become the preeminent pediatric urologic imaging modality because it is noninvasive, painless, does not expose the child to radiation, and produces excellent images. Because US examination is without risk, it can be used routinely in all children who have enuresis to reassure parent and physician. On the other hand, some selectivity is reasonable, in that as many as 20% of children are enuretic and the great majority of them do not have a urologic abnormality.

All children who have urinary tract infection require imaging, however. If enuresis persists after infection is treated and cured, they can be placed into the appropriate subgroup for treatment.

Distinguishing patterns of enuresis yields, as noted, three subgroups. Each, in turn, has its own indications for further imaging study and treatment.

Sleep Enuresis

Children who wet only when asleep, void normally during the day, and are normal on physical examination constitute the largest subgroup. They may have mild symptoms of urgency during the day, particularly after several hours without voiding, but they do not void with undue frequency or have significant enuresis when awake.

Sleep enuresis is more common in boys than in girls. Typically, urinary tract imaging does not reveal any abnormality and bladder capacity and function are normal. UTI is uncommon.

Based on our, and others', experience,[5,6] we do not recommend imaging study for children who have sleep enuresis. Exceptions are a history of UTI and significant voiding symptoms. Consider the findings of a review of 300 consecutive children (192 boys and 108 girls) aged 5 to 18 years old who had sleep enuresis and were evaluated at our institution.

For this study, routine evaluation included US. Voiding cystourethrogram (VCUG) was performed only when UTI had been documented. US was normal in 253 of 268 children (32 refused study). Clinically insignificant abnormalities were observed in 9 children (caliectasis or ureterectasis, or both, without reflux or obstruction in 5; ectopic or solitary kidney in 2; minor renal parenchymal abnormalities in 2). Significant anatomic abnormalities were found in only 4 children (ureteropelvic junction obstruction in 1; caliectasis secondary to vesicoureteral reflux in 2; a gallstone in 1).

Urgency Syndrome

These children, in addition to wetting at night, have significant daytime symptoms of urgency, frequency, and urge incontinence. They do not have UTI. Often, children do not feel the need to void one minute, then are overwhelmed by a severe urge to void the next—and either wet on their way to the bathroom or squat on their heels trying to prevent urine leakage. Some even wet without knowing it.

Children in this subgroup always have a dry interval of at least 30 to 60 minutes, even though parents often report that the child leaks urine continuously. Physical examination does not demonstrate spinal deformities or orthopedic or neurologic abnormalities.

We recommend routine renal and bladder US for children who have urgency syndrome. Again, reserve VCUG for those who have UTI, fecal soiling, or orthopedic problems, or for when any of the abnormalities mentioned in the following paragraphs are detected during the physical examination or screening US. This recommendation is based in part on the findings of a study at our hospital of 143 children (105 girls and 38 boys) who had urgency syndrome (made at the time the 300 children who had sleep enuresis were evaluated).

In this study, abdominal US was recommended for all children, but VCUG was routine only when the history included UTI. None of the children had evidence of neurologic disease. In 82 (74 girls, 8 boys), UTI was documented.

Anatomic abnormalities were common in this group. They included vesicoureteral reflux found on VCUG (30 patients), a thickened, trabeculated bladder (15), and hydronephrosis (10). In six children, the bladder deformity was significant enough to suggest a neuropathy and justify urodynamic studies, myelography, and magnetic resonance imaging. Overall, however, whenever neurologic examination and lumbosacral spine films were normal, neurologic abnormality was not found.

Structural Abnormality

Management of this kind of problem is beyond the scope of this article. Note, however, that when 16 children who were evaluated for a complaint of enuresis at our hospital were found to have a structural abnormality, it was the office evaluation that raised initial concern about a structural lesion and guided the choice of testing.

The 16 were seen during the time the other two groups were. In each, a significant anatomic abnormality was discovered. Six had an ectopic ureter; five, an unsuspected deformity of the sacrum; three, posterior urethral valves; and two (girls), epispadias.

Continuous urinary dribbling with a normal voiding pattern was characteristic of all six children who had an ectopic ureter. The ectopic ureter was associated with the upper pole of a duplex collecting system and was easily demonstrated on the renal US. Physical examination was normal and the history did not include UTI.

The five children who had a sacral abnormality had daytime and nocturnal enuresis and a history of UTI, fecal soiling, orthopedic deformity, or gait problem, or an abnormality detected on physical examination. Neurologic abnormality was suspected in all cases before any imaging study; VCUG and renal US were confirmatory.

The three boys in whom urethral valves were found had daytime and nocturnal enuresis; in two, it was more common during the day. In all three, US demonstrated degrees of hydroureteronephrosis and thickening of bladder muscle. The VCUG was diagnostic.

The two girls who had epispadias reported continuous daytime and nocturnal urinary incontinence and did not have a normal voiding pattern. They had normal bowel control and did not have UTI. Physical examination was normal, except for a bifid clitoris in one. Both leaked urine obviously in response to suprapubic pressure. Imaging study was normal. Cystoscopy demonstrated a markedly patulous and foreshortened urethra.

What causes Enuresis?

Many theories[7,8] have tried to account for enuresis that occurs in the absence of an anatomic abnormality: improper toilet training, deep sleep pattern, sleep disorder, emotional disturbance, small bladder capacity, occult urethral obstruction, developmental delay, and excessive nocturnal urine production, among others. No one is generally accepted, but several observations about characteristics of enuretics are important.

Most parents report that their enuretic child is a very deep sleeper; no evidence suggests, however, that enuretic children are more difficult to awaken than nonenuretic children. Enuresis occurs in all stages of non-rapid-eye-movement sleep,[9] and the potential for an episode is not a function of the specific stage of sleep but the time spent in that stage.[10]

Keep in mind that most normal children do not awaken at night to void. The problem with an enuretic child, therefore, is not that he fails to respond to a bladder stimulus by getting up to void, but that his bladder empties inappropriately when he is asleep. Indeed, it is just as abnormal for a child to arise regularly from sleep to void as it is for him to wet the bed. Furthermore, psychological factors are more often secondary to, and not the cause of, enuresis.[11]

A reasonable theory is that enuresis reflects a maturational delay[12] in an otherwise normal child. At birth, bladder emptying is a simple reflex mediated through sacral segments 2, 3, and 4, uninhibited by the higher centers. When the time comes for the child to be toilet trained, he must learn several new skills (sphincter control, appreciation of bladder fullness and the continuous inhibition of reflex bladder contractions) to perform a complex neurologic event.

The facility with which a child can master these skills depends upon the quality of the training, his willingness to learn, and his physiologic readiness. As with all learning, the ability to accomplish this task comes at different ages. Genetics plays an important role, too; the risk of enuresis is related to how many of the child's blood relatives are, or were, enuretic, and how closely related they are.[13]

Another theory has emerged from the finding that the release of vasopressin normally increases during sleep. This hormone, by enhancing resorption of water in the distal tubule, progressively decreases urine volume during the night.[14] We know that some children do not release vasopressin in normal amounts; the hypothesis, therefore, is that overnight production of urine increases, the volume of urine eventually exceeds the child's functional bladder capacity, and he wets the bed.

Who should be Treated?

Enuresis does not cause longterm physical problems, but it can be a source of significant emotional disturbance for the child and his family. He can feel ashamed, guilty, frustrated, and that he is a failure. Self-esteem can deteriorate. His parents may see enuresis as a hostile gesture or as their failure to be good parents.[15] Typically, child and parents try to keep the bedwetting a secret, rather than risk humiliation each by their peers.

A simple comment from the physician—about the high incidence of bedwetting, its involuntary nature, or the potential for spontaneous cure—is helpful. It may, in fact, be all that the family needs to cope.

Certainly, successful treatment of enuresis improves some children's self-image,[16] but this does not justify universal treatment. Furthermore, the decision to treat—or not to treat—should be made by family, patient, and physician jointly: How often the child wets, how old he is, whether he wets during the day, and the effect of the condition on him are important questions to answer first.

In general, a 5-year-old child has significantly less of a need to be treated than a 12-year-old; a child who wets only at night, less than one who wets day and night; and a child who wets a few times a month, less than one who wets daily. I recommend treatment for most children who wet frequently during the day, but, in general, those who have sleep enuresis only do not need to be treated before 8 years of age unless they have a secondary emotional problem. Of the 300 children who had sleep enuresis in the series at our hospital, for example, 157 were treated.

Choices for Treatment

Over the years, a confusing array of treatments for enuresis have been proposed.[17,18] They include bladder retention training exercises, motivational therapy, conditioning devices, psychotherapy, hypnotherapy, drugs, manipulation of diet, fluid restriction, and lifting and awakening.

Treatments can be divided into two basic categories: behavioral and pharmacologic. Purported success of any treatment must be viewed cautiously because the placebo effect is at least 15% to 20% annually as these children grow up.

Behavioral Approaches

The success of behavioral modification techniques is difficult to evaluate. Because a true control group is impossible, success in treated patients is usually compared with the spontaneous resolution rate of an age-matched group—who receive none of the attention paid the treatment group.

Because behavioral techniques are very labor intensive, the treatment group is to a certain extent self-selected by the patient and family's willingness to participate. At least part of the success of the these programs, therefore, has to be attributed to the increased attention given the child; his participation in the treatment process; his knowledge that many other people (perhaps even his parents) had a similiar problem and that the enuresis is not his fault; the emotional support of his parents, other family members and physician; and reassurances that his problem will, eventually, resolve.

A behavior modification program can draw from several possible components in varying combinations. These include retention control training[19]; positive reinforcement, verbally or materially, for each dry night; and the bell-and-pad alarm system.[20]

The urine alarm is the centerpiece of most behavioral techniques. Its purpose is conditioning the child to awaken in response to the stimulus of bladder distension, suppress micturition, rise, and go to the toilet to void. The child must awaken and void as soon as the alarm is triggered; if he does not do so spontaneously, his parents must rouse him immediately and take him to the toilet to complete bladder emptying.

The alarm must be used every night, often for several months, if the method is to succeed. A 70% success rate is reported in the literature[19,20]; at least one third of children relapse, however. This technique requires a highly motivated family because the child may need to be awakened several times a night, and such nocturnal activity can cause problems when others in the household are awakened—and perhaps not the patient.

A procedure called Dry-Bed Training, described in 1974, uses the urine alarm, withholding urination, increased social motivation, and other components in an intensive, all-night program, sometimes employing an outside trainer in the home.[21] It is superior to standard conditioning techniques,[22] but is very labor intensive.

We have offered behavioral therapy to all sleep enuresis patients; 50 families have tried it. Thirteen children achieved a dry bed, and six reduced wet nights by 75%. Many children who had a good result reported that they now awakened spontaneosly at night to void; the device may thus condition the child, not the bladder.

Other families in our program discontinued using the urine alarm because the child did not awaken spontaneously and because they did not see significant improvement. We have not had success with the alarm in patients who have the urgency syndrome.

Drug Therapy

The tricyclic antidepressant imipramine hydrochloride [Tofranil] and desmopressin [DDAVP] are valuable treatments for sleep enuresis only. Oxybutynin [Ditropan] is useful only in patients who have the urgency syndrome. A few children respond to a combination of the medications.

Alone, imipramine and desmopressin sometime produce a dry bed after a single dose; in this circumstance, their use can be limited to special occasions when staying dry is particularly important, such as sleep-over parties.

These drugs do not cure enuresis. They simply control the condition until the child outgrows it, so to speak. (To say that relapse can occur after therapy stops is, therefore, inappropriate.) Their major advantages are simplicity and rapid action.

Imipramine. This drug has been used extensively for many years to treat enuresis.[23] At first, its mechanism of action was believed to involve an antidepressant effect, an influence on sleep patterns, or an anticholinergic action, but none of these mechanisms have proved responsible. Today, despite innumerable studies, the exact antienuretic mechanism remains unknown.

In my experience, only children who have sleep enuresis respond to imipramine. Those who have the urgency syndrome do not demonstrate significant response.

Imipramine is administered as a single dose of 1 to 2 mg/kg, 1 hour before bed. Higher dosages increase side effects without enhancing efficacy. Typically, the patient is given a 25 mg starting dose for 1 week, which can be increased as needed by 25 mg each week to a maximum of 100 mg, depending on the child's weight.

When treatment succeeds, imipramine is continued for 6 months. It is then reduced gradually—over the course of 3 or 4 weeks—because abrupt discontinuation after prolonged treatment can cause nausea, anxiety, and malaise. If bedwetting persists, additional 6-month blocks of treatment are possible.

The drug should be discontinued if significant side effects develop, including personality changes, cardiac arrhythmias, sleep disorders, and mild gastrointestinal problems, or if the maximum dose does not provide significant improvement. All families should be warned about the potential for accidental acute overdose and the need to monitor the drug carefully at home—in particular, keeping it out of reach of younger children.

Imipramine was used to treat 117 of the 300 children studied at our hospital who had primary nocturnal enuresis. Sixty reported a dry bed, 22 had at least 75% fewer wet nights, and 35 did not have a significant response.

Desmopressin. This synthetic vasopressin analogue is superior to placebo in treating sleep enuresis.[24-26] Although it can be effective only for enuretics whose lower-than-normal nocturnal vasopressin concentration results in polyuria, vasopressin levels and urine volume are not measured in practice.

Desmopressin is administered by nasal spray in a dose of 10 to 40 μg (each spray is 10 μg) before bedtime. Typically, the child starts with one spray; if necessary, the dose is gradually increased to four sprays during a 2-week trial. Once treatment succeeds, the dose is stabilized and maintained for 6 months.[27] The medication is then withdrawn gradually. Additional 6-month treatments may be needed.

Few side effects of desmopressin have been reported; headache is the most common. Success varies—40% to 70%—directly with the size of the dose; I find its relative efficacy and that of imipramine to be the same. Of 15 children whom we have treated with desmopressin, 10 report that the number of wet nights has decreased by more than 75%.

The principal drawback to the use of desmopressin is its expense. As a result, we generally reserve it for rhildren in whom imipramine is ineffective, although the pros and cons of both drugs are discussed with parents and patient and the choice can be theirs.

Oxybutynin. This drug is useful in enuretic children who have the urgency syndrome.[1] In our experience, oxybutynin is not, however, generally helpful for children who have pure sleep enuresis.[28]

The effective dose of oxybutynin—ranging from 2.5 mg twice daily to 10 mg four times daily—must be determined operationally, not calculated on the basis of weight. The starting dose of 2.5 mg twice a day is gradually increased as needed, the endpoint being succcess or intolerable side effects.

Typically, at effective doses a child has some facial flushing and a dry mouth and feels warm to the touch. But these side effects do not necessarily indicate that the drug should be discontinued or the dosage reduced. Blurred vision, behavioral disturbance, and hyperthermia indicate excessive dosage; if any of these are noted, the dosage should be reduced or the medication stopped.

To enhance the success of oxybutynin therapy, the child must void every 2 to 4 hours—even if he does not feel the need to do so. Likewise, fluid intake must be limited to reasonable amounts. Using this management program, we have found that approximately 80% of our patients obtain excellent daytime dryness, although only 50% of them are dry at night.

Treatment Failures

Some enuretic children fail to respond to any therapy. For reasons not well understood, however, they may have a good result a year or so after failure.

Whenever a child fails to respond to any therapy for enuresis, it is important to recognize the risk of additional consequences. Consider that perhaps treatment was started because a younger sibling is already dry; perhaps a family member or friend who does not understand the nature of the problem questioned or criticized the parents; or perhaps the child really wanted to be dry. If treatment succeeds, the pressure of these situations may vanish, but when the child does not respond or relapses, these problems may reemerge or become acccentuated.

When that happens, physician and family must be supportive and guide the child away from dwelling on failure. Emphasize a positive attitude; let the child know that failure is not his fault and that although many children are enuretic, very few adults are. Last, the parents must look beyond the present problem and work to ensure that the child does not sustain a long-lasting emotional wound.

Bedwetting: Helping Your Child At Home

Self-awakening

The most straightforward approach to bedwetting is teaching your child to awaken at night. In theory, awakening is the quickest way to cure the problem because it can make up for production of a large amount of urine or a small bladder. The smaller a child's bladder, the more important is it for him to learn to awaken at night.

An important thing you should know about bedwetting is that many children do not realize that they need to get up at night. They go to bed telling themselves to "hold it until morning"—an impossible assignment for those who have a small bladder. Instead, they need to tell themselves to "wake up every night and use the toilet." Many families are surprised to hear that children need to be given this goal.

One technique to teach self-awakening is to ask your child to rehearse a particular sequence of events every night before going to sleep. He (or she, of course) lies in bed with his eyes closed and pretends that it is the middle of the night and his bladder is trying to wake him up by starting to hurt. He then runs to the bathroom and empties his bladder.

At the end of the rehearsal, your child can remind himself that he should get up the same way if he needs to urinate during the night. Many children are surprised to learn that their bladder sends the same signal when it becomes full at night as it does during the day.

Your child may benefit from a picture book meant to teach bedwetters to awaken at night (*Dry All Night* by Allison Mack; Little, Brown & Co., 1989).

The Alarm Clock

If your child cannot awaken himself at night and you choose not to use a bed-wetting alarm, teach him to use an alarm clock or clock radio. Set it for three or four hours after your child goes to bed. Put it beyond arm's reach.

Encourage your child to practice responding to the alarm during the day while lying on the bed with his eyes closed. Have him set the aiarm each night. Prepare him for getting up at night even if he is not dry in the morning.

Dry-bed Training

This is a more labor-intensive technique for teaching children to awaken at night. For it to succeed, you must be committed and consistently available. Here is what you must do:

- On the first night, wake the child once an hour until 1 a.m. Use the least effort or prompt necessary, from turning on the light on up to saying his name or touching him. Make sure he is awake enough to walk and talk coherently. If he is dry, praise him and ask, "Do you need to go to the toilet or can you wait another hour?" He must walk to the toilet on his own. If he is wet, encourage him to change his pajamas and bedding. At the 1 a.m. awakening, tell him to void even if he is dry.

- For the next five nights, wake the child only once. On the first night, wake him 3 hours after he falls asleep. The next night, wake him 2 1/2 hours after he falls asleep. Keep diminishing the interval, so that on the fifth night you wake him an hour after he falls asleep. On the sixth night, tell him to wake himself from then on.

- If the child relapses—that is, if he has three consecutive wet nights—repeat the six nights of awakening.

How to Use the Bedwetting Alarm

Several portable, transistorized conditioning alarms that are worn on the body (brand names include Nite-Train'r, Nytone, Wet-Stop) can help teach children to awaken to the sensation of a full bladder. They are convenient, comfortable, inexpensive, and easy for the child to set up without help. They should replace the older, bell-and-pad type of alarm.

Enuresis alarms are often effective; almost 60% of children who use them are reported cured. Some children relapse after they stop using the alarm, but many of them are cured after a second course.

The disadvantage of an enuresis alarm is that it takes a lot of your time. It also requires your child and you to be motivated and to be willing to learn how to use it properly and continue to use it for 2 or 3 months.

An alarm is especially frustrating when, time and again, a child does not awaken to the buzzer. You must remind your child at bedtime to wake up before the buzzer sounds, and you must use a program that teaches self-awakening along with the alarm. By having your child awaken as quickly as possible to the alarm, the goal is to have him eventually learn, by conditioning or guessing, to awaken to the feeling of a full bladder. Most children who are successful with an alarm learn to awaken at night.

Almost all children who wet the bed need to get up during the night to urinate. A bedwetting alarm, activiated by moisture, can help your child learn to awaken in time to go to the bathroom. The new models are light and easy for him to operate.

What to Tell Your Child

Give your child the following instructions:

- This is your alarm. It can help you wake up if you use it correctly. Remember, the alarm will not help you unless you listen for it carefully and respond to it quickly.

- Hook up the alarm system by yourself. Make the buzzer go off a few times by touching the sensors with a wet finger, then practice going to the bathroom as you are going to do if it goes off during the night.

- Turn on your nightlight before you go to sleep, or keep a flashlight near your bed so you can see what you are doing when the alarm sounds.

- Try to beat the buzzer. Wake up when your bladder feels full, but before any urine leaks out and sets off the alarm. If the buzzer does go off, try to wake up and stop urinating as soon as

397

you think you hear it—even if you think you are hearing it in a dream.

- As soon as you hear the alarm, jump out of bed and stand up. Once you are standing and awake, turn off the buzzer by removing the metal strip from the little pocket in your underwear (for the Wet-Stop model) or disconnect the clips (for the Nytone model) and dry them off.

- Hurry to the bathroom. Empty your bladder to see how much urine you were able to hold back.

- Put on dry underwear and pajamas, and hook up the alarm again. Put a dry towel over the wet spot on your bed. Remind yourself to get up before the alarm buzzes next time and think over your plan again.

- In the morning, write on your calendar DRY (the alarm didn't buzz), WET SPOT (you got up after the alarm buzzed), or WET (you did not get up even though the alarm buzzed).

- Use the alarm every night until you go 3 or 4 weeks without wetting the bed. This usually takes 2 or 3 months to do, so try to be patient.

Your Role

First, remember that while your child is using the bedwetting alarm he must also practice a self-awakening program at bedtime.

If your child does not awaken immediately to the sound of the buzzer on the bedwetting alarm, he needs your help. You may need to be involved every night for the first 2 or 3 weeks. Here is what to do:

- Go to the child's room when the buzzer rings, turn on the light, and say loudly, "Get out of bed and stand up."

- If that does not work, sit him up in bed and run a cold washcloth over his face to bring him out of deep sleep.

- When he is on his feet, remind him to turn off the alarm. Do not do it for him. Your child must learn to carry out this step himself.

- Make sure your child is wide awake and walks into the bathroom before you leave him. If necessary, ask him questions to help him wake up.

- Your goal is to help your child awaken immediately and get out of bed when the buzzer sounds. Try to remove yourself from the alarm program gradually. Making sure your child goes to bed at a reasonable hour, with the radio off and a night light on, can help him respond faster to the alarm.

Where to Obtain an Alarm

Alarms and instructions can be ordered from:

Nite Train'r Enuresis Alarm: Koregon Enterprises Inc, 9735 SW Sunshine Ct, Suite 100, Beaverton, OR 97005 (800-544-4240).
Nytone Enuretic Alarm: Nytone Medical Products, 2424 S 900 West, Salt Lake City, UT 84119 (801-973-4090).
Wet-Stop Alarm: Patco Laboratories,1595 Soquei Dr Santa Cruz, CA 95065 (800-346-4488).

References

1. Kass EJ, Diokno AC, Montealegre A: Enuresis: principles of management and result of treatment. *J Urol* 1979;121:796–796
2. Forsythe W, Redmond A: Enuresis and spontaneous cure rate study of 1,129 enuretics. *Arch Dis Chld* 1974;49:259–269
3. Enfield C: Enuresis. *Med J Aust* 1976;2:908
4. Hawkins DN: Enuresis: a survey. *Med J Aust* 1962;1:979
5. Redmond JF, Seibert JJ: The uroradiogrsphic evaluation of the enuretic child. *J Urol* 1979;122:799
6. American Academy of Pediatrics Committee on Radiology: Excretory urography for evaluation of enuresis. *Pediatrics* 1980;65:644
7. Novello AC, Novello R: Enuresis. *Pediatric Clin North Am* 1987;34:719–733
8. Norgaard JP, Rittig S, Djurhuus JC: Nocturnal enuresis: an approach to treatment based on pathogenesis. *J Pediatr* 1989;114:705–710
9. Norgaard JP, Hansen JH, Wildschiotz G. et al: Sleep cystometries in children with nocturnal enuresis. *J Urol* 1989;141:1156–1159

10. Mikkelson EJ. Rapoport JL: Enuresis: psychopathology. sleep stage and drug response. *Urol Clin North Am* 1980;9:361–377

11. Fergusson DM, Horwood LT, Sannon FT: Factors related to the age of attainment of nocturnal bladder control: an 8-year longitudinal study. *Pediatrics* 1986;78:884–890

12. McKendry JBJ, Stewart DA: Enuresis. *Pediatr Clin North Am* 1974;21:1019

13. Bakwin H; The genetics of enuresis, in Kolvin I, MacKeith RC, Meadow SR (eds): Bladder Control and Enuresis. Philadelphia, J.B. Lippincott. 1973, pp 73–78

14. Norgaard JP, Pederson EB. Djurhuus. JC: Diurnal antidiuretic hormone levels in enuresis. *J Urol* 1985;134:1029

15. Foxman B, Valdez RB, Brook RH: Childhood enuresis; prevalence, perceived impact and prescribed treatments. *Pediatrics* 1986;77:482–487

16. Mottan MEK, Kato C, Pless IB; Improvements in self-concept after treatments of nocturnal enuresis: randomized controlled trials. *J Pediatr* 1987;110:647–652

17. Cohen MW; Symposium on behavioral pediatrics: enuresis. *Pediatr Clin North Am* 1975;22:545

18. Rushton HG: Nocturnal enuresis; epidemiology, evaluation, and currently available treatment options. *J Pediatr* 1989;114:691–696

19. Starfield B, Mellits ED: Increases in functional bladder capacity and improvements in enuresis. *J Pediatr* 1968;72:483–487

20. Forsythe WI, Butler RJ; Fifty years of enuretic alarms. *Arch Dis Child* 1989;64:879

21. Azrin NH, Sneed TJ, Foxx RM; Day-bed training: rapid elimination of childhood enuresis. *Behav Res Ther* 1974;12:147

22. Bollard J, Nettlebeck T: A component analysis of dry-bed training for treatment of bedwetting. *Behav Res Ther* 1982;20:383–390

23. Martin GI: Imipramine pamate in the treatment of childhood enuresis: a double-blind study. *Am J Dis Child* 1971:122:42

24. Klauber GT: Clinical efficacy and safety of desmopressin in the treatment of nocturnal enuresis. *J Pediatr* 1989;114:719–722

25. Fenie BG, MacFarlane J. Glen ES: DDAVP in young enuretic patients: a double-blind trial *Br J Urol* 1984;56:376–378

26. Meadow SR. Evans JH: Desmopressin for enuresis. *BMJ* 1989;298:1596–1597

27. Miller K: Nocturnal enuresis: experience with long-term use of intranasally administered desmopressin. *J Pediatr* 1989;114:723–726

28. Kass EJ: A practical approach to enuresis. Clinical Proceedings, Children's Hospital National Medical Center, Washington, D.C., 1981, 37(6):341–345

—by Evan J. Kass, MD

Section 33.3

Additional Resources on Enuresis

NKUDIC, Searches-On-File, Topics in Kidney and Urologic Diseases, July 1993.

Legend

TI Title
AU Author
CN Corporate Author
SO Source
AV Producer/Availability

TI **Approaching Enuresis in an Uncomplicated Way.**
AU Kass, E.J.
SO *Contemporary Urology*. 2(2): 15–16, 18–20, 22–24. February 1991.

TI **Bed-Wetting Child: Current Management of a Frustrating Problem.**
AU Rosenfeld, J.; Jerkins, G.R.
SO *Postgraduate Medicine*. 89(2): 63–65, 69–70. February 1, 1991.

TI *Bedwetting: Nocturnal Enuresis.*
SO Union, SC: Help for Incontinent People. 199x. 2 p.
CN Help for Incontinent People.
AV Available from Help for Incontinent People, Inc. (HIP). P.O. Box 544, Union, SC 29379. (803) 579-7900. PRICE: $1.00. Make check payable to HIP.

TI *Children and Kidney Disease.*
AU Alexander, S.R; Kennedy, J.E.
SO Rockville, MD: American Kidney Fund. 1987. 20 p.
AV Available from American Kidney Fund. 6110 Executive Boulevard, Rockville, MD 20852. (301) 881-3052 or (800) 638-8299.

TI *Controlling Bed-Wetting: A New Approach.*
SO Fort Washington, PA: Rorer Pharmaceuticals. 1990. 6 p.
CN Rorer Pharmaceuticals.
AV Available from Rorer Pharmaceuticals. Fort Washington, PA 19034. PRICE: Free.

TI **Drug Free Program For Nocturnal Enuresis.**
AU Long, B.C.
SO *Urologic Nursing*. 11(1): 15–16. March 1991.

TI **End to Enuresis.**
AU Hellerstein, S.
SO *Emergency Medicine*. 19(14): 25–43. August 15, 1987.

TI **Enuresis.**
AU Rushton, H.G.
SO In: Kher, K.K.; Makker, S.P., eds. *Clinical Pediatric Nephrology*. Blue Ridge Summit, PA: McGraw-Hill. 1992. p. 399–419.
AV Available from McGraw-Hill, Inc. 13311 Monterey Avenue, Blue Ridge Summit, PA 17294. (800) 262-4729. PRICE: $85.00 plus $3.00 for shipping and handling. ISBN: 0070345430.

TI *Enuresis: A Parenting Challenge.*
SO Kansas City, MO: Marion Laboratories, Inc. 1 p.
CN Simon Foundation. Marion Laboratories, Inc.
AV Available from Marion Laboratories, Inc. P.O. Box 9627, Kansas City, MO 64134.

TI **Frequent Urinary Tract Infections In Girls.**
AU Simon, G., et al.
SO *Pediatric Forum*. 142(4): 412–413. April 1988.

TI *How You Can Be Boss of the Bladder.*
AU Hall, J.
SO Wilmette, IL: Simon Foundation for Continence. 1989. 65 p.
AV Available from Simon Foundation for Continence. P.O. Box 835, Wilmette, IL 60091. (800) 237-4666 or (708) 864-3913. PRICE: $9.95. ISBN: 0731676734.

TI *If a Child Is A Bed Wetter.*
SO Ann Arbor, MI: National Kidney Foundation of Michigan, Inc. n.d. 6 p.
CN National Kidney Foundation of Michigan, Inc.
AV Available from National Kidney Foundation of Michigan, Inc. 2350 South Huron Parkway, Ann Arbor, MI 48104. (313) 971-2800 or (800) 482-1455.

TI **Incontinence in Childhood.**
AU Faller, N.
SO In: Jeter, K.F.; Faller, N.; Norton, C., eds. *Nursing for Continence*. Orlando, FL: W.B. Saunders Company. 1990. p. 91–107.
AV Available from W. B. Saunders Company. 6277 Sea Harbor Drive, Orlando, FL 32887. (800) 782-4479. PRICE: $31.95 plus shipping. ISBN: 0721628923.

TI *Information Packet on Urinary Incontinence and Enuresis.*
SO Kansas City, MO: Marion Laboratories, Inc. 8 p.
CN Marion Laboratories, Inc.
AV Available from Marion Laboratories, Inc. P.O. Box 9627, Kansas City, MO 64134.

TI *Now Hope For Your Bed-Wetting Child: Ask Your Doctor.*
SO Fort Washington, PA: Rorer Pharmaceuticals. 1990. 2 p.
CN Rorer Pharmaceuticals.
AV Available from Rorer Pharmaceuticals. Fort Washington, PA 19034. PRICE: Free.

TI   **Overnight Cure.**
AU   Newman, J.
SO   *American Health*. 9(6): 14. July-August 1990.

TI   *Pacific International Profile: A Professional Approach
to Bedwetting.*
AU   Draper, E.B.
SO   Nekoosa, WI: Pacific International, Ltd. 1988. 11 p.
CN   Pacific International, Ltd.
AV   Available from Pacific International, Ltd. 555 Birch Street,
Nekoosa, WI 54457. (800) 82S4875 or (800) 248-4098 (in Wis-
consin) or (800) 533-5237 (in Canada). PRICE: Single copy
free.

TI   **Promising Therapies for Urinary Incontinence.**
AU   Blaivas, J.G.
SO   *Contemporary Urology*. 3(1): 48, 51–52. January 1991.

TI   **Unstable Bladder in Childhood.**
AU   Meadow, S.R.
SO   In: Freeman, R. and Malvern, J. *Unstable Bladder*. Stoneham,
MA: Butterworth and Co., Ltd. 1989. p. 107–114.
AV   Available from Butterworth and Co. (Publishers) Ltd. Market-
ing Department, 80 Montvale Avenue, Stoneham, MA 02180-
9986. (617) 438-8464. PRICE: $135.00.

TI   *What Are Some of the Known Facts About Bedwetting?*
SO   Union, SC: Help for Incontinent People. 1 p.
CN   Help for Incontinent People.
AV   Available from Help for Incontinent People, Inc. (HIP). P.O.
Box 544, Union, SC 29379. (800) BLADDER. PRICE: $1.00.
Make check payable to HIP.

For More Information

CHID is available on-line through CDP Online. If you would like
references to materials on other topics, you may request a special literature search of CHID from a library that subscribes to CDP Online
or from the National Kidney and Urologic Diseases Information Clearinghouse, 3 Information Way, Bethesda, MD 20892-3580; (301) 654-
4415.

Chapter 34

Pinpoint Diagnosis: The Key to Managing Polyuria in Childhood

The history and physical exam can provide clues to the cause of excessive urinary volume, but definitive diagnosis requires laboratory testing of, among other parameters, urine and serum osmolality.

The causes of polyuria are numerous. Usually, the condition reflects an underlying neurologic, renal, or metabolic disorder. In this article, we review the origins of polyuria and offer a physiologic approach to evaluation and management.

What Causes Polyuria?

Polyuria is the result of a water diuresis or solute diuresis. Primary polydipsia or diabetes insipidus (DI) can cause a water diuresis.

Primary polydipsia may be the result of compulsive water drinking, medical treatment that involves drinking large quantities of water, or a defect in the thirst center.

Compulsive water drinking is rare in children. The disorder occurs most often in adolescents and adults who have a significant psychological disturbance.

As part of the treatment of such conditions as nephrolithiasis or when being given such drugs as cyclophosphamide, children may be instructed to drink large volumes of water, with resulting polyuria. The same is true for infants given milk or fluid as a pacifier.

Contemporary Urology, Volume 5 No. 12, December 1993.

Water diuresis

Primary polydipsia
  Compulsive water drinking
  Treatment with a high intake of water
  Defect of thirst center
Diabetes insipidus
  Neurogenic
    Primary
      Idiopathic
      Familial
    Secondary
      Head trauma
      Neurosurgery
      Infection (meningitis, encephalitis, CNS abscess)
      Tumor (craniopharyngioma, glioma, germinoma, metastasis)
      CNS granulomatous disease (histiocytosis X, sarcoidosis)
      Intracranial hemorrhage (aneurysm, thrombosis, embolus)
      Hypoxia
      Drugs (clonidine, alcohol)
  Nephrogenic
    Congenital
    Acquired
      Hypokalemia
      Hypercalcemia
      Drugs (lithium carbonate, demeclocycline, amphotericin B, phenytoin, nicotine, methoxyflurane)
      Renal parenchymal disorders (any cause of renal failure: any cause of diffuse cortical or medullary damage)

Solute (osmotic) diuresis

Organic solutes
  Glucose (diabetes mellitus, renal glucosuria, very large glucose load by IV)
  Urea (large protein intake, increased catabolism)
  Mannitol
Inorganic solutes
  Sodium chloride (oral or IV load, especially in combination with diuretics, salt-losing renal diseases, or mineralocorticoid deficiency)
  Ammonium chloride (with chronic metabolic acidosis)
  Potassium chloride
  Sodium or, possibly, potassium bicarbonate (alkali ingestion)

Table 34.1. Causes of polyuria in childhood.

Defects of the thirst center may be primary or may develop as a consequence of a lesion in the hypothalamus.

Diabetes insipidus is caused by failure of the neurohypophysis to synthesize or secrete adequate antidiuretic hormone (ADH) (neurogenic DI) or by failure of the kidney to respond appropriately to circulating ADH (nephrogenic DI).

Neurogenic DI results from any of a spectrum of deficiencies of ADH—from only mild, partial defects to complete absence. The condition occurs as a primary disorder or secondary to a number of other disorders.

Primary neurogenic DI can manifest at any age. Distribution is sporadic among most cases reported in children; the uncommon familial forms occur as an autosomal dominant or an X-linked recessive condition.

Secondary neurogenic DI is more common, and can be the result of any lesion that damages the neurohypophyseal system.

Nephrogenic DI is a congenital or an acquired condition. The congenital form is transmitted as an X-linked recessive trait; acquired nephrogenic DI is more common.

Accumulation of organic or inorganic solutes in the urine causes a solute diuresis. Common organic solutes that have been implicated are glucose and urea; inorganic solutes that play a role are salts of sodium, potassium, and, possibly, ammonium, in which the anion is usually chloride or bicarbonate.

The Differential Diagnosis

Polyuria must be distinguished from small-volume urinary frequency. Polyuria is almost always associated with frequency, but frequency is not always associated with polyuria. Furthermore, polyuria is usually associated with polydipsia; small-volume frequency is not.

Urinary frequency can occur secondary to cystitis; urethritis; urethral irritation from a chemical agent, such as bubble bath; urethral obstruction; and urethral trauma after catheterization, masturbation, sexual abuse, or straddle injury.

The daytime frequency syndrome is seen in healthy children, usually boys. It is characterized by frequency as severe as 20 to 40 times a day in the absence of an organic cause. Dysuria and enuresis are uncommon. The condition is usually self-limiting, with frequency subsiding in less than 3 months.

How to Evaluate

The presenting symptom of polyuria is an increasing trend in the volume voided. In an infant, this can take the form of frequent wet and excessively heavy diapers. The child may be irritable or cry excessively because of unrelieved thirst.

An older child may report enuresis. The absence of enuresis or nocturia in the presence of polyuria suggests excessive fluid intake, such as occurs with primary polydipsia.

Another notable observation is that the onset of water drinking that is compulsive in nature is, typically, more gradual than it is in DI. When frequency is secondary to polyuria, the patient reports copious, pale, water-like urine; when frequency is unrelated to polyuria, the volume of urine is low.

If the basic diagnosis is in doubt, a 24-hour collection of urine may be necessary to establish the diagnosis. A good assessment of the completeness of a 24-hour urine collection is to measure urine creatinine, which should be at least 15 mg/kg/d.

Thirst is generally associated with polyuria; an exception is polyuria secondary to iatrogenic fluid or solute overload. Most children who have neurogenic or nephrogenic DI exhibit an intense thirst, particularly for cold water. In contrast, a preference for cold water is not a feature of primary polydipsia or a solute diuresis.

The history may suggest clues to the cause of the polyuria. In addition, specific features of the physical examination are helpful in evaluating children who have polyuria.

Assessment of extracellular fluid (ECF) volume is important in the workup of polyuria because ECF volume contraction can result from the loss of sodium and chloride that occurs in polyuria. Polyuria secondary to primary polydipsia or sodium chloride load is marked by a normal ECF volume, whereas polyuria caused by an osmotic diuresis is usually marked by a reduction of ECF volume.

Selecting Therapy

Any underlying disease should be recognized and treated: Correcting hypokalemia and hypercalcemia, treating diabetes mellitus and renal disease, and discontinuing an offending drug, for example, may cause polyuria to resolve. Children who have DI should have unrestricted access to fluids to prevent severe contraction of the intracellular fluid.

If the history is remarkable for	The cause of polyuria may be
Family history	
Neurogenic diabetes insipidus (DI)	Neurogenic DI
Nephrogenic DI	Nephrogenic DI
Diabetes mellitus	Diabetes mellitus
Abrupt onset	Neurogenic DI
Increased appetite and weight loss	Diabetes mellitus
Recent head trauma or intracranial infection	Neurogenic DI or defect of thirst center
Headache or visual loss	Neurogenic DI or defect of thirst center
Drugs	
Lithium carbonate, demeclocycline, amphotericin B, phenytoin, nicotine, methoxyflurane	Nephrogenic DI
Clonidine, alcohol	Neurogenic DI
Diuretic, mannitol	Solute diuresis
Recurrent pyelonephritis or past renal parenchymal disease	Nephrogenic DI
Parenteral fluid therapy	Solute or water diuresis
Behavioral disturbance or psychiatric illness	Compulsive water drinking
Muscle weakness or constipation	Hypokalemia
Kidney stones	Hypercalcemia

Table 34.2. *How the history aids the evaluation of polyuria.*

If the examination reveals	The cause of polyuria may be
Pallor	Chronic renal failure
Growth failure	Neurogenic diabetes insipidus (DI) Nephrogenic DI
Precocious puberty	Neurogenic DI
Neurologic deficits, bitemporal hemianopsia, optic atrophy, or papilledema	Neurogenic DI
Weak urinary stream or large kidneys and bladder	Obstructive uropathy
Acetone on the breath	Diabetes mellitus
Extracellular fluid volume contraction	Osmotic diuresis (diabetes mellitus or increased catabolism)

Table 34.3. *Interpreting physical findings in the evaluation of polyuria.*

409

In neurogenic DI, replacement therapy with ADH or its analogue, arginine vasopressin, produces a satisfactory response in almost all children. Intranasal DDAVP, 5 to 20 μg, once or twice a day, is highly effective.

The dose should be individualized based on renal response. If the drug is given once a day, an evening dose is preferable because it avoids nocturia.

DDAVP has fewer pressor effects than ADH, and maintains the antidiuretic effect. It has a relatively long duration of action, and absorption from the nasal mucosa is excellent. Excess nasal mucus caused by allergic or infectious rhinitis may, however, interfere with absorption of DDAVP. Side effects are uncommon, but headache and hypertension secondary to water retention have been reported when the dosage exceeds 40 μg/d.

Vasopressin tannate in oil, 2 to 5 U every 24 to 72 hours given intramuscularly, can also be used to treat neurogenic DI. When using this drug, the child's weight, serum concentration of sodium, and serum osmolality should be monitored—weekly at first, then with decreasing frequency—to ensure that the dose is appropriate. Once these parameters are stable, they should still be monitored every 3 months.

The combination of a diuretic such as hydrochlorothiazide, 1-2 mg/kg/d, and dietary salt restriction may help lower the urine volume in a patient who has nephrogenic DI. The price of this reduction, however, is contracted ECF volume; maintaining the child in a state of mild ECF volume contraction enhances reabsorption of sodium chloride and water, thus minimizing polyuria. Hypokalemia can be prevented by increasing dietary intake of potassium.

Compulsive water drinking is a formidable therapeutic challenge. Psychotherapy is usually required to control the problem.

ECF volume contraction, which can result from the polyuria of an osmotic diuresis, requires treatment with sodium chloride—at a rate that provides a positive balance of sodium and returns the ECF volume to normal. Sufficient water must be given to ensure that the serum sodium concentration does not rise appreciably.

—by Alexander K.C. Leung, MBBS, FRCPC, FRCP(Edin),
FRCP(Glasg), FRCPI, FMP, FRSH, DCH(Lond), DCH(I);
William Lane M. Robson, MD, FRCPC, FRSH; and
Mitchell L. Halperin. MD, FRCPC.

Chapter 35

Urinary Reflux in Children

Chapter Contents

Section 35.1

Reflux Disorders in Children

Kidney and Urology Facts, ©1992 National Kidney Foundation.
Used by permission.

What Is Reflux? What Causes It?

Your child can be born with a problem valve in the bladder. The valve is found where the bladder joins the urine tube (ureter) that comes from the kidney. The valve does not close properly so urine backs up (refluxes) from the bladder to the kidney. The amount of reflux can be large or small.

Other problems, called voiding disorders, cause problems controlling urine and may also cause reflux. Some of these will go away as your child gets older.

How Is Reflux Diagnosed? Are There Signs to Alert Parents to the Problem?

This problem is usually found when you take your child to see the doctor after a urinary tract infection. About 50 percent of babies and 30 percent of older children with infections will have reflux. The backflow of urine to the kidney can cause a urinary infection to spread to the kidney, which can make your child very sick and can lead to kidney damage. You may see that your child:

- goes to the bathroom more often
- says "It burns or hurts" when passing urine
- says "My belly hurts"
- has a fever

You need to take your child to a doctor who will get a urine culture if he suspects an infection.

How Is Reflux Treated?

It can be corrected by surgery. However, most children will get better as they grow older. Therefore, your child may be treated with special medicines (antibiotics) to prevent infection. Only one child in ten will get an infection when taking medicine.

Sometimes, it is hard to decide what is best for your child. If your doctor suggests surgery, you may want to get a second opinion from a doctor who specializes in the care of reflux, called a pediatric urologist. Most American children's hospitals have one of these doctors.

It is important for the doctor to evaluate other possible causes of reflux, such as voiding disorders, which usually cause problems with wetting. Some children's hospitals have training programs to help children develop better urine control.

Do Children with This Problem Generally Do Okay or Do They Tend to Have Serious Problems Later?

Children with this problem usually do very well. Once the problem is corrected, it is very rare for it to happen again. However, if the kidneys have been damaged, high blood pressure may occur later in life. The risk of high blood pressure is about 10 percent if one kidney has been damaged and about 20 percent if both kidneys have been damaged. Most children do not have serious kidney damage from reflux. However, some do. A small number will go on to have kidney failure in later life.

Is Research Being Done to Find Better Ways of Preventing and Treating This Problem?

Yes. Researchers are trying to find easier ways to correct the reflux. In the future, surgery may be done without an incision through a tube that allows the doctor to look into the bladder. This type of surgery would be done on an outpatient basis so that your child does not need to stay in the hospital.

Is There Anything Else That Parents Should Know about This Problem?

Yes. If your child gets a fever, complains about belly pain or pain when urinating, or if the child goes to the bathroom more often than usual, he or she may have a urinary infection. A urine culture should always be done and most doctors will also order x-rays to detect reflux, which is a common problem in children with urinary tract infections.

What Is the National Kidney Foundation and How Does it Help?

Twenty million Americans have some form of kidney or urologic disease. Millions more are at risk. The National Kidney Foundation, Inc., a major voluntary health organization, is working to find the answers through prevention, treatment and cure. Through its 50 Affiliates nationwide, the Foundation conducts programs in research, professional education, patient and community services, public education and organ donation. The work of The National Kidney Foundation is funded entirely by public donations.

Section 35.2

Additional Resources on Urinary Reflux Disorders in Children

Searches-On-File, Topics in Kidney and Urologic Disease, NKUDIC.

Legend

TI   Title
AU   Author
CN   Corporate Author
SO   Source
PD   Product
AV   Producer/Availability

TI   Imaging: Nuclear Medicine.
AU   Taylor, C.M.; Chapman, S.
SO   In: Taylor, C.M. and Chapman, S. *Handbook of Renal Investigations in Children.* Stoneham, MA: Butterworth and Co., Ltd. 1989. p. 128–149.
AV   Available from Butterworth and Co. (Publishers) Ltd. Marketing Department, 80 Montvale Avenue, Stoneham, MA 02180-9986. (617) 438-8464. PRICE: $65.00.

TI   Imaging: Contrast Radiology.
AU   Taylor, C.M.; Chapman, S.
SO   In: Taylor, C.M. and Chapman, S. *Handbook of Renal Investigations in Children.* Stoneham, MA: Butterworth and Co., Ltd. 1989. p. 69–97.
AV   Available from Butterworth and Co. (Publishers) Ltd. Marketing Department, 80 Montvale Avenue, Stoneham, MA 02180-9986. (617) 438-8464. PRICE: $65.00.

TI   **Managing Vesicoureteral Reflux in Children.**
AU   Drosieko, A.G.; Hiott, K.
SO   *Journal of Urological Nursing.* 11(4): 255–266. October-November-December 1992.

TI   **Methodologic Limitations in the Literature on Vesicoureteral Reflux: A Critical Review.**
AU   Shanon, M.; Feldman, W.
SO   *Journal of Pediatrics.* 117(2 Part 1): 171–178. August 1990.

TI   ***Problems in Pediatric Nephrology.***
AU   Gauthier, B.
SO   Chapel Hill, NC: Health Sciences Consortium. 1991. (computer-assisted instruction program).
PD   Computer assisted instruction program for IBM and Apple II computers, 8 diskettes (5 1/4 in or 3 ½ in), with instructions. IBM format requires IBM PC, PC/XT, PC/AT, PS/2 or 100 percent compatibles, running IBM/MS DOS 2.0 and higher. Apple format requires AppleII plus, Apple IIe, or 100 percent compatible computers with 48K bytes of RAM and at least two floppy disk drives.
AV   Available from Health Sciences Consortium (HSC). 201 Silver Cedar Court, Chapel Hill, NC 27514. (919) 942-8731. PRICE: $1,056.00 (non-members) or $748.00 (HSC members) plus $5.00 shipping and handling for IBM version. Order Number: IBM A890-MC-020I. Contact HSC for price and ordering information for Apple format software.

TI   ***Reflux Disorders in Children.***
SO   New York, NY: The National Kidney Foundation, Inc. 1992. 2 p.
CN   The National Kidney Foundation, Inc.
AV   Available from The National Kidney Foundation, Inc. 30 East 33rd Street, New York, NY 10016. (800) 622-9010. PRICE: Single copy free from State Affiliates. Order Number 02-25NN.

TI   **Urinary Tract Infection in Children: A Review.**
AU   Cepero-Akselrad, A.; Ramirez-Seijas, F.; Castaneda, A.M.
SO   *International Pediatrics.* 8(3): 314–325. 1993.

TI **Urinary Tract Infection.**
AU Kher, K.K.; Leichter, H.E.
SO In: Kher, K.K.; Makker, S.P., eds. *Clinical Pediatric Nephrology.* Blue Ridge Summit, PA: McGraw-Hill. 1992. p. 277–321.
AV Available from McGraw-Hill, Inc. 13311 Monterey Avenue, Blue Ridge Summit, PA 17294. (800) 262-4729. PRICE: $85.00 plus $3.00 for shipping and handling. ISBN: 0070345430.

TI **Urinary Tract Infections in the Pediatric Patient.**
AU Wilson, D.; Killion, D.
SO *Nurse Practitioner.* 14(7): 38, 41–42. July 1989.

TI **Urodynamic Investigations.**
AU Taylor, C.M.; Chapman, S.
SO In: Taylor, C.M. and Chapman, S. *Handbook of Renal Investigations in Children.* Stoneham, MA: Butterworth and Co., Ltd. 1989. p. 150–159.
AV Available from Butterworth and Co. (Publishers) Ltd. Marketing Department, 80 Montvale Avenue, Stoneham, MA 02180-9986. (617) 438-8464. PRICE: $65.00.

TI **Urological Workup of the Child With Renal and Urinary Tract Disease.**
AU Treiger, B.F.; Jeffs, R.D.
SO In: Barakat, A.Y. *Renal Disease in Children: Clinical Evaluation and Diagnosis.* Secaucus, NJ: Springer-Verlag. 1990. p. 329–339.
AV Available from Springer-Verlag. Order Department, 44 Hartz Way, Secaucus, NJ 07094. (800) 777-4643 or (212) 460-1500 ext. 599. PRICE: $85.00. ISBN: 0387970363.

TI **Vesicoureteral Reflux.**
AU Harmon, T.W.
SO *Journal of Urological Nursing.* 8(4): 732–739. October-December 1989.

TI **Vesicoureteric Reflux and Renal Injury.**
AU Arant, B.S.
SO *American Journal of Kidney Diseases.* 17(5): 491–511. May 1991.

For Additional Information

CHID is available on-line through BRS Online, a division of CD-Plus Technologies. If you would like references to materials on other topics, you may request a special literature search of CHID from a library that subscribes to BRS or the National Kidney and Urologic Diseases Information Clearinghouse, Box NKUDIC, 9000 Rockville Pike, Bethesda, MD 20892; (301) 654-4415.

Part Nine

Understanding Adult Urinary Tract Disorders

Chapter 36

Adult Urinary Incontinence

Chapter Contents

Section 36.1

Urinary Incontinence in Adults

DHHS, AHCPR. Pub. No. 92–0041.

Abbreviations

BPH   Benign prostatic hyperplasia
CIC   Clean intermittent catheterization
CMG   Cystometrogram
DI   Detrusor instability
DH   Detrusor hyperreflexia
DHIC Detrusor hyperactivity with impaired bladder contractility
DSD   Detrusor external sphincter dyssynergia
ISD   Intrinsic sphincter deficiency
MS   Multiple sclerosis
PSA   Prostate specific antigen
PVR   Post-void residual volume
UI   Urinary incontinence

How Your Body Makes, Stores and Releases Urine

When you eat and drink, your body absorbs the liquid. The kidneys filter out waste products from the body fluids and make urine.

Urine travels down tubes called ureters into a muscular sac called the urinary bladder, which stores the urine.

When you are ready to go to the bathroom, your brain tells your system to relax.

Urine travels out of your bladder through a tube called the urethra. You release urine by relaxing the urethral sphincter and contracting the bladder muscles. The urethral sphincter is a group of muscles that tightens to hold urine in and loosens to let it out.

422

Many people lose urine when they don't want to. When this happens enough to be a problem, it is called urinary incontinence.

Urinary incontinence is very common. But some people are too embarrassed to get help. The good news is that millions of men and women are being successfully treated and cured.

Reading this information will help you. But it is important to tell your health care provider (such as a doctor or nurse) about the problem.

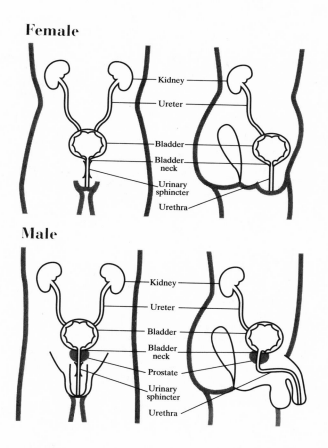

Female

- Kidney
- Ureter
- Bladder
- Bladder neck
- Urinary sphincter
- Urethra

Male

- Kidney
- Ureter
- Bladder
- Bladder neck
- Prostate
- Urinary sphincter
- Urethra

Figure 36.1.1.

Causes of Urinary Incontinence

Urinary incontinence is not a natural part of aging. It can happen at any age, and can be caused by many physical conditions. Many causes of incontinence are temporary and can be managed with simple treatment. Some causes of temporary incontinence are:

- Urinary tract infection
- Vaginal infection or irritation
- Constipation
- Effects of medicine

Incontinence can be caused by other conditions that are not temporary. Other causes of incontinence are:

- Weakness of muscles that hold the bladder in place
- Weakness of the bladder itself
- Weakness of the urethral sphincter muscles
- Overactive bladder muscles
- Blocked urethra (can be from prostate enlargement)
- Hormone imbalance in women
- Neurologic disorders
- Immobility (not being able to move around)

In almost every case, these conditions can be treated. Your health care provider will help to find the exact cause of your incontinence.

Types of Incontinence

There are also many different types of incontinence. Some people have more than one type of incontinence. You should be able to identify the type of incontinence you have by comparing it to the list below.

Urge Incontinence

People with urge incontinence lose urine as soon as they feel a strong need to go to the bathroom. If you have urge incontinence you may leak urine:

- When you can't get to the bathroom quickly enough
- When you drink even a small amount of liquid, or when you hear or touch running water

You may also go to the bathroom very often; for example, every two hours during the day and night. You may even wet the bed.

Stress Incontinence

People with stress incontinence lose urine when they exercise or move in a certain way. If you have stress incontinence, you may leak urine:

- When you sneeze, cough, or laugh
- When you get up from a chair or get out of bed
- When you walk or do other exercise

You may also go to the bathroom often during the day to avoid accidents.

Overflow Incontinence

People with overflow incontinence may feel that they never completely empty their bladder. If you have overflow incontinence, you may:

- Often lose small amounts of urine during the day and night
- Get up often during the night to go to the bathroom
- Often feel as if you have to empty your bladder but can't
- Pass only a small amount of urine but feel as if your bladder is still partly full
- Spend a long time at the toilet, but produce only a weak, dribbling stream of urine

Some people with overflow incontinence do not have the feeling of fullness, but they lose urine day and night.

Finding the Cause of Urinary Incontinence

Once you tell your health care provider about the problem, finding the cause of your urinary incontinence is the next step.

Your health care provider will talk with you about your medical history and urinary habits. You probably will have a physical examination and urine tests. You may have other tests, as well. These tests will help find the exact cause of your incontinence and the best treatment for you.

425

Treating Urinary Incontinence

Once the type and cause of your urinary incontinence is known, treatment can begin. Urinary incontinence is treated in one or more of three ways: behavioral techniques, medication, and surgery.

Behavioral Techniques

Behavioral techniques teach you ways to control your own bladder and sphincter muscles. They are very simple and work well for certain types of urinary incontinence. Two types of behavioral techniques are commonly used—bladder training and pelvic muscle exercises. You may also be asked to change the amount of liquid that you drink. You may be asked to drink more or less water depending on your bladder problem.

Bladder Training. Bladder training is used for urge incontinence, and may also be used for stress incontinence. Both men and women can benefit from bladder training. People learn different ways to control the urge to urinate. Distraction (thinking about other things) is just one example. A technique called prompted voiding—urinating on a schedule—is also used. This technique has been quite successful in controlling incontinence in nursing home patients.

Pelvic Muscle Exercises. Pelvic muscle exercises called Kegel exercises are used for stress incontinence. The Kegel exercises help to strengthen weak muscles around the bladder.

Medication

Some people need to take medicine to treat conditions that cause urinary incontinence. The most common types of medicine treat infection, replace hormones, stop abnormal bladder muscle contractions, or tighten sphincter muscles. You will be told if you need medication and how and when to take it.

Surgery

Surgery is sometimes needed to help treat the cause of incontinence. Surgery can be used to:

- Return the bladder neck to its proper position in women with stress incontinence
- Remove tissue that is causing a blockage
- Replace or support severely weakened pelvic muscles
- Enlarge a small bladder to hold more urine

There are many different surgical procedures that may be used to treat incontinence. The type of operation you may need depends on the type and cause of your incontinence. Your doctor will discuss the specific procedure you might need.

Be sure to ask questions so that you fully understand the procedure.

Some other products can be used to help manage incontinence. These include pads and catheters. Catheters are used when a person cannot urinate. A catheter is a tube that is placed in the bladder to drain urine into a bag outside the body. The catheter usually is left inside the bladder, but some catheters are not left in. They are put in and taken out of the bladder as needed to empty it every few hours. Condom catheters (mostly used in men) attach to the outside of the body and are not placed directly in the bladder. Specially designed pads are available to help men and women with incontinence.

Catheters and pads are not the first and only treatment for incontinence. They should only be used to make other treatments more effective or when other treatments have failed.

What to Do Next

Your health care provider will tell you about the type of incontinence you have and will recommend a treatment. While you are being treated, be sure to:

- Ask questions
- Follow instructions
- Take all of your medicine
- Report side effects of your medicine, if any
- Report any changes, good and bad, to your health care provider

And remember, incontinence is not a natural part of aging. In most cases, it can be successfully treated and reversed.

Common Tests Used to Diagnose Urinary Incontinence

Blood Tests. Examines blood for levels of various chemicals.

Cystoscopy. Looks for abnormalities in bladder and lower urinary tract. It works by inserting a small tube into the bladder that has a telescope for the doctor to look through. Because you may be uncomfortable during part of this test, you may be given some medication to help relax you.

Post-void Residual (PVR) Measurement. Measures how much urine is left in the bladder after urinating by using ultrasound (sound waves).

Stress Test. Looks for urine loss when stress is put on bladder muscles usually by coughing, lifting, or exercise.

Urinalysis. Examines urine for signs of infection, blood, or other abnormality.

Urodynamic Testing. Examines bladder and urethral sphincter function (may involve inserting a small tube into the bladder; x-rays also can be used to see the bladder).

Risks and Benefits of Treatment

Three types of treatment are recommended for urinary incontinence:

- Behavioral techniques
- Medicine
- Surgery

How well each of these treatments works depends on the cause of the incontinence and, in some cases, patient effort. The risks and benefits described below are based on current medical knowledge and expert opinion. How well a treatment works may also depend on the individual patient. A treatment that works for one patient may not be as effective for another patient. Therefore, it is important to talk with a health care provider about treatment choices.

Behavioral techniques. Between 54 and 95 percent of persons using behavioral treatment show significant improvement in their incontinence. Between 12 and 16 percent of persons are cured. There are no risks for this type of treatment.

Medicine. As much as 77 percent of patients who need medicine to treat their incontinence show significant improvement, and 44 percent are cured. As with most drugs, there is a risk of having a side effect. If you are taking medicine for other conditions, the drugs could react with each other. Therefore, it is important to work with the health care provider and report all of your medicines and any side effects as soon as they happen.

Surgery. Approximately 78 to 92 percent of patients who need surgery to treat their incontinence are cured. With any surgery there is a possibility of a risk or complication. It is important to discuss these risks with your surgeon.

Coping with Incontinence

Several national organizations help people with urinary incontinence. They may be able to put you in touch with local groups that can give you more information, ideas, and emotional support in coping with urinary incontinence.

Alliance for Aging Research
(Information on bladder training program)
2021 K Street, N.W.
Suite 305
Washington, DC 20006

Help for Incontinent People
P.O. Box 544
Union, SC 29379
(803) 579-7900

Simon Foundation for Continence
Box 835
Wilmette, IL 60091
(800) 23-SIMON

Clinicians' Highlights of Patient Management

Editor's note: The following section is from the Quick-Reference Guide for Clinicians on Urinary Incontinence in Adults *from the U.S. Department of Health and Human Services. While it is geared toward professional health care workers, the information presented may also have value for the non-professional. Please discuss the following information with your physician.*

For this [chapter], urinary incontinence (UI) is defined as involuntary loss of urine sufficient to be a problem. This quick-reference guide addresses acquired incontinence in ambulatory patients in the outpatient and inpatient settings. The following items summarize a step-wise process of patient management.

Question patient about continence.

Use open-ended questions such as, "Do you have trouble with your bladder?" and "Do you have trouble holding your urine (water)?" Follow these with specific questions such as, "Do you ever lose urine when you don't want to?" and "Do you ever wear a pad or other protective device to collect your urine?"

Investigate patients who complain of incontinence.

It is important to follow through on patient complaints. Patients complaining of problems with continence must be evaluated.

Evaluate patient with a history, physical examination, and urinalysis.

Patients complaining of UI should be evaluated in the following manner:

1. Basic evaluative history with focused medical, neurologic, and genitourinary history and medication review, including non-prescription medications, and a detailed exploration of the UI-associated symptoms and factors:

    *   Duration and characteristics of the incontinence
    *   Frequency, timing, and amount of continent and incontinent voids

- Precipitants of incontinence (situational antecedents, abdominal pressure, surgery, trauma, disease)
- Other lower urinary tract symptoms (nocturia, dysuria, hesitancy, straining, interrupted stream, hematuria, pain, frequency, urgency, increased leakage)
- Fluid intake pattern
- Alterations in bowel habit or sexual function
- Previous treatment and effects on UI
- Use of pads, briefs, or other protective devices

2. Physical examination, which includes:

- Abdominal examination to detect masses, fullness, tenderness, and estimation of PVR volume
- Genital examination in men to detect abnormalities of foreskin, glans penis, and perineal skin
- Pelvic examination for atrophy, prolapse, skin condition, tenderness, muscle tone, hypermobility, etc.
- Rectal examination to test for rectal sensation, tone, fecal impaction, masses; bimanual estimation of PVR; and estimation of prostatic contour and consistency
- General examination, if indicated, to detect comorbid conditions such as edema and to assess cognition and manual dexterity if functional UI is suspected.

3. Urinalysis

Simple tests of urinary tract function may be required to clarify symptoms, identify abnormalities, and guide initial therapy.

4. Voiding diary

5. PVR values as follows:

- 200 mL—abnormal
- 50-199 mL—clinical judgment
- <50 mL—normal

6. Provocative stress testing

7. Blood tests

8. Urine cytology

9. Additional assessments (e.g., environmental and social factors)

Identify and manage transient causes of UI and exclude serious underlying conditions.

Following the basic evaluation, all incontinent patients with identified transient (reversible) causes of UI should be managed appropriately (see Table 36.1.1). Following such management, a decision should be made whether to pursue further evaluation or to initiate therapy.

Table 36.1.1
Common Causes of Transient Urinary Incontinence

Potential Causes

Delirium (confusional state). In the delirious patient, incontinence is usually an associated symptom that will abate with proper diagnosis and treatment of the underlying cause of confusion.

Infection (symptomatic urinary tract infection). Dysuria and urgency from symptomatic infection may defeat the older person's ability to reach the toilet in time. Asymptomatic infection, although more common than symptomatic infection, is rarely a cause of incontinence.

Atrophic urethritis or vaginitis. Atrophic urethritis may present as dysuria, dyspareunia, burning on urination, urgency, agitation (in demented patients), and occasionally as incontinence. Both disorders are readily treated by conjugated estrogen administered either orally (0.3-1.25 mg/d) or locally (2 g or fraction/d).

Pharmaceuticals as Potential Causes

Sedative Hypnotics. Benzodiazepines, especially long-acting agents, such as flurazepam and diazepam, may accumulate in elderly patients and cause confusion and secondary incontinence. Alcohol, frequently used as a sedative, can cloud the sensorium, impair mobility, and induce a diuresis, resulting in incontinence.

Diuretics. A brisk diuresis induced by loop diuretics can overwhelm bladder capacity and lead to polyuria, frequency, and urgency, thereby precipitating incontinence in a frail older person. The loop diuretics include furosemide, ethacrynic acid, and bumetanide.

Anticholinergic agents (Antihistamines, Antidepressants, Antipsychotics, Disopyramide, Opiates, Antispasmodics [dicyclomine and Donnatal], Anti-parkinsonian agents [trihexyphenidyl and benztropine mesylate]). Nonprescription (over-the-counter) agents with anticholinergic properties are taken commonly by older patients for insomnia, coryza, pruritus, and vertigo, and many prescription medications also have anticholinergic properties. Anticholinergic side effects include urinary retention with associated urinary frequency and overflow incontinence. Besides anticholinergic actions, antipsychotics such as thioridazine and haloperidol may cause sedation, rigidity agents and immobility.

Alpha-adrenergic agents, Sympathomimetics (decongestants) and Sympatholytics (e.g., prazosin, terazosin, and doxazosin). Sphincter tone in the proximal urethra can be decreased by alpha antagonists and increased by alpha agonists. An older woman, whose urethra is shortened and weakened with age, may develop stress incontinence when taking an alpha antagonist for hypertension. An older man with prostate enlargement may develop acute urinary retention and overflow incontinence when taking multicomponent "cold" capsules, which contain alpha agonists and anticholinergic agents, especially if a nasal decongestant and a nonprescription hypnotic antihistamine are added.

Calcium-channel blockers. Calcium-channel blockers can reduce smooth muscle contractility in the bladder and occasionally can cause urinary retention and overflow incontinence.

Psychological. Severe depression may occasionally be associated with incontinence, but is probably less frequently a cause in older patients.

Excessive urine production. Excess intake, endocrine conditions that production cloud the sensorium and induce a diuresis (e.g., hypercalcemia, hyperglycemia, and diabetes insipidus); expanded volume states such as congestive heart failure, lower extremity venous insufficiency, drug-induced ankle edema (e.g., nifedipine, indomethacin); and low albumen states cause polyuria and can lead to incontinence.

Restricted mobility. Limited mobility is an aggravating or precipitating cause of incontinence that can frequently be corrected or improved by treating the underlying condition (e.g., arthritis, poor eyesight, Parkinson's disease, or orthostatic hypotension). A urinal or bedside commode and scheduled toileting often help resolve the incontinence that results from hospitalization and its environmental barriers (e.g., bed rails, restraints, and poor lighting).

Stool impaction. Patients with stool impaction present with either urge or overflow incontinence and may have fecal incontinence as well. Disimpaction restores continence.

Adapted from Winograd, C.H. and Resnick, N.M. (1991). Incontinence. In Rubenstein, E. and Federman, D.D. (eds)., Scientific American Medicine, Volume IX. Disorders in Geriatric Patients (p.6). New York: Scientific American Press.

Identify the type of UI.

Individuals who do not have transient UI or whose incontinence persists may have incontinence that can be classified as stress, urge, or overflow.

1. Stress incontinence: Involuntary loss of urine during coughing, sneezing, laughing, or other physical activity. The symptom may be confirmed by observing urine loss during activities that incur increased abdominal pressure (stress).

2. Urge incontinence: Involuntary loss of urine associated with an abrupt and strong desire to void (urgency). Urge UI is usually associated with urinary frequency, urgency, or a complaint of "I'm unable to make it to the bathroom on time." At times, urine loss is massive and sudden, occurring with little or no warning at all.

3. Overflow incontinence: Involuntary loss of urine associated with overdistension of the bladder (overflow). This type of UI

may have a variety of presentations including frequent or constant dribbling, or may include urge or stress UI symptoms.

4. Mixed incontinence: It is not unusual for patients to present with a combination of urge and stress incontinence. Many frail elderly patients have components of both urge and stress UI. When dealing with mixed symptoms, use the algorithm for the type of incontinence that predominates.

Identify need for further evaluation by a specialist.

Patients requiring further evaluation include those who meet one of the following criteria:

1. Uncertain diagnosis and inability to develop a reasonable management plan based on the basic diagnostic evaluation — possibly due to lack of correlation between symptomatology and clinical findings

2. Failure to respond to an adequate therapeutic trial

3. Hematuria without infection

4. The presence of other comorbid conditions, such as:

    *   Incontinence associated with recurrent symptomatic urinary tract infections
    *   Severe symptoms of difficult bladder emptying
    *   Severe symptomatic pelvic prolapse
    *   Prostate nodule
    *   Abnormal PVR urine volume.

Note: Referral is not suggested for patients in whom further investigation is not feasible.

Identify treatment options.

The three major categories of treatment are behavioral, pharmacologic, and surgical. Patients should be informed of all the treatment options including their risks, benefits, and outcomes. As a general rule, the least invasive and least dangerous procedure that is appropriate for the patient should be the first choice. For many forms of UI, behavioral techniques meet these criteria. However, an informed patient's preference must be respected.

Tables 36.1.2, 36.1.3, and 36.1.4 summarize outcomes of the various treatment options for patients with stress and urge UI undergoing behavioral, pharmacologic, and surgical treatments.

Behavioral techniques.

Before implementing behavioral therapy, patients should have the basic evaluation completed. The basic evaluation should rule out overflow UI that would preclude a behavioral intervention, but identification of specific voiding dysfunctions is often not needed. Behavioral interventions usually include:

- Bladder training for urge and stress UI
- Habit training for urge UI
- Prompted toileting in frail or cognitively impaired persons
- Pelvic muscle exercises for urge and stress UI

Pharmacologic treatment.

1. Drugs for incontinence due to detrusor overactivity.

    - Anticholinergic/antispasmodic agents. The purpose of these drugs is to relax the bladder and increase bladder capacity. *Note: All anticholinergic drugs are contraindicated in patients with narrow-angle but not wide-angle glaucoma.*

    - Propantheline. Recommended at 7.5–30 mg in the fasting state, t.i.d.-q.i.d. (higher dosages may be needed).

    - Oxybutynin. *Recommended at 2.5–5 mg, p.o., t.i.d.

    - Tricyclic agents. Imipramine and doxepin may be beneficial at 10–100 mg, p.o./d, initially in divided doses.

    - Dicyclomine hydrochloride. Clinical experience suggests that this drug is as effective as other anticholinergic agents in controlling detrusor overactivity. Dose is 10–20 mg, t.i.d., p.o.

2. Drugs for incontinence due to urethral sphincter insufficiency.

    - Alpha-adrenergic agonist agents. These drugs increase urethral resistance by stimulation of urethral smooth muscle acting on alpha-adrenergic receptors in the urethra.

    - Phenylpropanolamine (PPA). The recommended dose is 25–75 mg, p.o., q. 12h.

    - *Note: These drugs should be used with caution in patients with hypertension, hyperthyroidism, cardiac arrhythmias, and angina.*

3. Estrogen supplementation therapy.

    Estrogen replacement in postmenopausal woman may restore urethral mucosal coaptation. Estrogen replacement should be given with a progestin when endometrial tissue is present. (Atrophic vaginitis should be treated cyclically with conjugated estrogen, 0.3–1.25 mg/d, p.o., or vaginally, 2 g or fraction/d). Progestin 2.5–10 mg/d continuous or intermittent.

4. Combined alpha-adrenergic agonist and estrogen supplementation therapy.

    Based on three well-controlled studies and clinical experience to date, combination therapy may be considered when an initial single drug therapy fails.

5. Imipramine.

    Imipramine may be beneficial in the treatment of stress and urge UI at the recommended dose of 10–100 mg, p.o./d, initially in divided doses. *Note: Imipramine is officially approved by the FDA for enuresis in children but not for adults.*

    *Drugs marked with a single asterisk have been officially approved by the FDA for the indicated use. The remainder are not approved but are commonly used.

Surgical management.

Presurgical assessment requires a comprehensive clinical evaluation, including estimation of surgical risk, objective confirmation of diagnosis and severity, correlation of anatomic and physiologic findings with surgical plan, and estimation of impact of proposed surgery on patient quality of life. See chart which follows.

Table 36.1.2
Outcome of Stress Incontinence Treatments

Behavorial Technique

Pelvic Muscle Exercise. 12% Cured, 75% Improved, No side effects or complications.

Bladder Training. 16% Cured, 54% Improved. No side effects or complications.

Pharmacologic Treatment

Alpha-agonist. 0–14% Cured, 19–60% Improved. Minimal to 20% had side effects. 5–33% had complications.

Surgical Technique

Retropubic suspension. 78% Cured, 5% Improved. 20% reported complications.

Needle suspension. 84% Cured, 4% Improved. 20% reported complications.

The figures used represent the average reported outcome within a given management option (e.g., behavioral, pharmacologic) based on the literature review. The figures do not apply equally across specific treatments within a given management option (e.g., pelvic muscle exercise vs. oxybutynin) because the studies lack uniformity in many critical issues including outcome criteria, types of subjects used, treatment protocol, follow up period, analytical method, etc.

Table 36.1.3
Outcome of Urge Incontinence Treatments

Behavorial Technique: Bladder Training

Outcome: 12% Cured, 75% Improved, no side effects.

Pharmacologic Anticholinergic

Outcome: 0–44% Cured, 0–83% Improved, 0–70% side effects.

The figures used represent the average reported outcome within a given management option (e.g., behavioral, pharmacologic) based on the literature review. The figures do not apply equally across specific treatments within a given management option (e.g., pelvic muscle exercise vs. oxybutynin) because the studies lack uniformity in many critical issues including outcome criteria, types of subjects used, treatment protocol, follow up period, analytical method, etc.

Table 36.1.4
Surgical Outcome for Female Intrinsic Sphincter Deficiency

Treatment Options

Bulking Technique

Teflon: 59% Cured, 16% Improved, 75% Cured/Improved, 6% complications.

Collagen: 69% Cured, 25% Improved, 94% Cured/Improved, no complications.

Sling Operation

89% Cured, 6% Improved, 95% Cured/Improved, 31% complications.

Artificial Urinary Sphincter

92% Cured, 4% Improved, 96% Cured/Improved, 32% complications.

The figures used represent the average reported outcome within a given management option (e.g., behavioral, pharmacologic) based on the literature review. The figures do not apply equally across specific treatments within a given management option (e.g., pelvic muscle exercise vs. oxybutynin) because the studies lack uniformity in many critical issues including outcome criteria, types of used, treatment protocol, follow up period, analytical method, etc.

For Further Information

The information in this chapter was taken from the *Clinical Practice Guideline on Urinary Incontinence in Adults*. The guideline was developed by an expert panel of doctors, nurses, other health care providers, and consumers sponsored by the Agency for Health Care Policy and Research. Other guidelines on common health problems are being developed and will be released in the near future. For more information about the guidelines or to receive additional copies of this booklet, contact:

Agency for Health Care Policy and Research
Publications Clearinghouse
Post Office Box 8547
Silver Spring, MD 20907
(800) 358-9295
(301) 495-3453

Section 36.2

Incontinence Comes Out of the Closet

FDA Consumer, March 1987.

Unless 9-year-old Linda is wakened for a trip to the bathroom several times a night, she wets the bed. She's afraid to go on "sleep-overs" with friends, and time after time she comes home with her sweater tied around her hips to hide the fact that she's wet her clothes.

Greg, a successful young businessman, quit his job right after being promoted. The new position involved travel and, on the road, he was required to share hotel rooms. But he couldn't face his co-workers' finding out about his incontinence. Greg settled for a lower-paying job elsewhere.

Marion, age 72, dreads returning to her dentist. She wet the dental chair during her last visit because her appointment took longer than she had anticipated.

For Linda, Greg, Marion, and others who suffer from urinary incontinence, or the involuntary passing of urine, here's good news: Incontinence can be treated and often cured, even in the elderly.

The National Institute on Aging estimates that over 12 million Americans are incontinent. In nursing homes, more than 50 percent of patients over 65 are so affected; in fact, incontinence is the second most common reason for institutionalizing older people. (Dementia, or mental deterioration, is the first.) Outside nursing homes, incontinence afflicts about 17 percent of elderly men and 37 percent of elderly women. It's particularly troubling for older women because they generally live longer than men.

Incontinence is costly, in dollars and in psychological trauma. U.S. Surgeon General C. Everett Koop has estimated that, in nursing homes alone, the annual cost of caring for incontinent people is nearly $8 billion. And though incontinence isn't life-threatening, the stigma attached to clothes-wetting, bed-wetting, and the resultant odor can inflict profound consequences: humiliation, depression and social with-drawal. Even in the lives of people with only mild leakage, inconti-nence can be a ruling force.

Sad to say, only one in 12 people with incontinence seeks medical help—a fact perhaps due to embarrassment, isolation, or the mistaken notion that incontinence is normal with aging.

"Incontinence is no more a normal part of aging than is chest pain or diabetes," said Dr. Neil Resnick, of the Harvard Medical School, at a national conference sponsored in 1986 by the Food and Drug Ad-ministration and the Public Health Service Coordinating Committee on Women's Health Issues.

Normally, the urinary system removes waste products from the body in a well-coordinated fashion. Through nerve pathways, the brain synchronizes the individual housecleaning tasks that nature has as-signed to different body parts: The two kidneys move wastes from the blood into the urine, tubes called ureters (one per kidney) channel the urine to the sac-like muscle called the bladder for storage, and then, as needed, two sphincter muscles open and close the bladder outlet to control urine flow to the outside via a tube known as the urethra.

But sometimes the system doesn't work the way it's supposed to. As Harvard's Resnick put it: "Either the bladder contracts when it should not, leading to the patient's being wet, or it fails to contract when it should, so that urine builds up and spills over.... Either the outlet is open when it ought to be closed or it is closed when it ought to be open." Resnick added that such factors generally associated with aging, such as illness, medicines, and the weakening of the urinary system, can increase a person's risk of incontinence.

Incontinence occurs when one of those working parts is adversely affected—by an obstruction in the urethral tube, for instance, or by an abnormality in the sphincter muscle, bladder muscle, or both. It may result from a condition as common as chronic constipation, par-ticularly if stool is impacted, or from the lack of nearby toilets, as may be the case for some patients in institutions. It may develop after a hysterectomy or prostate, rectal, or lower intestinal surgery. Obesity and childbirth also can contribute to incontinence. Other causes in-clude drug side effects, multiple sclerosis, cancer, spinal cord injury, diabetes mellitus, stroke, Parkinson's or Alzheimer's disease, and birth defects—80 percent to 90 percent of children born with spina bifida are incontinent.

When acute (relatively severe, but of short duration) incontinence occurs, it's generally the result of another acute medical problem. For instance, a heart attack or some type of infection may cause a mental state called delirium, in which consciousness can become so clouded that the patient has difficulty controlling the bladder. Persistent incontinence, on the other hand, is not associated with an acute medical problem; it often worsens over time and can occur in different ways:

- **Stress incontinence.** Minor physical stress such as coughing, sneezing, laughing or lifting results in small amounts of urine leakage. This is common in older women, but is usually not seen in men unless there has been sphincter damage during surgery.

- **Overflow incontinence.** The person doesn't feel the urge to void or isn't able to urinate normal amounts ("normal" generally being 8 to 20 ounces), so the bladder overfills and spills small amounts of urine.

- **Urge incontinence.** The person feels a strong desire to urinate, but can't get to a toilet before the bladder empties.

- **Primary enuresis.** This is the term most commonly used for bed-wetting in children beyond the age (5 years) when they should be capable of bladder control and in adults who never gained nighttime control.

- **Reflex incontinence.** The bladder fills and empties without the person's having any mental control over it at all.

The key weapon in the psychological and physical battle to stay dry is: Tell your physician about the incontinence, so that a correct diagnosis can be made and treatment options can be discussed. Ask whether you should consult a specialist in treating incontinence (for children, for example, a urologist who specializes in pediatric problems; for adults, a geriatrician, gynecologist or urologist). Early diagnosis and treatment are important for many reasons, but they can be life-saving when the incontinence is the first sign of a serious medical condition, such as a tumor. If help isn't forthcoming, see another doctor.

To begin the medical investigation, the physician usually takes a patient's history and performs an examination. Urine and blood specimens are collected, and tests are performed—how many and what type depend on the patient's symptoms and history.

Patients may be asked to undergo procedures called "urodynamic" tests to help the physician pinpoint whether the problem lies in the urinary system and, if so, where. They're done on an outpatient basis. One such test measured the speed of urine flow from the bladder as the person urinates into a special toilet connected to a machine. An obstruction would cause the flow to be slower than normal. Other procedures test the sphincter and bladder muscles, as follows: One end of a catheter (a small plastic tube) is passed up the urethra to the bladder, and an electrode carried by the catheter is attached to the sphincter. Then, electrical impulses coming from the sphincter muscles and pressure changes within the bladder are recorded. The physician evaluates the readings to see whether the muscles are functioning normally.

Other types of tests may be ordered as well.

Physicians treat incontinence by treating its underlying cause. Treatments include:

- **Battery-operated alarm.** Used for bed-wetting, the alarm is triggered by the wetting. Initially, for children, it may be necessary for someone in the household to respond to the alarm and waken the patient. Once patients become conscious of the alarm, they should waken on their own when it rings. Eventually, the patients are supposed to become so used to waking when wetting occurs that they start waking beforehand.

- **Scheduled voiding regimens.** For urge incontinence, patients may be asked to wait longer before urinating, gradually increasing the "waiting period," or to urinate only at assigned intervals. Mentally impaired patients may be prompted to stay dry by simply being asked if they need to urinate and, if so, helped to the toilet. What works for one incontinence problem may not work for another, so it's best to get medical advice before beginning a regimen. And, generally, women shouldn't put off urinating, as that can promote bladder infections.

- **"Kegel" exercises.** In 1948 Arnold Kegel, M.D., who was practicing in Los Angeles at that time, introduced exercises to strengthen the pelvic floor muscles in women with stress incontinence and, so, to preserve or regain bladder control. It's possible to feel where these muscles are, at one end of the pelvic floor, by interrupting the flow several times during urination and, at the other end, by drawing in the muscle around the anus as if to stop a bowel movement. The patient is supposed to repeat the exercises—interrupting each urination and tightening the pelvic floor muscles from back to front—many times throughout the day.

Harvard's Resnick advises that all women who aren't pregnant practice Kegel exercises to strengthen the pelvic floor muscles, which, in turn, may help ward off incontinence later in life. But, he says, people usually need professional instruction to do them correctly.

- **Drugs.** Estrogen therapy is prescribed for women with estrogen deficiency. The condition can cause the tissue lining of the urethra to become inflamed, and the irritated tissue can cause or worsen urge incontinence. The antispasmodic drug flavoxate is prescribed to treat incontinence associated with such conditions as cystitis (inflammation of the bladder). Flavoxate decreases muscle spasms in the bladder. However, the large dosages that are often required can be hazardous to other tissue, and the patient may have to contend with undesirable side effects, such as dry mouth, constipation, and blurred vision.

- **Reevaluation of drug therapy.** Incontinence may be due to drugs the person is taking for some other condition: Sedatives or tranquilizers may dull the senses so much that the urge to urinate isn't felt; anticholinergics prescribed for bowel spasm can decrease the bladder's ability to contract; diuretics, often given to lower blood pressure, increase urine production; and cold medicines may increase the bladder outlet's resistance so that the bladder doesn't completely empty. Upon reevaluation, the physician may find that a different drug will work without causing incontinence.

- **Surgical procedures.** Even frail, elderly patients can easily tolerate a number of newer corrective procedures, says Resnick. Deep abdominal surgery is usually not required; rather, the surgeon works through the vagina or a tiny abdominal incision and uses an endoscope (a narrow tube-like instrument inserted via the urethra or the incision) to see inside the bladder. This way, the surgeon can relieve an obstruction, tie up pelvic floor tissues to return a sagging urethra or bladder to a normal position, or

445

repair a constantly opening bladder outlet so that it closes properly. The hospital stay is usually only a day or two; a younger person may be in and out of the hospital the same day. Other surgical options may be to implant an artificial sphincter or to reconstruct the bladder.

Sometimes the underlying cause of the incontinence can't be cured, but the situation is still far from hopeless. There are many measures to help a person stay dry: more frequent trips to the toilet, a portable commode for invalids, and self-catheterization (after proper instructions) to empty the bladder several times a day. There are urine collection devices and disposable pads and pants available from medical supply stores, certain drugstores, and home health-care catalogs. One product may work better than another, so a person may want to try several. Also, oral deodorant tablets can be taken as an aid to reduce urinary odor. The active ingredient, chlorophyllin copper complex, helps to mask the odor.

Incontinence will probably never lead the list of tea-time topics of conversation. But health professionals, public health officials, women's groups, the media, makers of incontinence-related products, and others personally acquainted with the difficult problem are erasing the incontinence stigma. Actress June Allyson, appearing in ads that promote disposable absorbent pants, unashamedly acknowledges that her mother became incontinent after a stroke and that they're dealing with it. By being so frank, Allyson also promotes the idea that it's all right to talk about incontinence. Two support groups for incontinent patients were incorporated in 1983: HIP, or Help for Incontinent People, and The Simon Foundation, whose founder-director is herself incontinent. The groups offer information about such topics as recovery after prostate surgery, cleaning urine stains from clothing, incontinence-treatment products, and treatment options. To receive an information packet (there may be a charge), send the request and a stamped, self-addressed, business-size envelope to:

- HIP, P.O. Box 544, Union, S.C. 29379 (phone 803-585-8789), or
- The Simon Foundation, P.O. Box 835, Wilmette, III. 60091 (phone 1-800-23SIMON).

—by Dixie Farley

Section 36.3

NIH Consensus on Adult Urinary Incontinence

NIH Consensus Statement, October 1988.

Introduction

Urinary incontinence, the involuntary loss of urine so severe as to have social and/or hygienic consequences, is a major clinical problem and a significant cause of disability and dependency. Urinary incontinence affects all age groups and is particularly common in the elderly. At least 10 million adult Americans suffer from urinary incontinence, including approximately 15 to 30 percent of community-dwelling older people and at least one-half of all nursing home residents. The monetary costs of managing urinary incontinence are conservatively estimated at $10.3 billion annually, and the psychosocial burden of urinary incontinence is great.

Urinary incontinence is a symptom rather than a disease. It appears in a limited number of clinical patterns, each having several possible causes. In some cases, the disorder is transient, secondary to an easily reversed cause such as a medication or an acute illness like urinary tract infection. Many cases are chronic, however, lasting indefinitely unless properly diagnosed and treated.

There is a persistent myth that urinary incontinence is a normal consequence of aging. While normal aging is not a cause of urinary incontinence, age-related changes in lower urinary tract function predispose the older person to urinary incontinence in the face of additional anatomic or physiologic insults to the lower urinary tract or by systemic disturbances such as illnesses common in older people.

Even frail nursing home residents or persons being cared for by family caregivers often have urinary incontinence that can be significantly improved or cured. Persons with urinary incontinence should be alerted to the importance of reporting their symptoms to a health

447

care professional and of asserting their right to proper assessment, diagnosis, and treatment. The first steps to treatment are acknowledgment of the problem and appropriate assessment and diagnosis.

Knowledge of the occurrence, causes, consequences, and treatment of the specific forms of urinary incontinence has increased. While new diagnostic tests have been developed, well-defined guidelines are needed for their application. Similarly, despite numerous new potential therapies, opinions differ widely concerning the best approach to many specific forms of the disorder. The most common treatments include pelvic muscle exercises and other behavioral treatments, local and systemic drug therapies, and a variety of surgical approaches.

The number of patients with urinary incontinence who are not successfully treated remains surprisingly high. This is due to several factors, including under reporting by patients; under recognition as a significant clinical problem by health providers; lack of education of health providers regarding new research findings; inadequate staffing in the long-term care setting; and the persistent major gaps in our understanding of the natural history, pathophysiology, and most effective treatments of the common forms of urinary incontinence. The amount of basic research as well as research focusing on prevention is meager.

To resolve issues regarding the incidence, causes, and consequences of urinary incontinence in adults, the National Institute on Aging and the Office of Medical Applications of Research of the National Institutes of Health, in conjunction with the National Institute of Diabetes and Digestive and Kidney Diseases, the National Center for Nursing Research, the National Institute of Neurological and Communicative Disorders and Stroke, and the Veterans Administration, convened a Consensus Development Conference on Urinary Incontinence in Adults on October 3-5, 1988. After a day and a half of presentations by experts in the relevant fields involved with urinary incontinence, a consensus panel consisting of representatives from geriatrics, urology, gynecology, psychology, nursing, epidemiology, basic sciences, and the public considered the evidence and developed answers to the following central questions:

- What is the prevalence and clinical, psychological, and social impact of urinary incontinence among persons living at home and in institutions?

- What are the pathophysiological and functional factors leading to urinary incontinence?

- What diagnostic information should be obtained in assessment of the incontinent patient? What criteria should be employed to determine which tests are indicated for a particular patient?

- What are the efficacies and limitations of behavioral, pharmacological, surgical, and other treatments for urinary incontinence? What sequences and/or combination of these interventions are appropriate? What management techniques are appropriate when treatment is not effective or indicated?

- What strategies are effective in improving public and professional knowledge about urinary incontinence?

- What are the needs for future research related to urinary incontinence?

What Is the Prevalence and Clinical, Psychological, and Social Impact of Urinary Incontinence Among Persons Living at Home and in Institutions?

Occurrence and Risk

Estimates of the occurrence of urinary incontinence depend on the nature of the study population and definition of the disorder. Prevalence rates range from 8 to 51 percent; an estimate of 15 to 30 percent for community-dwelling older persons seems reasonable, and of these, 20 to 25 percent may be classified as severe. Prevalence rates are twice as high in women as in men, and are higher in older than in younger adults. Though these community rates are alarmingly high, rates in nursing homes are even higher. Half or more of the 1.5 million Americans in nursing homes suffer from urinary incontinence.

Little is known about the natural history of urinary incontinence, including age at onset, incidence rates, progression, and spontaneous remission. Limited data exist on associated morbidity and functional impairment. To date, most studies have been conducted in whites, and data are needed on the occurrence in nonwhite ethnic groups.

Though urinary incontinence is a symptom of many conditions, defining risk factors would be extremely useful for identifying high-risk persons and remediable environmental causes. While age, gender, and parity are established risk factors, many other factors have been suggested but not rigorously proven. These include urinary infection, menopause, genitourinary surgery, lack of postpartum exercise, chronic illnesses, and various medications. Risk factor identification is essential for a concerted effort at prevention.

Clinical, Psychological, and Social Impact

In the Community

Because only about half of the people with incontinence in the community have consulted a doctor about the problem, the true extent and clinical impact of urinary incontinence is not known. Rashes, pressure sores, skin and urinary tract infections, and restriction of activity are some of the problems that could be prevented or treated if the underlying incontinence were brought to medical attention. Many people with incontinence turn prematurely to the use of absorbent materials without having their difficulty properly diagnosed and treated.

The psychosocial impact of incontinence in the community falls on individuals and their care providers. Studies of women show that the condition is associated with depressive symptoms and leads to embarrassment about appearance and odor, although such reactions may be related more to illness than to incontinence. Excursions outside the home, social interactions with friends and family, and sexual activity may be restricted or avoided entirely in the presence of incontinence. Spouses and other intimates also may share the burden of this condition. A highly conservative estimate of the direct costs of caring for persons with incontinence of all ages in the community is $7 billion annually in the United States.

In Nursing Homes

Many physicians fail to recognize the clinical impact of urinary incontinence in nursing homes, and very few nursing home residents with incontinence have had any type of diagnostic evaluation. In this setting, fecal incontinence, physical and mental impairment, pressure sores, and urinary tract infections are commonly associated with urinary incontinence, but cause-and-effect relationships are not clear. Many nursing home residents who are incontinent are managed with indwelling catheters, which carry an increased risk of significant urinary tract infection, and the use of such devices varies widely. The odor of urine that permeates many nursing homes can be repellent to residents, staff, and potential visitors. Managing those with incontinence presents a major problem to insufficient and often untrained staff. The annual direct cost of caring for incontinence among nursing home patients is approximately $3.3 billion.

What Are The Pathophysiological and Functional Factors Leading to Urinary Incontinence?

Continence requires a compliant bladder and active sphincteric mechanisms, such that maximum urethral pressure always exceeds intravesical pressure. Normal voiding requires sustained and coordinated relaxation of the sphincters and contraction of the urinary bladder.

These functions are regulated by the central nervous system through autonomic and somatic nerves. The system requires the integration of visceral and somatic muscle function and involves control by voluntary mechanisms originating in the cerebral cortex. These voluntary mechanisms are learned and culturally prescribed (i.e., toilet training).

Incontinence can be produced by any pathologic, anatomic, or physiologic factor that causes intravesical pressure to exceed maximum urethral pressure. Intravesical pressure can be raised by involuntary detrusor contractions (unstable bladder or detrusor hyperreflexia), by acute or chronic bladder overdistension (urinary retention with overflow), or by an increase in intra-abdominal pressure. Similarly, a decrease in urethral pressure may occur as a result of uninhibited sphincter relaxation (unstable urethra), loss of pelvic floor support (genuine stress incontinence), and urethral wall defects from trauma, surgery, or neurologic disease.

Subtypes of Urinary Incontinence

The most commonly encountered clinical forms of urinary incontinence in adults are stress incontinence, urge incontinence, overflow incontinence, and a mixed form. In stress incontinence, dysfunction of the bladder outlet leads to leakage of urine as intra-abdominal pressure is raised above urethral resistance while coughing, bending, or lifting heavy objects. Volume of urine leakage is generally modest at each occurrence and, in uncomplicated cases, postvoid residual volume is low. Stress incontinence has many causes, including direct anatomic damage to the urethral sphincter (sphincteric incontinence), which may lead to severe, continuous leakage, and weakening of bladder neck supports, as is often associated with parity.

Urge incontinence occurs when patients sense the urge to void (urgency) but are unable to inhibit leakage long enough to reach the toilet. In most, but not all, cases, uninhibited bladder contractions contribute to the incontinence. Urine loss is moderate in volume, occurs at several hour intervals, and postvoid residual volume is low at several hour intervals. Among the causes of urge incontinence are central nervous system lesions such as stroke or demyelinating disease, which impair inhibition of bladder contraction, and local irritating factors such as urinary infection or bladder tumors. In many cases of urge incontinence, no specific etiology can be identified despite detailed clinical and laboratory evaluation.

An important variant of urge incontinence is reflex incontinence, in which urine is lost due to uninhibited bladder contractions in the absence of the symptoms of urgency. In addition, many persons suffer from very frequent symptoms of urgency and are only able to remain continent by conducting their activities in the proximity of restrooms.

Overflow incontinence occurs when the bladder cannot empty normally and becomes overdistended, leading to frequent, sometimes nearly constant, urine loss. Causes include neurologic abnormalities that impair detrusor contractile capacity, including spinal cord lesions, and any factor that obstructs outflow, including medications, tumors, benign strictures, and prostatic hypertrophy.

Many cases of urinary incontinence fall into the mixed category, displaying some aspects of more than one of the major subtypes, both clinically and on extensive laboratory evaluation.

The term "functional" incontinence is applied to those cases in which the function of the lower urinary tract is intact, but other factors such as immobility or severe cognitive impairment result in urinary incontinence.

It should be clear that urinary incontinence can be caused by multiple and often interacting conditions. Of particular importance are the transient or reversible factors such as infection, delirium, and drugs. These causes, which may be common in the elderly patient, should be carefully considered in the pathophysiology of urinary incontinence.

There are age-related changes in the lower urinary tract that increase its vulnerability to both chronic and transient factors. Increases in uninhibited contractions, nocturnal fluid excretion, and prostate size, accompanied by decreases in bladder capacity and flow rate, all lead to greater susceptibility to urinary incontinence in the face of stresses associated with disease, functional impairment, or environmental factors. In older persons, cognitive decline, musculoskeletal impairments, and restricted access to toilets may all convert the marginally continent system to incontinence.

What Diagnostic Information Should Be Obtained in Assessment of the Incontinent Patient? What Criteria Should Be Employed to Determine Which Tests Are Indicated for a Particular Patient?

Evaluation and therapy must be tailored to the individual, taking into account clinical, cognitive, functional, and residential status in addition to the potential for correcting the problem. Just as a child is not simply a young adult, octogenarians differ from persons in their forties. Patients with stress urinary incontinence are quite dissimilar from those with uninhibited contractions and unstable bladders. Proper diagnosis and active case finding are imperative.

Evaluation

History

The evaluation of all patients with incontinence requires a thorough history, including medical, urologic, gynecologic, and neurologic assessment, with particular attention to those factors that influence bladder function. The duration, frequency, volume, and type of incontinence should be described and validated by a voiding diary. Other important information includes associated illnesses, previous operations, and current medications.

Physical Examination

Physical examination is required, with emphasis on mental status; mobility and dexterity; and neurologic, abdominal, rectal, and pelvic findings. A provoked full-bladder stress test is recommended. Since prostate enlargement is often asymmetric, the size of the prostate as estimated on rectal exam may be misleading when evaluating the possible contribution of prostatic hypertrophy to urinary obstruction.

In addition to the history and physical examination, core measurements to be obtained in all patients are urinalysis, serum creatinine or blood urea nitrogen, and postvoid residual urine volume. Other tests such as urine culture, blood glucose, and urinary cytology may be useful.

Based on the findings from the core evaluation, a decision for treatment or more definitive evaluation is made, taking into consideration the type and degree of incontinence.

Specialized Studies

The tests currently available for specialized study include:

- Cystometrogram—to be used as the basic study in cases requiring more than core evaluation, should be accompanied by measurement or estimation of abdominal pressure.
- Electrophysiologic sphincter testing (EMG).
- Ultrasound of the bladder or kidneys may detect residual urine or hydronephrosis.
- Cystourethroscopy with or without cytology is indicated in patients with hematuria or the recent onset of urgency or urge incontinence who are at increased risk for carcinoma.
- Uroflowmetry has wide application in the evaluation of obstructive disease in men but a limited role in the evaluation of women.
- Videourodynamic evaluation requires special expertise. Its role is limited to the more elusive incontinence problems.
- Urethral pressure profilometry is a controversial test. Its predictive value has been questioned, and it requires further validation before it can be recommended for widespread use.

These numerous noninvasive and invasive tests must be used selectively. Examples of patients rarely requiring further diagnostic testing after the core examination include the young woman with classic stress incontinence or the 80-year-old woman with a recent stroke and the new onset of urge incontinence. Patients with stress incontinence and a significant urge component or those in whom previous operations have failed may require combined cystography and fluoroscopy with a complete urodynamic evaluation. Some patients with urge or mixed incontinence, or those who are not helped by empiric therapy or operation, also will require more complete urodynamic testing. Some patients may not be candidates for sophisticated studies due to inability to cooperate or a poor prognosis for correction. Armed with this information, the investigating physician should be able to reach an accurate diagnosis leading to appropriate therapy.

What Are the Efficacies and Limitations of Behavioral, Pharmacological, Surgical, and Other Treatments For Urinary Incontinence? What Sequences and/or Combination of These Interventions Are Appropriate?

General Principles of Treatment

- All persons with incontinence should be considered for evaluation and treatment.
- Treatment decisions should be based on a diagnosis made after a reasonable evaluation of anatomy and function of urine storage and emptying.
- Treatment for incontinence is given to a specific individual, whose personality, environment, expectations, and clinical status are important determinants of treatment modalities to be used and the order of their application.
- The patient requires sufficient information and explanation to be able to make a choice among therapeutic options.
- Environmental constraints in the community or in an institution that may impede treatment are common, and strategies to circumvent impediments are a part of the therapy.
- In particular, availability of adequate numbers of properly constructed public toilets is an important adjunct to incontinence management.

Pharmacologic Treatment

Most drugs currently used in managing the varied causes of urinary incontinence have not been studied in well-designed clinical trials. Nevertheless, it has been suggested that many agents are beneficial, especially for urge incontinence due to uninhibited detrusor contractions. For these patients, drugs that increase bladder capacity can be helpful. One attendant risk is the precipitation of retention. Accordingly, outlet obstruction or a weak detrusor should be looked for as possible contraindications to these agents.

Bladder Relaxants

These agents are generally used for urge incontinence:

Anticholinergics

Anticholinergic agents inhibit detrusor contraction, and may produce increased bladder capacity and delay and reduction in amplitude of involuntary contractions. Propantheline is frequently effective, although high doses may produce unacceptable side effects such as dry mouth, dry eyes, constipation, confusion, or precipitation of glaucoma.

Direct Smooth Muscle Relaxants

These antispasmodics work directly on bladder muscle, but they have a mild anticholinergic effect as well. A randomized, double-blind, placebo-controlled study has shown benefit with oxybutynin in patients with detrusor instability, some but not all of whom were incontinent. Favorable reports also exist about flavoxate and dicyclomine, the other two agents in this class.

Calcium Channel Blockers

These agents, used clinically for cardiovascular indications, have a depressant effect on the bladder as well, but they have not been studied rigorously for the treatment of urge incontinence in comparison with other agents. In the patient being considered for treatment for heart disease, the bladder effects of calcium antagonists must be kept in mind for both their potential benefit as well as risk of retention.

Imipramine

This tricyclic antidepressant has anticholinergic and direct relaxant effects on the detrusor and an alpha adrenergic enhancing (contracting) effect on the bladder outlet, all of which enhance continence. Although imipramine is commonly used, potential side effects of postural hypotension and sedation as well as all peripheral anticholinergic effects make caution imperative when considering this agent in older persons.

Bladder Outlet Stimulants

Alpha adrenergic agonists, used in treatment of stress incontinence, produce smooth muscle contraction at the bladder outlet and may improve continence. Pseudoephedrine and ephedrine both are active, but phenylpropanolamine has been used most often, and objective benefit by urodynamic study has been shown.

Estrogens

Because urinary incontinence increases in women with increasing age, and because menopause results in estrogen deficiency, estrogen replacement has been thought to be helpful for urinary incontinence. Several studies have shown no improvement in stress incontinence, but women with postmenopausal urge incontinence, urgency, and frequency have shown improvement. Long-term use should be considered in view of other risks and benefits.

Surgery

Surgery is particularly effective in treatment of pure stress incontinence associated with urethrocoele. A variety of surgical techniques for the transvaginal or transabdominal suspension of the bladder neck yield a success rate between 80 and 95 percent in appropriately selected patients with stress incontinence at 1-year follow up. Long-term results require study. When incontinence in men is secondary to outflow obstruction and chronic retention is secondary to prostatic enlargement, it is best treated with prostatectomy.

In addition, there are several specialized and more extensive surgical procedures. When incontinence is due to intrinsic sphincter dysfunction, which may occur after the surgical trauma of radical prostatectomy or sphincter denervation, the compressive action of the sphincter is lost. An implantable prosthetic sphincter can restore this compression. Continence is restored in 70 to 90 percent of patients in various series. A complication rate greater than 20 percent includes erosion of the urethra, infection, and mechanical failure. Reoperations are frequently required.

Urethral sling procedures pass a ribbon of fascia or artificial material beneath the urethra. The sling, fixed to the anterior body wall, serves to elevate and compress the urethra, restoring continence in 80 percent of patients. Bladder augmentation with isolated bowel segments will increase bladder capacity and vent excessive bladder pressure. This procedure is limited to certain specific bladder problems such as the contracted bladder of neurologic disease or tuberculosis. Bladder replacement with continent diversion can also be offered to the cystectomy patient.

There are no simple procedures to control bladder instability or sensory urgency. When incontinence is due to a mixture of stress and urge, pharmacologic or behavioral treatment may be employed in conjunction with surgery, but results are not as good as when stress incontinence exists alone.

Selection of patients for surgical procedures depends upon the diagnosis and upon the condition of the patient. The frailty of the patient, the condition of tissues, and the state of nutrition bear on the ability to heal. The severity of symptoms must be considered in relation to the risk the patients must undertake for their surgical correction. Finally, such factors as the durability of the treatment and the incidence of complications must also be considered in choosing a treatment option.

Behavioral Techniques

Behavioral techniques increase the patient's awareness of the lower urinary tract and environment and can enhance control of detrusor and pelvic muscular function. Such techniques are participatory, relatively noninvasive, and generally free of side effects, and they do not limit future options. They do require time, effort, and continued practice. Some patients become dry, while a larger number experience important reduction of wetness, and others receive no benefit. Those who appear to benefit most are highly motivated individuals without cognitive deficits. Men and women with stress and urge incontinence have benefitted, whereas patients with severe sphincter damage (such as in postradical prostatectomy with constant leakage) generally do not benefit.

Behavioral techniques should be offered as a choice to patients who are motivated to put in the time and effort and wish to avoid a more invasive procedure. Commonly employed techniques include:

Pelvic Muscle Exercises. Pelvic muscle exercises strengthen the voluntary periurethral and pelvic floor muscles, the contraction of which exerts a closing force on the urethra. These techniques have been emphasized for women with stress incontinence but appear to be useful in men as well. Benefit has been reported in 30 to 90 percent of women, but criteria for improvement differ among studies. Patients with mild symptoms may improve most. Continued exercise is required for continued benefit.

Biofeedback. Biofeedback is a learning technique to exert better voluntary control over urine storage. Biofeedback uses visual or auditory instrumentation to give patients moment-to-moment information on how well they are controlling the sphincter, detrusor, and abdominal muscles. After such training, successful patients typically learn to perform the correct responses relatively automatically. Patients with urinary incontinence are trained to relax the detrusor and abdominal muscles and/or contract the sphincter, depending upon the form of incontinence. When used in patients with stress and/or urge incontinence, biofeedback has been shown to result in complete control of incontinence in approximately 20-25 percent of patients and to provide important improvement in another 30 percent. There are two caveats: the degree of improvement is variable, and long-term follow up data are not available. It is important to recognize that biofeedback requires sophisticated equipment and training. The benefit of adding biofeedback to pelvic muscle exercise regimens has not been adequately evaluated.

Bladder Training. Bladder training instructs patients to void at regular short intervals, usually hourly during the day, and then at progressively longer intervals of up to 3 hours over a training period of a few to a dozen weeks. Bladder training appears to be effective in reducing the frequency of stress and urge incontinence. Studies have indicated cure rates of 10-15 percent and improvement in the majority of patients.

Behavioral Techniques in the Nursing Home. For institutionalized elderly, almost any consistent attention to the problem, including bladder training and frequent scheduled checks for dryness appears to reduce incontinence in at least some patients. Another technique applicable in the nursing home is prompted voiding, in which frequent (1 to 2 hourly) checks for dryness are made, reminding the patient to void and praising success.

Staging of Treatment

As a general rule, the least invasive or dangerous procedures should be tried first. For many forms of incontinence, behavioral techniques meet this criterion. When behavioral techniques do not achieve the desired result, pharmacologic treatment can be initiated. Clear indications for surgical intervention must be respected, however, and surgical treatment should not be withheld inappropriately. Overflow incontinence due to prostatism and urge incontinence due to carcinoma of the bladder or prostate must be recognized and treated promptly. After having been informed of surgical and nonoperative options, the patient who is a surgical candidate and wants prompt treatment (e.g., as in the case of stress incontinence) should be operated on. In patients with mixed incontinence, a combination of surgery, behavioral techniques, and pharmacotherapy may be helpful.

What Management Techniques Are Appropriate When Treatment Is Not Effective or Indicated?

For patients who have not been successfully treated, management plans must be developed to maximize their well-being. Even when permanent improvement is not expected, techniques such as frequent toileting and reminders may be useful in reducing the impact of the patient's incontinence. Careful evaluation of the timing and pattern of incontinence may suggest helpful changes such as bedtime fluid restriction, provision of easier access to toilet facilities, and temporary or permanent arrangements for protection of the patients, their clothing, and environment.

Currently available modes of protection include absorbent pads or garments, indwelling catheters, and external collection devices such as condom catheters. Absorbent pads or garments provide comfort and convenience when used temporarily in conjunction with therapy; no method is entirely satisfactory for long-term use. For long-term use with incapacitated patients, absorbent materials are expensive, require personnel time, and can be associated with pressure sores when circumstances prevent meticulous attention to prompt changes.

For men, external collection devices are less expensive and less time-consuming for patient and caregiver, but they are associated with increased incidence of urinary tract infection and other complications. Practical external collection devices for women are not generally available.

Indwelling urethral or suprapubic catheters may be necessary for selected patients, but almost invariably lead to bacteriuria within a few weeks and have been associated with sepsis.

What Strategies Are Effective in Improving Public and Professional Knowledge about Urinary Incontinence?

There have been limited efforts to inform the public and professionals about urinary incontinence. The effectiveness of these strategies has not been evaluated. Incontinence education, therefore, must rely on methods that have been used in other areas of health education. Effective strategies to improve public and professional awareness need to be developed, implemented, and evaluated.

Negative societal attitudes about urinary incontinence have been a barrier to increasing public and professional knowledge. The scientific study of incontinence and the dissemination of research findings will help professionals and laypersons realize that loss of continence need not be a condition that is inevitable or shameful.

Strategies for Improving Public Knowledge

Providing accurate information on the management of incontinence to persons with this problem and their families is a challenging and important task. Studies suggest that only half of the people with incontinence report their condition to a physician. Strategies that will reach the largest number of people will be effective in encouraging them to seek professional help. These include informative newspaper and magazine articles, radio and television programs, and special educational programs in senior centers.

One innovative suggestion that deserves consideration is the mandatory labeling of all absorbent products, informing the public that persistent urinary incontinence should be evaluated and that effective treatments are available.

Strategies for Improving Professional Knowledge

There is an urgent need to educate professionals and paraprofessionals about urinary incontinence.

First and foremost, information on urinary incontinence should be included in the core curricula of undergraduate and graduate professional schools. Schools of nursing should consider the feasibility of educating specialists on incontinence care, who can serve as expert advisers to health care professionals.

To increase practitioners' knowledge of this important condition, continuing education courses focusing on the types of incontinence and

461

appropriate diagnostic measures and treatment should be offered. Professionals most likely to provide care to people with incontinence should be encouraged to attend these courses.

Education on the topic of urinary incontinence should also be a part of the training programs for paraprofessional students such as licensed vocational nurses, nurses aides, and auxiliary workers in the community. Because urinary incontinence is a problem of great magnitude in long-term care settings, special emphasis should be placed on educating nurses aides.

Last, coordinated care for people with incontinence will be facilitated by encouraging alliances among all professionals responsible for caring for people with incontinence.

What Are the Needs for Future Research Related to Urinary Incontinence?

The Consensus Development Conference on Urinary Incontinence in Adults has provided an overview of current knowledge on the etiology, pathophysiology, sequelae, and management of this prevalent clinical problem. Although information on incontinence is increasing, this field has long been neglected, and numerous gaps exist in our knowledge. While many controversies were addressed, numerous questions were identified that await answers and thus serve as the focus for future research directions. These issues will require the collaborative input of investigators from the spectrum of relevant disciplines and the rigorous application of appropriate research principles.

Directions for future research:

- Basic research on the mechanisms underlying the etiology, exacerbation, and response to treatment of specific forms of urinary incontinence and urgency.

- Epidemiologic studies with emphasis on elucidation of risk factors for development of urinary incontinence, its occurrence in specific populations (particularly males and nonwhites), and the natural history of the various clinical and physiologic subtypes.

- Studies of strategies to prevent urinary incontinence.

- Randomized clinical trials, including longitudinal studies in well-specified populations, of algorithms for the systematic assessment of patients with incontinence and of specific behavioral, pharmacologic, and surgical treatment, either alone or in combination.

- Development of new therapies, including pharmacologic agents with greater specificity for the urinary tract and new behavioral and surgical strategies and other innovative techniques, including electrical stimulation.

Conclusions

- Urinary incontinence is very common among older Americans and is epidemic in nursing homes.
- Urinary incontinence costs Americans more than $10 billion each year.
- Urinary incontinence is not part of normal aging, but age-related changes predispose to its occurrence.
- Urinary incontinence leads to stigmatization and social isolation.
- Of the 10 million Americans with urinary incontinence, more than half have had no evaluation or treatment.
- Contrary to public opinion, most cases of urinary incontinence can be cured or improved.
- Every person with urinary incontinence is entitled to evaluation and consideration for treatment.
- Most health care professionals ignore urinary incontinence and do not provide adequate diagnosis and treatment.
- Inadequate nursing home staffing prohibits proper treatment and contributes to the neglect of nursing home residents.
- Medical and nursing education neglect urinary incontinence. Curriculum development is urgent.
- A major research initiative is required to improve assessment and treatment for Americans with urinary incontinence.

Copies of this statement and bibliographies prepared by the National Library of Medicine are available from the Office of Medical Applications of Research, National Institutes of Health, Federal Building, Room 618, Bethesda, MD 20892.

Section 36.4

Additional Resources on Urinary Incontinence

NKUDIC, Searches-On-File, Urinary Incontinence, February 1995.

Legend

TI   Title
AU Author
CN Corporate Author
SO Source
AV Producer/Availability
PD Product

TI   *About Prostate Surgery.*
AU Jeter, K.F.
SO Union, SC: HIP (Help for Incontinent People), Inc. 1992. 2 p.
CN HIP (Help for Incontinent People), Inc.
AV Available from HIP, Inc. P.O. Box 544, Union, SC 29379. (803) 579-7900 or (800) BLADDER. PRICE: Free.

TI   *Active Living: Your Complete Incontinence Care Product Catalog.*
SO South Burlington, VT: Laborie Medical Technologies Corporation. 1993. 56 p.
CN Laborie Medical Technologies Corporation.
AV Available from Laborie Medical Technologies Corporation. 7 Green Tree Drive, Number 4, South Burlington, VT 05403. (800) 522-3394. PRICE: $3.00.

TI *Age Page: Urinary Incontinence.*
SO Bethesda, MD: National Institutes of Health. 1991. 2 p.
CN National Institute on Aging.
AV Available from the National Kidney and Urologic Diseases Information Clearinghouse. 3 Information Way, Bethesda, MD 20892-3580. (301) 654-4415. PRICE: 1–25 copies free; quantities over 25, $.10 per copy.

TI *Answers to Your Questions About Urinary Incontinence: Loss of Bladder Control.*
SO Baltimore, MD: Bladder Health Council. 1993. 16 p.
CN Bladder Health Council.
AV Available from Bladder Health Council. c/o American Foundation For Urologic Disease, 300 West Pratt Street, Suite 401, Baltimore, MD 21201. (800) 242-2383. Free.

TI **Artificial Urinary Sphincter.**
AU Hughes, R.
SO *HIP Report.* Help for Incontinent People Report. 11(2): 1–2. Spring 1993.
AV Available from Help for Incontinent People, Inc. P.O. Box 544, Union, SC 29379. (803) 579-7900 or (800) BLADDER. PRICE: Free.

TI **Better Way Than Diapers.**
AU Burgio, K.L.; Pearce, K.L.; Lucco, A.J.
SO *Johns Hopkins Magazine.* 42(6 Supplement 2): p. 1–8. December 1990.

TI **Biofeedback: What Is It? How Does It Work?**
AU Woolner, B.F.
SO *HIP Report.* Help For Incontinent People. 12(1): 7. Winter 1994.
AV Available from HIP (Help For Incontinent People). P.O. Box 544, Union, SC 29379. (800) BLADDER.

TI **Cigarette Smoking and Incontinence in Women.**
AU Bump, R.C.; McClish, D.K.
SO *HIP Report.* Help for Incontinent People Report. 11(3): 1. Summer 1993.
AV Available from Help For Incontinent People, Inc. P.O. Box 544, Union, SC 29379. (803) 579-7900 or (800) BLADDER. PRICE: Free.

TI *Continent Surgical Procedures for Ileostomy and Urostomy.*

SO Irvine, CA: United Ostomy Association Inc. 1993. 2 p.

CN United Ostomy Association Inc.

AV Available from United Ostomy Association Inc. 36 Executive Park, Suite 120, Irvine, CA 92714. (800) 826-0826. PRICE: Single copy free.

TI **Correcting Myths About Incontinence.**

AU Jeter, K.F.

SO *HIP Report.* Help for Incontinent People Report. 11(4): 1. Fall 1993.

AV Available from HIP-Help for Incontinent People, Inc. P.O. Box 544, Union, SC 29379. (803) 579-7900 or (800) BLADDER. PRICE: Free.

TI *Facts About Urinary Incontinence.*

SO McGaw Park, IL: Baxter Health care Corporation. 1991. 4 p.

CN Baxter Health Care Corporation.

AV Available from Baxter Health care Corporation. Customer Service, Health Care Communications, 1500 Waukegan Road, McGaw Park, IL 60085. (800) 766-3646. PRICE: Bulk orders only. 50 copies for $20.00 plus $2.00 shipping. Order number HIP 220-032.

TI *Femina: The Easy Way to do Kegel Exercises.*

SO Minneapolis, MN: Dacomed Corporation. 1990. (pelvic floor muscle training weights).

CN Dacomed Corporation.

PD Set of five cone-shaped weights.

AV Available from Dacomed Corporation. 1701 East 79th Street, Minneapolis, MN 55425. (800) 328-1103 or (612) 854-7522. PRICE: $99.00 per set plus $5.00 handling. MN residents add 6 percent sales tax. Product brochure available free of charge.

TI **Help for Urinary Incontinence.**

AU Aaberg, R.A.

SO *Diabetes Self-Management.* 8(2): 4749. March-April 1991.

AV Available from R.A. Rapaport Publishing, Inc. 150 West 22nd Street, New York, NY 10011. (800) 234-0923.

TI *Home Delivery Incontinent Supplies Catalog.*
SO Ferguson, MO: Home Delivery Incontinent Supplies Co., Inc. 1992. 47 p.
AV Available from Home Delivery Incontinent Supplies Co., Inc. 325 Paul Avenue, Ferguson, MO 63135. (314) 521-1380 or (800) 538-1036; FAX (314) 521-3257. Free.

TI **I Will Manage: A Program Designed Just For You.**
SO *The Informer*. p. 1, 3. Spring/Summer 1991.
CN Simon Foundation.
AV Available from Simon Foundation. P.O. Box 815, Wilmette, IL 60091. (800) 23-SIMON.

TI **Incontinence in Women.**
SO *Postgraduate Medicine*. 93(2): Inside Back Cover. February 1, 1993.
AV Available from McGraw-Hill, Inc. 1221 Avenue of the Americas, New York, NY 10020. (612) 832-7869.

TI *Incontinence: Why We Should Talk About It.* **rev. ed.**
SO Neenah, WI: Kimberly-Clark Home Health Care. 1991. 2 p.
CN Kimberly-Clark Corporation.
AV Available from Kimberly-Clark Home Health Care. P.O. Box 2002, Neenah, WI 54956. (800) 558-6423 or (800) 242-6463 (in Wisconsin). PRICE: Free.

TI *Incontinence: Everything You Wanted to Know But Were Afraid to Ask.*
SO Washington, DC: Alliance for Aging Research. 1990. 4 p.
CN Alliance for Aging Research.
AV Available from Alliance for Aging Research. 2021 K Street, N.W., Suite 305, Washington, DC 20006. (202) 293-2856. PRICE: Up to 50 copies free; additional copies $0.20 each.

TI *Insurance and Your Implant.*
SO Minneapolis, MN: American Medical Systems. 1990. 2 p.
CN American Medical Systems.
AV Available from American Medical Systems. Consumer Information, Department R, P.O. Box 9, Minneapolis, MN 55440. (800) 253-6469. PRICE: Single copy free. Publication Number 40229.

TI **Learning to Live Again: Controlling Incontinence.**
SO *Advances: Newsletter of the Robert Wood Johnson Foundation.* 4(1): 2–3. Spring 1991
CN Robert Wood Johnson Foundation, Communications Office.
AV Available from Robert Wood Johnson Foundation. College Road, P.O. Box 2316, Princeton, NJ 08543-2316. (609) 243-5925. Free.

TI *Let Us Tell You About HIP.*
SO Union, SC: Help For Incontinent People, Inc. 19 p.
CN Help For Incontinent People, Inc.
AV Available from Help for Incontinent People, Inc. (HIP). P.O. Box 544, Union, SC 29379. (803) 579-7900. PRICE: Free.

TI **Most Cases of Urinary Incontinence Curable.**
AU Blaivas, J.G.
SO *Kidney '91.* 8(3): 6–8. Winter 1991.
AV Available from National Kidney Foundation, Inc. Medical Department, 30 East 33rd Street, New York, NY 10016. (800) 622-9010 or (212) 889-2210.

TI **Needle Bladder Suspension for the Treatment of Stress Urinary Incontinence in Women.**
AU Payne, C.K.; Raz, S.
SO *HIP Report.* Help for Incontinent People Report. 11(2): 4. Spring 1993.
AV Available from Help for Incontinent People, Inc. P.O. Box 544, Union, SC 29379. (803) 579-7900 or (800) BLADDER. Free.

TI *NKF Science Writers News Briefing: News Briefing for Science Writers on Transplantation, Dialysis, and Kidney Research* **(press packet).**
SO New York, NY: National Kidney Foundation, Inc. August 1990. 55 p.
CN National Kidney Foundation, Inc.
AV Available from the National Kidney Foundation, Inc. 30 East 33rd Street, New York, NY 10016. (212) 889-2210 or (800) 622-9010. PRICE: Free.

TI *Resource Guide of Continence Products and Services,
6th ed.*
SO Union, SC: Help for Incontinent People, Inc. 1992. 70 p.
CN Help for Incontinent People, Inc.
AV Available from Help for Incontinent People, Inc. (HIP). P.O.
Box 544, Union, SC 29379. (800) BLADDER. PRICE: $10.00
plus shipping and handling. Make check payable to HIP.

TI **Save Your Skin.**
AU Krasner, D.
SO *To Life!* p. 13. Summer 1990.
AV Available from Kimberly-Clark. Department KC-790, 2100
Winchester Road, Neenah, WI 54956. (800) 558-6423.

TI **Seeking Treatment for Incontinence: When, Why, and
Who?**
AU Jeter, K.F.
SO *HIP Report* (Help For Incontinent People). 12(1): 1–3. Winter
1994.
AV Available from HIP (Help For Incontinent People). P.O. Box
544, Union, SC 29379. (800) BLADDER.

TI *Shield Mail Order Medical Supply Catalog.*
SO Santa Clarita, CA: Shield Health Care. 1993. 64 p.
AV Available from Shield Health Care. P.O. Box 922, Santa
Clarita, CA 91380. (800) 232-7443. Free.

TI **Straight Talk About Incontinence.**
AU McKee, S.
SO *American Health.* 13(8): 54–59. October 1994.

TI *Toobie: Self-Cath Coloring Book for Boys and Girls.*
AU Field, J.
SO Santa Barbara, CA: Mentor Urology. October 1992. 26 p.
AV Available from Mentor Urology. 5425 Hollister Avenue, Santa
Barbara, CA 93111. (805) 681-6000 or (800) 328-3863. Free.

TI   *Undercare: Men's and Women's Incontinence Underwear.*
SO   Bridgeport, CT: Visa-Therm Products, Inc. 1990.
CN   Visa-Therm Products, Inc.
PD   Incontinence underwear for men and women.
AV   Available from Visa-Therm Products, Inc. P.O. Box 486, Bridgeport, CT 06604. (203) 334-4560.

TI   *Urinary Incontinence in Adults: A Patient's Guide.*
SO   Rockville, MD: Department of Health and Human Services. 1992. 6 p.
CN   Department of Health and Human Services.
AV   Available from Agency for Health Care Policy and Research. Publications Clearinghouse, P.O. Box 8547, Silver Spring, MD 20907. (800) 358-9295. PRICE: Single copy free. Agency approval is required for requests for 100 or more brochures. Publication No. AHCPR 92-0040. Spanish Version: Publication No. AHCPR 92-0089.

TI   **Urinary Incontinence.**
AU   Petrucci, K.
SO   *Diabetes Forecast.* 43(1): 3941. January 1990.
AV   Available from American Diabetes Association, Inc. 1660 Duke Street, Alexandria, VA 22314. (800) 232-3472.

TI   *Urinary Incontinence.*
SO   Washington, DC: American College of Obstetricians and Gynecologists. December 1990. 4 p.
CN   Committee on Patient Education, American College of Obstetricians and Gynecologists.
AV   Available from American College of Obstetricians and Gynecologists. 409 12th Street, SW, Washington, DC 20024-2188. (202) 638-5577. PRICE: Single copy free; 50 for $15.

TI   *Urinary Incontinence: Treating Loss of Urine Control.*
SO   New York, NY: National Kidney Foundation, Inc. 1991. 4 p.
CN   National Kidney Foundation, Inc.
AV   Available from National Kidney Foundation, Inc. 30 East 33rd Street, New York, NY 10016. (800) 622-9010. Free.

TI ***What You Should Know About Urinary Incontinence: Loss of Urine Control.***

SO West Haven, CT: Miles, Inc., Pharmaceutical Division. 1992. 4 p.

CN Miles, Inc., Pharmaceutical Division.

AV Available from Miles, Inc. Pharmaceutical Division, 400 Morgan Lane, West Haven, CT 06516. (800) 468-0894. Free.

For Additional Information

CHID is available on-line through CDP Online. If you would like references to materials on other topics, you may request a special literature search of CHID from a library that subscribes to CDP Online or from the National Kidney and Urologic Diseases Information Clearinghouse, 3 Information Way, Bethesda, MD 20892-3580; (301) 654-4415.

Chapter 37

Interstitial Cystitis

This text is for people who have interstitial cystitis and for their family, friends, and co-workers who want to understand the experiences and challenges associated with the disorder. Information is included on the causes, diagnosis, and treatment of interstitial cystitis as well as information on current research studies that aim to understand and treat the disorder.

Basic and clinical research is advancing our knowledge of interstitial cystitis, but the disorder still poses many questions that scientists cannot answer. Only further research and the efforts of patients and doctors working together will shed light on improved treatments and, ultimately, a cure for this debilitating disorder.

Interstitial Cystitis: A Bladder Disorder

The urinary system consists of the kidneys, ureters, bladder, and urethra. The kidneys, a pair of purplish-brown organs, are located below the ribs toward the middle of the back. The kidneys remove liquid waste from the blood in the form of urine, keep a stable balance of salts and other substances in the blood, and produce erythropoietin, a hormone that aids the formation of red blood cells. Narrow tubes called ureters carry urine from the kidneys to the bladder, a triangle-shaped chamber in the lower abdomen. Like a balloon, the bladder's elastic walls relax and expand to store urine and contract

NIDDK; NIH Publication No. 94–3220.

and flatten when urine is emptied through the urethra. The typical adult bladder can store about 1 ½ cups of urine.

Adults pass about a quart and a half of urine each day. The amount of urine varies, depending on the fluids and foods a person consumes. The volume formed at night is about half that formed in the daytime.

Normal urine is sterile. It contains fluids, salts and waste products, but it is free of bacteria, viruses and fungi. The tissues of the bladder are isolated from urine and toxic substances by a coating that discourages bacteria from attaching and growing on the bladder wall.

People with interstitial cystitis (IC) have an inflamed, or irritated, bladder wall. This inflammation can lead to scarring and stiffening of the bladder, decreased bladder capacity, glomerulations (pinpoint bleeding) and, in rare cases, ulcers in the bladder lining.

IC, also known as painful bladder syndrome and frequency-urgency-dysuria syndrome, is a complex, chronic disorder that has baffled doctors for as long as it has been recognized.

Estimates of the number of people who have IC run as high as 500,000, but no one knows for sure how many people have it. About 90 percent of IC patients are women. While people of any age can be affected, about two-thirds of patients are in their twenties, thirties, or forties. IC is rare in children. In a few cases, IC has afflicted both mother and daughter, but there is no evidence that the disorder is hereditary, or genetically passed from parent to child.

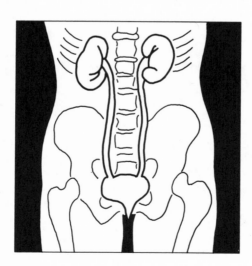

Figure 37.1. The urinary tract.

Two Types of IC

Because IC varies so much in its symptoms and severity, most researchers believe that it is not one but several diseases. Two types of IC are usually described; they are mainly distinguished by whether ulcers have formed on the bladder wall. Most researchers believe that IC does not generally progress from the nonulcerative to the ulcerative form.

Nonulcerative IC

This disorder is the most common type of IC. It usually affects young to middle-age women who have a normal, near normal, or increased bladder capacity when measured under general anesthesia. Glomerulations can be seen in the bladder wall.

Ulcerative IC

This type of IC tends to be found in middle-age to older women. Bladder capacity is low (less than 1 ½ cups) when measured under general anesthesia. The decrease is thought to result in part from fibrosis, the formation of threadlike tissue that makes the bladder stiff and small. Cracks, scars, and Hunner's ulcers (star-shaped sores) in the bladder wall may bleed when the bladder is filled to capacity during a cystoscopy.

Cause

No one knows what causes IC, but doctors studying the disorder believe it is a real, physical problem—not a result, symptom, or sign of an emotional problem.

One area of research on the cause of IC has focused on the lining of the bladder called the glycocalyx, made up primarily of substances called mucins and glycosaminoglycans (GAGs). This layer normally protects the bladder wall from toxic effects of urine and its contents. Researchers at the University of California, San Diego, found that this protective layer of the bladder was "leaky" in about 70 percent of IC patients they examined and may allow substances in urine to pass into the bladder wall and trigger IC symptoms. The researchers also found that patients with Hunner's ulcers had "leakier" bladders than patients without the ulcers.

475

Some people are diagnosed with IC after taking antibiotics for a presumed urinary tract infection. Therefore, it has been suggested that antibiotics may damage the bladder wall and make it "leaky." This idea has been studied carefully, but antibiotics have never been found to harm the bladder wall. Thus, other ideas are more likely to explain why some IC patients are diagnosed after a urinary tract infection. It is possible that the infection started an autoimmune response against the bladder, the patient's original symptoms were from IC all along, or an infecting organism is in bladder cells but is not detectable through routine tests.

Symptoms

The symptoms of IC vary greatly from one person to another but have some similarities to those of a urinary tract infection:

- decreased bladder capacity
- an urgent need to urinate
- frequently day and night
- feelings of pressure, pain, and tenderness around the bladder, pelvis, and perineum (the area between the anus and vagina or anus and scrotum), which may increase as the bladder fills and decrease as it empties
- painful sexual intercourse
- in men, discomfort or pain in the penis and scrotum.

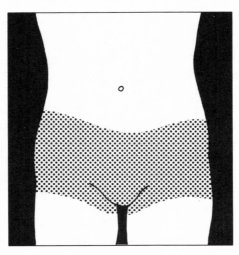

Figure 37.2. Area of pain and pressure.

In most women, symptoms usually worsen around the menstrual cycle. As with many other illnesses, stress may also intensify symptoms but does not cause them.

Diagnosis

Because the symptoms of IC are similar to those of other disorders of the urinary system, and because there is no definitive test to identify IC, doctors must rule out other conditions before considering a diagnosis of IC. Among these disorders are urinary tract or vaginal infections, bladder cancer, bladder inflammation or infection caused by radiation to the abdomen, eosinophilic and tuberculous cystitis, kidney stones, endometriosis, neurological disorders, sexually transmitted diseases, low-count bacteriuria, and, in men, chronic bacterial and abacterial prostatitis.

The diagnosis of IC in the general population is based on:

- presence of urgency, frequency or pelvic/bladder pain,
- cystoscopic evidence (under anesthesia) of bladder wall inflammation and glomerulations or Hunner's ulcers,
- absence of other diseases that may cause the symptoms.

Medical tests that help identify other conditions include a urinalysis, urine culture, cystoscopy, biopsy of the bladder wall and, in men, laboratory examination of prostate secretions.

Urinalysis and Urine Culture

These tests can detect and identify the most common organisms in the urine that may be causing symptoms. There are, however, organisms such as the bacteria chlamydia that can't be detected with these tests, so a negative culture does not rule out all types of infection. A urine sample is obtained either by catheterization or by the "clean catch" method. For a "clean catch," the patient washes the genital area before collecting urine "midstream" in a sterile container. White and red blood cells and bacteria in the urine may indicate an infection of the urinary tract, which can be treated with an antibiotic. If urine is sterile for weeks or months while symptoms persist, a doctor may consider a diagnosis of IC.

Culture of Prostate Secretions

In men, the doctor will obtain prostatic fluid from the patient. This fluid will be examined for signs of an infection, which can be treated with antibiotics.

Cystoscopy Under Anesthesia With Bladder Distension

During cystoscopy to diagnose IC, the doctor uses a cystoscope—an instrument made of a hollow tube about the diameter of a drinking straw with several lenses and a light—to see inside the bladder and urethra. The doctor will also distend or stretch the bladder to its capacity by filling it with a liquid or gas. Because bladder distension is painful in IC patients, before the doctor inserts the cystoscope through the urethra into the bladder, the patient must be given either regional or general anesthesia. These tests can detect inflammation; a thick, stiff bladder wall; Hunner's ulcers; and glomerulations (pinpoint bleeding) that may be seen only after the bladder is stretched.

The doctor may also test the patient's maximum bladder capacity, the amount of liquid or gas the bladder can hold under anesthesia. Without anesthesia, capacity is limited by either pain or a severe urge to urinate. Many people with IC have normal or large maximum bladder capacities under anesthesia. However, a small bladder capacity under anesthesia helps to support the diagnosis of IC.

Biopsy

A biopsy is a microscopic examination of tissue. Samples of the bladder and urethra may be removed during a cystoscopy and examined with a microscope later. A biopsy helps rule out bladder cancer and confirm bladder wall inflammation.

Treatment

Scientists have not yet found a cure for IC, nor can they predict who will respond best to which treatment. Symptoms may disappear without explanation or coincide with an event such as a change in diet or treatment. Even when symptoms disappear, however, they may return after days, weeks, months, or years. Scientists do not know why.

Because doctors do not know what causes IC, treatments are aimed at relieving symptoms. Most people are helped for variable periods of time by one or a combination of treatments, many of which are described briefly in this booklet. However, as researchers learn more about IC, the list of potential treatments may change. Patients should discuss treatment options with a doctor.

Bladder Distension

Because some patients have noted an improvement in symptoms after a bladder distension done to diagnose IC, the procedure is often thought of as one of the first treatment attempts. Researchers are not sure why distension helps, but some believe that the procedure may increase bladder capacity and interfere with pain signals transmitted by nerves in the bladder. Symptoms may temporarily worsen 24 to 48 hours after distension, but should then return to predistension levels or improve after 2 to 4 weeks.

Bladder Instillation

This procedure may also be called a bladder wash or bath. During a bladder instillation, the bladder is filled with a solution that is held for varying periods of time, from a few seconds to 15 minutes, before being drained through a narrow tube called a catheter.

The only drug approved by the U.S. Food and Drug Administration (FDA) for bladder instillation is dimethyl sulfoxide (DMSO, RIMSO-50). With DMSO treatments a narrow tube (catheter) is guided up the urethra into the bladder. A measured amount of DMSO is passed through the catheter into the bladder, where it is retained for about 15 minutes before being expelled. Treatments are given every week or two for 6 to 8 weeks, and repeated as needed. Most people with IC who respond to DMSO notice improvement of symptoms 3 or 4 weeks after the first 6- to 8-week cycle of treatments. Highly motivated patients who are willing to catheterize themselves may, after consultation with their doctor, be able to have DMSO treatments at home. Self-administration of DMSO is less expensive and more convenient than going to the doctor's office.

Doctors think DMSO works in several ways. Because it passes into the bladder wall, DMSO may more effectively reach tissue to reduce inflammation and block pain. It may also prevent muscle contractions that may cause pain, frequency, and urgency.

A bothersome but relatively insignificant side effect of DMSO treatments is a garlic-like taste and odor from the breath and skin. This may last up to 72 hours after a treatment. Long-term DMSO treatments have caused cataracts in animal studies, but this side effect has not appeared in humans. Blood tests, including a complete blood count and kidney and liver function tests, should be done about every 6 months.

A variety of other drugs have been used experimentally for bladder washes, including silver nitrate, sodium oxychlorosene (Clorpactin WCS-90), heparin, and pentosanpolysulfate (Elmiron).

Silver nitrate and oxychlorosene sodium are thought to work by first attacking the bladder lining. This triggers the body's immune system to step in and start the healing process. Some patients have been successfully treated with these drugs, but the frequent, painful treatments usually must be done under general anesthesia. Neither drug can be used in people who have urinary reflux, a condition in which urine flows backward up the ureters into the kidneys.

Heparin and pentosanpolysulfate are thought to work by replacing or repairing the "leaky" bladder lining.

Oral Drugs

There are no oral drugs approved by the FDA specifically for the treatment of IC, but a variety of drugs such as aspirin, ibuprofen, antihistamines, and the urinary tract pain reliever phenazopyridine (available by prescription as Pyridium and over-the-counter as Azo-Standard) may help lessen symptoms.

A blend of atropine, hyoscyamine, methenamine, methylene blue, phenyl salicylate and benzoic acid (Urised) may inhibit the growth of organisms in the urine and reduce bladder spasms that cause frequency, urgency, and nighttime trips to the bathroom. Drugs such as oxybutynin chloride (Ditropan) also may reduce bladder spasms. In separate studies of only a few patients each, hydroxyzine (Vistaril and Atarax), an antihistamine, and nifedipine (Procardia), a heart disease and high blood pressure treatment, have been reported to reduce symptoms in some IC patients. But, as stated by the authors of these reports, further studies are needed to determine the drugs' true value in IC patients. All of these drugs must be prescribed by a physician.

Amitriptyline (Elavil) is an FDA-approved tricyclic antidepressant, but its ability to block pain and reduce bladder spasms makes it helpful in treating IC. Amitriptyline may cause drowsiness but can be taken at night to reduce this effect. Most people who respond to this drug show improvement 3 or 4 weeks after starting treatment. The dose may need adjustment for the best possible results.

The experimental drug sodium pentosanpolysulfate (Elmiron) is thought to repair the layer lining the bladder. In several studies, 19 percent to 65 percent of patients reported at least partial symptom relief. Most people who respond to pentosanpolysulfate see improvement within 6 to 8 weeks after starting treatment. There are few side effects, but the most common is skin rash. Clinical trials have been completed, and the drug's manufacturer has requested FDA approval to market pentosanpolysulfate as a treatment for IC. Until approved by FDA, doctors can prescribe the drug only by first obtaining approval for compassionate use in individual patients, or by having patients participate in an FDA-approved clinical trial.

Another experimental drug, nalmefene hydrochloride (Incystene), blocks the body's receptors to pain, thus inhibiting the sensation of pain. Nalmefene is currently being evaluated in the treatment of IC in an FDA-approved clinical study sponsored by the drug's manufacturer.

Because drugs have side effects, patients should always consult a doctor before using any drug for an extended time.

TENS (Transcutaneous Electrical Nerve Stimulation)

With TENS, mild electric pulses enter the body for minutes to hours two or more times a day either through wires placed on the lower back or the suprapubic region, between the navel and the pubic hair, or through special devices inserted into the vagina in women or into the rectum in men. Although scientists don't know exactly how it works, it has been suggested that the electric pulses may increase blood flow to the bladder, strengthen pelvic muscles that help control the bladder, and trigger the release of hormones that block pain.

TENS is relatively inexpensive and allows the patient to take an active part in treatment. Within some guidelines, the patient decides when, how long, and at what intensity TENS will be used. TENS has been most helpful in relieving pain and decreasing frequency in IC patients who have Hunner's ulcers. Smokers do not respond as well as nonsmokers. If TENS is going to help, change usually occurs in 3 to 4 months.

Diet

There is no scientific evidence linking diet to IC, but some doctors and patients believe that alcohol, tomatoes, spices, chocolate, caffeinated and citrus beverages, and high-acid foods may contribute to bladder irritation and inflammation. Some patients also notice a worsening of symptoms after eating or drinking products containing artificial sweeteners. Patients may try eliminating such products from their diet and reintroduce them one at a time to determine which, if any, affect symptoms. It is important, however, to maintain a well-balanced and varied diet.

Smoking

Many IC patients feel that smoking worsens their symptoms. (Because smoking is the major known cause of bladder cancer, one of the best things a smoker can do for the bladder is to quit smoking.)

Exercise

Many IC patients feel that regular exercise helps relieve symptoms and, in some cases, hastens remission.

Bladder Training

People who have found some relief from pain may be able to reduce frequency using bladder training techniques. Methods vary, but basically the patient decides to void at designated times and use relaxation techniques and distractions to help keep to the schedule. Gradually, the patient tries to lengthen the time between the scheduled voids. A diary of voids is usually helpful in keeping track of progress.

Surgery

This option is considered only if an IC patient has failed all available treatments and the pain is severe. Most doctors are reluctant to operate because the outcome is unpredictable in individual patients—some people have surgery and still have symptoms.

Anyone considering surgery should discuss the potential risks and benefits, side effects, and long- and short-term complications with a surgeon and family, as well as with people who already have had the procedure. Surgery requires anesthesia, hospitalization, and weeks or months of recovery, and as the complexity of the procedure increases, so do the chances for complications and failure.

To locate a surgeon experienced in performing specific procedures, check with your doctor.

Transurethral fulguration and resection of ulcers. Fulguration involves burning Hunner's ulcers using electricity or a laser. When the area heals, the dead tissue and the ulcer fall off, leaving new, healthy tissue behind. Resection involves cutting around and removing the ulcers. Both treatments, done under anesthesia, use special instruments inserted into the bladder through a cystoscope. Laser surgery in the urinary tract should only be done by doctors who have the special training and expertise needed to perform the procedure.

Denervation. Denervation is a complicated procedure done by surgeons who have special training and expertise. Rarely used in the treatment of IC, it involves cutting some of the nerves to the bladder, interfering with pain signals. Many approaches and techniques are used, each of which has its own advantages and complications that should be discussed with the surgeon.

Augmentation. Augmentation makes the bladder larger, most often by adding a section of the patient's small intestine, a tube-like structure that absorbs and transports nutrients from food for use by the body. With this treatment, scarred, ulcerated and inflamed sections of the patient's bladder are removed, leaving only healthy tissue and the base of the bladder. A piece of the patient's small intestine is removed, reshaped, and attached to what remains of the bladder. After the incisions heal, the patient may be able to void normally.

Even in carefully selected patients—those with small, contracted bladders—the pain, frequency, and urgency may remain or return after surgery and the patient may have additional problems with infections in the new bladder and difficulty absorbing nutrients from the shortened intestine. Some patients are incontinent while others cannot void at all and must insert a catheter into the urethra to empty urine from the bladder.

Bladder Removal (Cystectomy). Different methods can be used to reroute urine once the bladder has been removed. In most cases, the ureters are attached to a piece of bowel that opens onto the skin of the abdomen, called a stoma. Urine empties through the stoma into a bag outside the body. This procedure is called a urostomy. Some urologists are using a technique that also requires a stoma but allows urine to be stored in a pouch inside the abdomen. At intervals throughout the day, the patient puts a catheter into the stoma and empties the pouch. Patients with either type of urostomy must use very clean, or sterile, steps to prevent infections in and around the stoma.

With a third method, a new bladder is made from a piece of the patient's bowel (large intestine) and attached to the urethra in place of the removed bladder. After a time of healing, the patient may be able to empty the bladder by voiding at scheduled times or may insert a catheter into the urethra. Few surgeons have the special training and expertise needed to perform this procedure.

Even after total bladder removal, some patients still experience variable symptoms of IC. Therefore, the decision to undergo a cystectomy should only be undertaken after serious deliberation on the potential outcome.

Electrical Nerve Stimulation. This surgical treatment is a variation of TENS, described previously, but involves permanent implantation of electrodes and a unit that emits continuous electrical pulses. This relatively new procedure has variable short-term results, unknown long-term effects and, therefore, is not widely used.

Special Concerns

Cancer

There is no evidence that IC increases the risk of bladder cancer. However, the long-term effects of IC require further observation and research.

Pregnancy

Researchers have little information about pregnancy and IC, but believe that the disorder does not affect fertility or the health of the fetus. Some women have a remission from IC during pregnancy, while others have more pain and pressure during the third trimester, possibly due to the weight of the fetus on the bladder.

Working

Symptom flare-ups that result in frequent absences from work may make it difficult to get or keep a job. The Social Security Administration provides information on Social Security Disability benefits. The National Organization of Social Security Claimants' Representatives can refer you to a lawyer experienced with Social Security claims. (See "Other Resources.")

Coping

The emotional support of family, friends, and other people with IC is very important in helping patients cope with the disorder. Studies have found that IC patients who learn about the disorder and become involved in their own care do better than patients who do not. The Interstitial Cystitis Association can provide the address and phone number of the nearest support group.

Other coping tips:

- Find a health care team that is sympathetic, helpful, and receptive.
- Understand that your health care team does not know all the answers and may be as frustrated as you are.
- Don't become isolated from family and friends.
- Involve your family in treatment decisions.
- Do not allow IC to become the center of your life.
- Try to put IC in perspective—worse could happen.
- Talk to other people with IC about their experiences and ways of coping.
- Trust yourself.

Research

Although answers may seem slow in coming, researchers are working every day to solve the painful riddle of IC. Some scientists receive funds from the Federal Government to help support their research, and some receive support from other sources such as their employing institution, drug companies, and the Interstitial Cystitis Association. Researchers and doctors around the country, regardless of who funds their work, may competently diagnose and treat IC.

The National Institute of Diabetes and Digestive and Kidney Diseases (NIDDK), a part of the National Institutes of Health (NIH), leads the Federal Government's research efforts on IC. Most studies funded by the NIDDK are a result of unsolicited grant applications sent to NIH by scientists at universities and medical centers throughout the United States. Other NIDDK-funded studies result from solicitations issued to encourage increased research on a certain topic.

By law, all applications sent to NIH are first reviewed by non-Government experts in the field of the proposed research for scientific merit and feasibility before being reviewed by the NIDDK's National Advisory Council. The council is made up of non-Government scientists, health professionals, and individuals who represent voluntary groups with an interest in the research of the institute. Approved applications are eligible for funding based on a scientific merit rating, or priority score, assigned by the initial reviewers. Applications are usually funded in priority score order, with the best applications funded first.

The NIDDK's investment in scientifically meritorious IC research has grown considerably since 1987, largely due to special solicitations. We now support research across the country that is looking at various aspects of IC, such as how urine contents may injure the bladder and what possible role organisms identified using nonstandard methods may have in causing IC. In addition to funding research, NIDDK sponsors scientific workshops where investigators share the results of their studies and discuss future areas for investigation.

Database

An important part of the NIDDK IC research program is the National IC Database Study, which will provide the first systematic, long-term look at a large number of people with IC. The database is expected to provide clues about how IC develops, how to diagnose and categorize patients, and how to treat the disorder more effectively.

Nine clinical centers and a data coordinating center have joined forces in this national project to collect and analyze dietary, diagnostic, symptom, treatment, and other information from more than 1,300 people with mild, moderate, or severe symptoms of IC. Patients may enroll at any listed center, regardless of where they live, but must be willing to travel to that center for evaluation and followup. Patients will be enrolled and monitored through April 1997.

National Interstitial Cystitis Database Study

Clinical Centers

University of California, San Diego Medical Center
Mail Code 8897
200 West Arbor
San Diego, CA 92103-8897
Research Coordinator: Diana LeBow, 619-543-5611

Northwestern University Medical School
707 North Fairbanks Court, Suite 618
Chicago, IL 60611
Research Coordinator: Mary Nieweglowski, R.N., 312-908-7019

William Beaumont Hospital Research Institute
3601 West 13 Mile Road
Royal Oak, MI 48073
Research Coordinator: Alexandre Afanasyev, M.D., 810-551-0885

Henry Ford Hospital
2799 West Grand Boulevard
Detroit, MI 48202
Research Coordinator: Michelle Fedon, R.N., 313-556-8265

University of Oklahoma
Health Sciences Center
920 Stanton L. Young Boulevard
Fifth Floor, Room 330
Oklahoma City, OK 73104
Research Coordinator: Linda Walker, R.N., 405-271-1693

Hospital of The University of Pennsylvania
Division of Urology, Fifth Floor Silverstein Pavilion
3400 Spruce Street
Philadelphia, PA 19104
Research Coordinator: Marilou Foy, R.N., 215-349-5874

The Graduate Hospital
1800 Lombard Street, Suite 606
Pepper Pavilion
Philadelphia, PA 19146
Research Coordinator: Marilou Foy, R.N., 215-349-5874

Temple University Hospital
Department of Urology
3401 North Broad Street
Parkinson Pavilion, Suite 350
Philadelphia, PA 19140
Research Coordinator: Marilou Foy, R.N., 215-349-5874

University of Wisconsin Hospital and Clinics
G5/348 CSC
600 Highland Avenue
Madison, WI 53792
Research Coordinator: Diane Pauk, B.S., 608-263-9721

Center for Biostatistics and Epidemiology
Hershey Medical Center
Pennsylvania State University College of Medicine
500 University Drive
Hershey, PA 17033

Diagnostic Criteria for Research Studies

Patients enrolled in NIDDK-supported research studies must fit strict diagnostic criteria so that researchers can reliably compare patients and study results. When too many variables are involved in research studies it is difficult, if not impossible, to clearly evaluate disease processes and potential treatments.

The diagnostic criteria for research studies were established in 1987 and refined in 1988 as a result of NIDDK-sponsored workshops that brought together basic and clinical researchers and patient groups. As our knowledge about IC develops, these criteria likely will be revised. Current criteria is as follows:

Patients must have:

- glomerulations (pinpoint bleeding) or Hunner's ulcers found by cystoscopy, and
- pain associated with the bladder, or urinary urgency.

Patients with ONE of the following are EXCLUDED from research studies:

- bladder capacity greater than 350 mL as demonstrated by a cystometrogram using either gas or liquid while the patient is awake
- no intense urge to void when the bladder is filled to 100 mL of gas or 150 mL of water with a medium rate of fill between 30 and 100 mL/minute
- demonstration of involuntary bladder contractions by cystometrogram with a medium rate of filling
- duration of symptoms less than 9 months
- absence of nocturia
- symptoms relieved by antimicrobials, antiseptics, anticholinergics, or antispasmodics
- frequency of urination while awake fewer than 8 times/day
- diagnosis of bacterial cystitis or prostatitis within 3 months— must have no bacteria for 3 months
- bladder or lower ureteral calculi
- active genital herpes
- uterine, cervical, vaginal, or urethral cancer
- urethral diverticulum
- cyclophosphamide, tuberculous, or radiation cystitis
- vaginitis
- benign or malignant bladder tumors
- younger than 18

Suggested Reading

The materials listed below may be found in medical libraries, many college and university libraries, through interlibrary loan in most public libraries, and at bookstores. Items are listed for information only; inclusion does not imply endorsement by the NIH.

Articles and Book Chapters

Bavendam, TG. "A Common Sense Approach To Lower Urinary Tract Hypersensitivity in Women."*Contemporary Urology*, 1992; 4(4):25–40.

Fleischmann, JD, et al. "Clinical and Immunological Response to Nifedipine for the Treatment of Interstitial Cystitis." *The Journal of Urology*, 1991; 146:1235–1239.

Hanno, PM, et al. "Diagnosis of Interstitial Cystitis." *The Journal of Urology*, 1990; 143(2):278–281.

Interstitial Cystitis Association. "IC and Social Security Disability." *ICA Update*, 1988; 3(3):1.

Messing, EM. "Interstitial Cystitis and Related Syndromes." *Campbell's Urology*. Eds. Walsh, PC, et al. Philadelphia, WB Saunders Company, 1986. 1070–1083.

Mosedale, L. "Embattled Bladders." *Health*, 1990; 22(5):40–78.

Parsons, CL. "Managing Interstitial Cystitis." *Contemporary Urology*, March 1990; 2:45–49.

Perez-Marrero, R, Emerson, LE. "Interstitial Cystitis." *The Canadian Journal of OB / GYN*, February 1990; 4–10.

Ratner, V, et al. "Interstitial Cystitis: A Bladder Disease Finds Legitimacy." *Journal of Women's Health*, 1992; 1(1):63–68.

Sant, GR. "Interstitial Cystitis: Pathophysiology, Clinical Evaluation, and Treatment." *Urology Annual*. Ed. Rous, SN. Connecticut, Appleton & Lange, 1989. 171–196.

Schmidt, RA, Vapnek, JM. "Pelvic Floor Behavior and Interstitial Cystitis." *Seminars in Urology*, 1991; 9(2):154–159.

Schmidt, RA. "Treatment of Unstable Bladder." *Urology*, 1991; 37(1):28–32.

Tanagho, EA. "Interstitial Cystitis." *General Urology*. Eds. Tanagho, EA, McAninch, JW. Connecticut, Appleton & Lange, 1988. 554–555.

Theoharides, TC. "Hydroxyzine for Interstitial Cystitis." *Journal of Allergy and Clinical Immunology*, 1993; 91:686–687.

Books and Booklets

Budish, AD. *Avoiding the Medicaid Trap: How To Beat the Catastrophic Costs of Nursing Home Care*. New York, Holt, 1989.

Chalker, R, Whitmore, KE. *Overcoming Bladder Disorders.* New York, Harper & Row, 1990.

Gillespie, L., Blakeslee, S. *You Don't Have To Live With Cystitis!* New York, Avon Books, 1986.

Hanno, PM, et al., ed. *Interstitial Cystitis.* New York, Springer, Verlag, 1990.

National Institutes of Health, Office of Clinical Center Communications. *Relieving Pain.* Single copies are available from NIH/OCCC, Relieving Pain/IC, Building 10, Room 1C255, 9000 Rockville Pike, Bethesda, MD 20892.

Pitzele, SK. *We Are Not Alone-Learning To Live With Chronic Illness.* Minneapolis, Thompson, 1985.

Sant, GR, Guest ed. "Interstitial Cystitis-1987." Supplement to *Urology.* 29(4). New Jersey, Hospital Publications, Inc., 1987.

Schrotenboer, K, Berkman, S. *The Woman Doctor's Guide To Overcoming Cystitis.* New York, Nal Penguin, Inc., 1987.

Other Resources

American Foundation for Urologic Disease
The Bladder Health Council
300 West Pratt Street, Suite 401
Baltimore, MD 21201
410-727-2908 or 1-800-242-2383

American Pain Society
5700 Old Orchard Road
Skokie, IL 60077
708-966-5595

American Uro-Gynecologic Society
401 North Michigan Avenue
Chicago, IL 60611-4267
312-644-6610

International Pain Foundation
909 Northeast 43rd Street, Suite 306
Seattle, WA 98105-6020
206-547-2157

Interstitial Cystitis Association of America, Inc.
P.O. Box 1553
Madison Square Station
New York, NY 10159-1553
212-979-6057 or 1-800-ICA-1626

National Chronic Pain Outreach Association
7979 Old Georgetown Road, Suite 100
Bethesda, MD 20814
301-652-4948

National Kidney Foundation
30 East 33rd Street
New York, NY 10016
212-889-2210 or 1-800-622-9010

National Kidney and Urologic Diseases Information Clearinghouse
3 Information Way
Bethesda, MD 20892-3580
301-654-4415

National Organization of Social Security Claimants' Representatives
6 Prospect Street
Midland Park, NJ 07432
201-444-1415 or 1-800-431-2804

Social Security Administration write or call your local office (found
in the telephone book under U.S. Government, Department of Health
and Human Services) or call 1-800-234-5772

United Ostomy Association
36 Executive Park, Suite 120
Irvine, CA 92714
714-660-8624

—by Mary M. Harris

Chapter 38

Overview of Urethral Stricture

Signs and Symptoms.

- Difficulty urinating
- Painful urination

Urethral stricture is a narrowing of the urethra (the narrow tube through the penis that transports urine and semen) to such a degree that the passage of urine is impeded. This is a rare condition. There are various causes of urethral stricture, including injury to the penis or disease that produces scar tissue which gradually shrinks and narrows the urethral passage. In extreme instances, the passage can even be blocked. Urethral stricture may become evident a number of years after an acute episode of gonorrhea.

The Diagnosis. Visit a urologist if you have difficulty or pain in urinating. A number of infections and conditions other than urethral stricture can be responsible. Your physician will examine your penis and may perform various tests, including examination of the urethra with a thin, flexible instrument called a Cystoscope.

How Serious Is Urethral Stricture? To restore the ability to urinate normally and painlessly, the urethral stricture must be

---

Larson, David E., ed. *Mayo Clinic Family Health Book* (New York: William Morrow and Company, 1990, p. 1121.

treated. Usually, the first approach is to stretch the urethra by dilating it with a thin instrument (called a sound) that is inserted into the urethra; local anesthesia is used. This treatment must be repeated a number of times. If the passageway does not remain adequate after repeated dilations, a surgical procedure may be necessary.

The severity of the stricture usually is monitored by using the cystoscope. If a surgical procedure is performed, it is done with special instruments through the cystoscope.

Chapter 39

Urinary Tract Infections

Chapter Contents

Section 39.1

Urinary Tract Infections in Adults

NIDDK; NIH Publication No. 91–2097, Revised September 1991.

Urinary tract infections are a serious health problem affecting millions of people each year.

Infections of the urinary tract are common—only respiratory infections occur more often. Each year, urinary tract infections (UTI's) account for about 8 million doctor visits. Women are especially prone

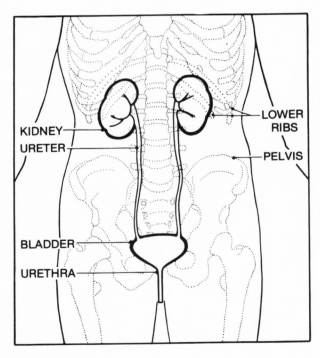

Figure 39.1.1.

to UTI's for reasons that are poorly understood. One woman in five develops a UTI during her lifetime.

The urinary system consists of the kidneys, ureters, bladder, and urethra. The key players in the system are the kidneys, a pair of purplish-brown organs located below the ribs toward the middle of the back. The kidneys remove liquid waste from the blood in the form of urine, keep a stable balance of salts and other substances in the blood, and produce a hormone that aids the formation of red blood cells. Narrow tubes called ureters carry urine from the kidneys to the bladder, a triangle-shaped chamber in the lower abdomen. Urine is stored in the bladder and emptied through the urethra.

The average adult passes about a quart and a half of urine each day. The amount of urine varies, depending on the fluids and foods a person consumes. The volume formed at night is about half that formed in the daytime.

Causes

Normal urine is sterile. It contains fluids, salts, and waste products, but it is free of bacteria, viruses, and fungi. An infection occurs when microorganisms, usually bacteria from the digestive tract, cling to the opening of the urethra and begin to multiply. Most infections arise from one type of bacteria, Escherichia coli (E. coli), which normally live in the colon.

In most cases, bacteria first begin growing in the urethra. An infection limited to the urethra is called urethritis. From there bacteria often move on to the bladder, causing a bladder infection (cystitis). If the infection is not treated promptly, bacteria may then go up the ureters to infect the kidneys (pyelonephritis).

Microorganisms called Chlamydia and Mycoplasma may also cause UTI's in both men and women, but these infections tend to remain limited to the urethra and reproductive system. Unlike E. coli, Chlamydia and Mycoplasma may be sexually transmitted, and infections require treatment of both partners.

The urinary system is structured in a way that helps ward off infection. The ureters and bladder normally prevent urine from backing up toward the kidneys, and the flow of urine from the bladder helps wash bacteria out of the body. In men, the prostate gland produces secretions that slow bacterial growth. In both sexes, immune defenses also prevent infection. Despite these safeguards, though, infections still occur.

Who is at Risk?

Some people are more prone to getting a UTI than others. Any abnormality of the urinary tract that obstructs the flow of urine (a kidney stone, for example) sets the stage for an infection. An enlarged prostate gland also can slow the flow of urine, thus raising the risk of infection.

A common source of infection is catheters, or tubes, placed in the bladder. A person who cannot void, is unconscious or critically ill, often needs a catheter that stays in place for a long time. Some people, especially the elderly or those with nervous system disorders who lose bladder control, may need a catheter for life. Bacteria on the catheter can infect the bladder, so hospital staff take special care to keep the catheter sterile and remove it as soon as possible.

People with diabetes have a higher risk of a UTI because of changes of the immune system. Any disorder that suppresses the immune system raises the risk of a urinary infection.

UTI's may occur in infants who are born with abnormalities of the urinary tract, which sometimes need to be corrected with surgery. UTI's are rarely seen in boys and young men. In women, though, the rate of UTI's gradually increases with age. Scientists are not sure why women have more urinary infections than men. One factor may be that a woman's urethra is short, allowing bacteria quick access to the bladder. Also, a woman's urethral opening is near sources of bacteria from the anus and vagina. For many women, sexual intercourse seems to trigger an infection, although the reasons for this linkage are unclear.

According to several studies, women who use a diaphragm are more likely to develop a UTI than women who use other forms of birth control. Recently, researchers found that women whose partners use a condom with spermicidal foam also tend to have growth of E. coli bacteria in the vagina.

Recurrent Infections

Many women suffer from frequent UTI's. Nearly 20 percent of women who have a UTI will have another, and 30 percent of those will have yet another. Of the last group, 80 percent will have recurrences.

Usually, the latest infection stems from a strain or type of bacteria that is different from the infection before it, indicating a separate infection. (Even when several UTI's in a row are due to E. coli, slight differences in the bacteria indicate distinct infections.)

Research funded by the National Institutes of Health (NIH) suggests that one factor behind recurrent UTI's may be the ability of bacteria to attach to cells lining the urinary tract. A recent NIH funded study has also shown that women with recurrent UTI's tend to have certain blood types. Some scientists speculate that women with these blood types are more prone to UTI's because the cells lining the vagina and urethra may allow bacteria to attach more easily. Further research will show whether this association is sound and proves useful in identifying women at high risk for UTI's.

Infections in Pregnancy

Pregnant women seem no more prone to UTI's than other women. However, when a UTI does occur, it is more likely to travel to the kidneys. According to some reports, about 2 to 4 percent of pregnant women develop a urinary infection. Scientists think that hormonal changes and shifts in the position of the urinary tract during pregnancy make it easier for bacteria to travel up the ureters to the kidneys. For this reason, many doctors recommend periodic testing of urine.

Symptoms

Not everyone with a UTI has symptoms, but most people get at least some. These may include a frequent urge to urinate and a painful, burning feeling in the area of the bladder or urethra during urination. It is not unusual to feel bad all over-tired, shaky, washed out—and to feel pain even when not urinating. Often, women feel an uncomfortable pressure above the pubic bone, and some men experience a fullness in the rectum. It is common for a person with a urinary infection to complain that, despite the urge to urinate, only a small amount of urine is passed. The urine itself may look milky or cloudy, even reddish if blood is present. A fever may mean that the infection has reached the kidneys. Other symptoms of a kidney infection include pain in the back or side below the ribs, nausea, or vomiting.

In children, symptoms of a urinary infection may be overlooked or attributed to another disorder. A UTI should be considered when a child or infant seems irritable, is not eating normally, has an unexplained fever that does not go away, has incontinence or loose bowels, or is not thriving. The child should be seen by a doctor if there are any questions about these symptoms, especially if there is a change in the child's urinary pattern.

Diagnosis

To find out whether you have a UTI, your doctor will test a sample of urine for pus and bacteria. You will be asked to give a "clean catch" urine sample by washing the genital area and collecting a "midstream" sample of urine in a sterile container. (This method of collecting urine helps prevent bacteria around the genital area from getting into the sample and confusing the test results.) Usually, the sample is sent to a laboratory, although some doctors' offices are equipped to do the testing.

In the urinalysis test, the urine is examined for white and red blood cells and bacteria. Then the bacteria are grown in a culture and tested against different antibiotics to see which drug best destroys the bacteria. This last step is called a sensitivity test.

Some microbes, like Chlamydia and Mycoplasma, can only be detected with special bacterial cultures. A doctor suspects one of these infections when a person has symptoms of a UTI and pus in the urine, but a standard culture fails to grow any bacteria.

When an infection does not clear up with treatment and is traced to the same strain of bacteria, the doctor will order a test that makes images of the urinary tract. One of these tests is an intravenous pyelogram (IVP), which gives x-ray images of the bladder, kidneys, and ureters. An opaque dye visible on x-ray film is injected into a vein, and a series of x-rays are taken. The film shows an outline of the urinary tract, revealing even small changes in the structure of the tract.

If you have recurrent infections, your doctor also may recommend an ultrasound exam, which gives pictures from the echo patterns of sound waves bounced back from internal organs. Another useful test is cystoscopy. A cystoscope is an instrument made of a hollow tube with several lenses and a light source, which allows the doctor to see inside the bladder from the urethra.

Treatment

UTI's are treated with antibacterial drugs. The choice of drug and length of treatment depends on the patient's history and the urine tests that identify the offending bacteria. The sensitivity test is especially useful in helping the doctor select the most effective drug. The drugs most often used to treat routine, uncomplicated UTI's are trimethoprim (Trimpex), trimethoprim/sulfamethoxazole (Bactrim, Septra, Cotrim), amoxicillin (Amoxil, Trimox, Wymox), nitrofurantoin (Macrodantin, Furadantin), and ampicillin.

Often, a UTI can be cured with 1 or 2 days of treatment if the infection is not complicated by an obstruction or nervous system disorder. Still, many doctors ask their patients to take antibiotics for a week or two to assure that the infection has been cured. Single-dose treatment is not recommended for some groups of patients, for example, those who have delayed treatment or have signs of a kidney infection, patients with diabetes or structural abnormalities, or men who have prostate infections. Longer treatment is also needed by patients with infections caused by Mycoplasma or Chlamydia, which are usually treated with tetracycline, trimethoprim/sulfamethoxazole (TMP/SMZ), or doxycycline. A followup urinalysis helps to confirm that the urinary tract is infection-free. It is important to take the full course of treatment because symptoms may disappear before the infection is fully cleared.

Severely ill patients with kidney infections may be hospitalized until they can take fluids and needed drugs on their own. Kidney infections generally require several weeks of antibiotic treatment. Researchers at the University of Washington found that 2-week therapy with TMP/SMZ was as effective as 6 weeks of treatment with the same drug in women with kidney infections that did not involve an obstruction or nervous system disorder. In such cases, kidney infections rarely lead to kidney damage or kidney failure unless they go untreated.

Various drugs are available to relieve the pain of a UTI. A heating pad or a warm bath may also help. Most doctors suggest that drinking plenty of water helps cleanse the urinary tract of bacteria. For the time being, it is best to avoid coffee, alcohol, and spicy foods. (And one of the best things a smoker can do for his or her bladder is to quit smoking. Smoking is the major known cause of bladder cancer.)

Recurrent Infections in Women

About 4 out of 5 women who have a UTI get another in 18 months. Many women have them even more often. A woman who has frequent recurrences (three or more a year) should ask her doctor about one of the following treatment options:

- Take low doses of an antibiotic such as TMP/SMZ or nitrofurantoin daily for 6 months or longer. (If taken at bedtime, the drug remains in the bladder longer and may be more effective.) NIH-supported research at the University of Washington has shown this therapy to be effective without causing serious side effects.

- Take a single dose of an antibiotic after sexual intercourse.

- Take a short course (1 or 2 days) of antibiotics when symptoms appear.

Dipsticks that change color when an infection is present are now available without prescription. The strips detect nitrite, which is formed when bacteria change nitrate the urine to nitrate. The test can detect about 90 percent of UTI's and may be useful for women who have recurrent infections.

Doctors suggest some additional steps that a woman can take on her own to avoid an infection:

- Drink plenty of water every day. Some doctors suggest drinking cranberry juice, which in large amounts inhibits the growth of some bacteria by acidifying the urine. Vitamin C (Ascorbic Acid) supplements have the same effect.

- Urinate when you feel the need; don't resist the urge to urinate;

- Wipe from front to back to prevent bacteria around the anus from entering the vagina or urethra;

- Take showers instead of tub baths;

- Cleanse the genital area before sexual intercourse;

- Avoid using feminine hygiene sprays and scented douches, which may irritate the urethra.

Infections in Pregnancy

A pregnant woman who develops a UTI should be treated promptly to avoid premature delivery of her baby and other risks such as high blood pressure. Some antibiotics are not safe to take during pregnancy.

In selecting the best treatments, doctors consider various factors such as the drug's effectiveness, the stage of pregnancy, the mother's health, and potential effects on the fetus.

Complicated Infections

Curing infections that stem from a urinary obstruction or nervous system disorder depends on finding and correcting the underlying problem, sometimes with surgery. If the root cause goes untreated, this group of patients is at risk of kidney damage. Also, such infections tend to arise from a wider range of bacteria, and sometimes from more than one type of bacteria at a time.

UTI's are unusual in men. They usually stem from an obstruction — for example, a urinary stone or enlarged prostate — or a medical procedure involving a catheter. The first step is to identify the infecting organism and the drugs to which it is sensitive. Usually, doctors recommended lengthier therapy in men than in women, in part to prevent infections of the prostate gland. Prostate infections (prostatitis) are harder to cure because antibiotics are unable to penetrate infected prostate tissue effectively. For this reason, men with prostatitis often need long-term treatment with a carefully selected antibiotic.

Research in Urinary System Disorders

The NIH conducts and supports a variety of research in diseases of the kidney and urinary tract. The knowledge gained from these studies is advancing scientific understanding of why UTI's develop and is leading to improved methods of diagnosing, treating, and preventing infections.

The National Institute of Diabetes and Digestive and Kidney Diseases, part of the NIH, has established six research centers around the country with the goal of reducing the major causes of kidney and urinary tract diseases through innovative research. The lead researchers, their institutions, and research focus are as follows:

George M. O'Brien Kidney and Urological Research Centers

Barry M. Brenner, M.D.
Division of Nephrology
Brigham and Women's Hospital
75 Francis Street
Boston, Massachusetts 02115
(617) 732-5850
Kidney Disease of Diabetes Mellitus and Kidney Transplant Rejection

Roger C. Wiggins, M.D.
Division of Nephrology
University of Michigan
3914 Taubman Center
1500 East Medical Center Drive
Ann Arbor, Michigan 48109-0364
(313) 936-5645
Glomerulonephritis

Harry R. Jacobson, M.D.
Vanderbilt University
School of Medicine
53223 Medical Center North
21st Avenue, South
Nashville, Tennessee 37232-2732
(615) 322-4794
Progressive Glomerular Sclerosis and Kidney Transplant Rejection

David G. Warnock, M.D.
Division of Nephrology
University of Alabama at Birmingham
Room 647 THT, UAB Station
Birmingham, Alabama 35294
(205) 934-3585
Effects of High Blood Pressure on the Kidney, Glomerulonephritis and
Interstitial Nephritis

Ahmad Elbadawi, M.D.
SUNY Upstate Center
750 East Adams Street
Syracuse, New York 13210
(315) 464-5737
Urinary Tract Obstruction

John T. Glayhack, M.D.
Department of Urology
Northwestern University Medical School
303 East Chicago Avenue
Chicago, Illinois 60611
(312) 908-8145
Prostate Enlargement

Suggestions for Additional Reading

The following materials can be found in medical libraries, many college and university libraries, and through interlibrary loan in most public libraries.

Corriere, Joseph N. Jr. et al., "Cystitis: Evolving Standard of Care," Patient Care, Feb. 29, 1988, pp. 3347.

Fowler, Jackson E. Jr., "Urinary Tract Infections in Women," Urologic Clinics of North America, Nov. 1986, pp. 673–683.

Gillenwater, Jay Y. et al., eds. Adult and Pediatric Urology, vol. 1. Chicago: Yearbook Medical Publishers, 1987.

Goldman, Peggy L. et al., "Evaluating Dysuria in the Era of STDs," Patient Care, January 15, 1991, pp. 51–69.

Hooton, Thomas M. et al., "Escherichia coli Bacteriuria and Contraceptive Method," Journal of the American Medical Association, January 2, 1991, pp. 64–69.

Krieger, John N., "Complications and Treatment of Urinary Tract Infections During Pregnancy," Urologic Clinics of North America, Nov. 1986, pp. 685–693.

Section 39.2

New Help for Urinary Tract Infections

FDA Consumer, June 1995.

Though men don't escape urinary tract infections—especially as they age and their prostates cause problems—women get the lion's share of UTIs, about 25 times more often than men. Most of these infections are uncomplicated: They occur in otherwise healthy women and girls who have normal urinary tracts and normal urinary functioning and no underlying physical problems.

The National Institute or Diabetes and Digestive and Kidney Diseases of the National Institutes of Health estimates that by age 30, half of all women experience at least one UTI, and about 20 percent of these women will have recurrent UTIs. Each year, UTIs are responsible for more than 6 million doctor visits and about $4.5 billion in health-care costs. Only upper respiratory tract infections account for more absenteeism in working women.

The urinary tract consists of the kidneys, ureters, bladder, and urethra. The kidneys—bean-shaped organs weighing about 4 to 6 ounces in the adult and located below the ribs toward the middle of the back—filter liquid waste from the blood that passes through them to produce urine. Urine passes from the kidneys down through two narrow tubes called ureters to the bladder, a triangular-shaped organ in the lower abdomen. The bladder acts as a reservoir for urine until it is emptied out through the urethra, a tube leading from the bladder to outside the body.

When limited to the urethra, an infection of the urinary tract is called urethritis. More often than not, however, bacteria travel up a woman's one-and-a-half-inch-long urethra to the bladder, where they may cause cystitis, the most common urinary tract infection. A more serious condition called pyelonephritis results when bacteria from the bladder ascend to the kidneys via the ureters.

Before the modern drug era, doctors prescribed the urinary anti-septic Mandelamine (methenamine mandelate), cranberry juice, and diets that acidified the urine to prevent and treat recurrent UTIs. In many cases, this treatment was ineffective, and women who had recurrent UTIs ultimately suffered kidney failure. By the 1940s, the antimicrobial sulfa drugs had been introduced and proved very effective in treating UTIs. The explosive development of broad-spectrum antibiotics that began about the same time with the discovery of penicillin—and continued with the development of tetracyclines, erythromycin and cephalosporins—provided more options in treating UTIs.

New Drugs

In the last few years, FDA has approved a group of drugs called quinolones (including ciprofloxacin [Cipro], enoxacin [Penetrex], norfloxacin [Noroxin], ofloxacin [Floxin], cinoxacin [Cinobac], and lomefloxacin [Maxaquin]) for treating both uncomplicated UTIs and more serious urinary tract disorders. Philip Hanno, M.D., chairman of the urology department and professor of urology at Temple University, Philadelphia, Pa., says that with quinolones, "... you don't have to bring people into the hospital to get good levels of antibiotics that can treat pseudomonas and other gram-negative organisms. Previously, we had to use parenteral antibiotics [intravenous medications]. I do think they're overused, though, and resistance to them is developing."

Each group of drugs affects bacteria in the urine differently, either by interfering with reproduction, or depriving them of certain enzymes necessary for their growth. Successful treatment depends on the concentration of the bacteria fighting drug in the urine.

Normal urine is sterile. An average adult passes about 3 pints of urine each day, but the amount varies, depending on how much food and drink are consumed.

The urinary system is constructed to repel infection. Valve-like structures at the lower ends of the ureters prevent urine from backing up (called vesicoureteral reflux) into the kidneys, where it could cause damage. When infection occurs, urination helps wash bacteria out of the bladder.

Symptoms of Infection

Sometimes a person can have a UTI without having symptoms. But usually UTIs are accompanied by such discomforts as pain and a burning sensation during urination, frequent urination—often passing no more than a few drops at a time—and a feeling that the bladder doesn't feel empty even after urinating. The urine may look cloudy, or may have a bloody tinge. A person with a UTI may feel tired and shaky, sick all over. Often, women feel pressure above the pubic bone and men feel fullness in the rectum. Chills and fever, flank pain, nausea, and vomiting suggest kidney involvement.

Common Culprits

Many bacteria can cause UTIs in women, but the most common are *Escherichia coli (E. Coli)*, responsible for over 80 percent of infections. Normally, these bacteria reside in the gastrointestinal tract, but they may also be present in the vaginal and rectal areas, and on the skin of the perineum, the band of flesh between the anus and the vagina. Sexually transmitted microorganisms *Chlamydia trachomatis* and T-mycoplasma *(Ureaplasma)* can cause UTIs in both men and women. These infections are usually confined to the urethra and reproductive organs.

Women can acquire UTIs after sexual intercourse. Many women have their first bout of cystitis after they become sexually active; in fact, "honeymoon cystitis" was once a common name for this affliction. Data from a variety of studies suggest that during sexual intercourse, bacteria in the vaginal area can be pushed into the urethral opening and move up into the bladder, making it one of the most important risk factors for developing uncomplicated UTIs.

Using a diaphragm for contraception can be an additional risk factor for UTIs. The diaphragm may press on the neck of the bladder, preventing it from emptying completely and leaving a pool of stagnant urine for bacteria to grow in. Bacteria may also enter the urinary tract when the diaphragm is inserted and removed and when it is left in place longer than recommended by the labeling or the doctor. Recently, researchers found an association between UTIs and sexual intercourse when women use a spermicide or a diaphragm/spermicide or when their partners use a condom with spermicidal foam. Thomas Hooton, M.D., and Walter Stamm, M.D., in the March 1991 issue of *Medical Clinics of North America* report that spermicides increase colonization of the vagina with bacteria, thus increasing risk of bladder infection.

Pregnant women get about the same number of UTIs as nonpregnant, sexually active women of childbearing age. However, when a pregnant woman gets a UTI, it is more likely to travel upwards to the kidneys. Since a woman can have bacteria in her urine, but no symptoms, it's important that urine cultures be performed on the first prenatal visit and at intervals thereafter. Studies have shown an association between bacteria in the urine in the first trimester and the subsequent development of acute pyelonephritis. Pregnant women with UTIs can be treated with antibiotics, but, as always, the drug's effectiveness, the stage of pregnancy, the mother's health, and the potential effects on the fetus have to be carefully considered.

Not all UTIs are a result of sexual activity. Another common source of infection is the catheter, a tube that is placed in the bladder to drain off urine when a patient is unconscious, very ill, recovering from surgery, or incontinent. About 900,000 UTIs are contracted in hospitals each year, and up to 90 percent of these infections are associated with indwelling catheters. Avoiding unnecessary catheterization is the best way to prevent such UTIs. When a catheter is necessary, strict antiseptic techniques must be used by medical personnel when inserting and maintaining this device to prevent the introduction of bacteria into the bladder.

Diabetics run a higher risk of UTIs because their immune systems are suppressed. Additionally, their urine is rich in glucose, which is a good growing medium for any bacteria that enter the bladder.

Diagnosis

Though a urinalysis can tell the doctor bacteria are present in the urine, only a urine culture can identify the particular organism. Which drug will be effective and the length of time it is used depend both on the patient's history and what the culture reveals. Since a UTI can cause excruciating discomfort—and since many medications are effective against a UTI—most doctors prefer to treat patients with symptoms without waiting the 48 hours or so for culture results. The medication can be changed at that time, if necessary.

Doctors may treat routine, uncomplicated UTIs with trimethoprim (Trimpex), trimethoprim/sulfamethoxazole (Bactrim, Septra, Cotrim), amoxicillin (Amoxil, Trimox, Wymox), nitrofurantoin (Macrodantin, Furadantin), ampicillin, and other drugs. Many of these drugs cause side effects, such as rash, itching, nausea, diarrhea, abdominal cramping, difficulty in breathing, and sensitivity to sunlight. Tetracyclines, cotrimoxazole, nitrofurantoin, and quinolones are not recommended for pregnant women. Patients should report all known allergies, such as an allergy to penicillin or sulfa drugs, to the doctor before treatment begins.

Types of Therapy

Doctors can use single-dose therapy, a three-day course of drugs, or a longer regimen. Studies have shown that a single dose of trimethoprim or cotrimoxazole, for instance, is effective in treating uncomplicated bacterial cystitis and asymptomatic bacterial infections in sexually active women and in girls with normal urinary tracts. Not only do single-dose therapies save money, but they are simple to take—thus promoting compliance—well-tolerated, and preferred by patients. In addition, they produce fewer side effects and less risk of developing resistant organisms. And, for pregnant women, a single dose of some drugs also poses less danger to the fetus.

Not all urologists like single-dose therapy. "I rarely use it," says Hanno, "unless it's someone who's very responsible and has not had symptoms for a long time—generally people who are on self-treatment programs—and won't panic if symptoms don't go away after one dose. Then they can take one dose of medicine and that's it. But since it usually takes two or three days for the symptoms to go away even if you sterilize their urine with one dose, you know that they're going to call you back after taking one pill. I find it makes more sense to put people on the three-day therapy."

Urologists deal with recurrent UTIs in several ways. When women have three or more symptomatic UTIs a year, some urologists may prescribe low doses of an antimicrobial drug, such as trimethoprim/sulfamethoxazole or nitrofurantoin, to be taken daily for six months or longer as a preventative. Taken at bedtime, the drug remains in the bladder the whole night and is thus more effective. Other urologists prefer to give their patients medications to be taken on alternate nights or even three nights a week. When sexual intercourse is the culprit, one dose of an antibiotic after sex has proved a safe, effective and inexpensive treatment for preventing recurrent urinary tract infections.

Since illness is apt to strike at inconvenient times, women subject to recurrent UTIs often panic when they feel symptoms coming on and don't have immediate access to a doctor. "What most urologists do, once we have established that it's a recurrent urinary infection from reinfection—which makes up about 99 percent of UTIs in women—is give them a prescription to keep with them," says Hanno. "At the first sign of infection they take antibiotics for three days. If symptoms don't get better in three days, then it's worthwhile to do a urine culture, to see if something unusual is going on."

UTIs in Men

Men have lower rates of uncomplicated UTIs than women for various reasons. The longer male urethras the greater distance between the urethral opening and the anus (the usual source of bacteria), and the drier environment surrounding the urethra present less opportunity for bacteria to enter the urinary tract. Another plus is that the prostate secretes fluid with antibacterial properties.

"UTIs are uncommon in men," says Hanno. "They usually reflect some anatomic abnormality or bladder dysfunction, and they're usually related to a deep-seated problem."

The male prostate is often involved in UTIs. An enlarged prostate can slow urine flow by squeezing the urethra, which it surrounds, thus setting the stage for a UTI. It works the other way, too. When the prostate is infected (prostatitis), the infection soon spreads to the bladder. UTIs in males are usually treated by long-course therapy of 14 to 21 days, especially when the prostate is involved.

When infections in either men or women persist despite treatment and are caused by the same strain of bacteria, the doctor checks for problems in the urinary system. The intravenous urogram (often incorrectly called the intravenous pyelogram) is an important diagnostic tool: The radiologist injects an iodine-containing liquid dye into the veins. As the dye concentrates in the kidneys and urine and flows through the ureters and bladder, x-ray pictures are taken that outline the urinary tract and reveal any abnormalities.

Another valuable test—especially for babies and people who cannot tolerate the dye used in the intravenous urogram—is done by ultrasound, which gives pictures from the echo patterns of sound waves bounced back from the urinary organs. Doctors may also perform a cystoscopy, where they look into the bladder with a cystoscope, an instrument made of a hollow tube with several lenses and a light source. The doctor can see tumors or other lesions in the bladder, or sediment from urinary stones.

Fortunately, most UTIs don't require such measures. Most healthy adults with normally functioning urinary tracts who have UTIs can be safely and effectively treated with a variety of medications. And, with prompt treatment, they will experience no long-term damage to the urinary system.

How Women Can Prevent UTIs

Here are some suggestions to help prevent UTIs:

- Drink at least eight glasses of water a day, in addition to the coffee, tea, cola drinks, and other beverages you normally drink. Frequent urination flushes bacteria out of the bladder and makes urinary symptoms, if you get a UTI, more bearable. Some doctors advise drinking large amounts of cranberry juice, which acidifies the urine and makes it less hospitable to bacteria.

- Wipe from front to back to prevent bacteria in the anal area from entering the vagina and urethra.

- Empty the bladder shortly before and after sex.

- Wash the genital area before sex with plenty of warm water. Bacteria from the vaginal, anal and perineal areas can be introduced into the urethra during sex.

- Check with your gynecologist if you suspect a diaphragm is contributing to your problems. You may need another size, or perhaps another method of birth control.

- Use some sort of water-soluble lubricant, such as a vaginal jelly (not petroleum jelly), if your vagina feels dry and uncomfortable during sex, especially if you're past menopause. Bruised tissues may become irritated, even infected.

- Avoid using feminine hygiene products, such as sprays, deodorants or douches, which may irritate the urethra.

- Change sanitary pads and tampons frequently during menstruation.

- Avoid using hot tubs—because the water is not hot enough to kill bacteria—and highly chlorinated pools, because too much chlorine may irritate the genital area.

- Don't use perfumed toilet paper, heavily scented soaps and powders in the vaginal area, or bubble baths. (Some bubble bath products warn that they can cause urinary tract irritation.) Some laundry detergents, bleaches, and fabric softeners leave residues that can be irritating or cause allergic reactions. Try unscented laundry detergents or soaps if you are sensitive.

- Take showers instead of baths, because showers wash bacteria away.

- Avoid wearing tight jeans, bodysuits and pantyhose. The heat generated by tight clothing makes it easier for bacteria in your genital area to grow. Replace nylon underclothing with cotton underwear.

— by Evelyn Zamula

Section 39.3

Additional Resources on Urinary Tract Infections

Searches-On-File, Topics in Kidney and Urologic Diseases, NKUDIC.

Legend

TI   Title
AU   Author
CN   Corporate Author
SO   Source
AV   Producer/Availability

TI   **Acute and Recurrent Symptomatic Urinary Tract Infections in Women.**
AU   Bruce, A.W.; Reid, G.
SO   *International Urogynecology Journal.* 4(4): 240–245. 1993.

TI   **Acute Urinary Tract Infection in Women: What Kind of Antibiotic Therapy is Optimal?**
AU   Elder, N.C.
SO   *Postgraduate Medicine.* 92(6): 159–162, 165–166, 172. November 1, 1992.

TI   **Asymptomatic Significant Bacteriuria in the Elderly.**
AU   Oreopoulos, D.G.; Lam, D.T.Y.
SO   *Geriatric Nephrology and Urology.* 1(1): 57–64. 1991.

TI   **Battle of the Bladder: The Pathogenesis and Treatment of Uncomplicated Cystitis.**
AU   Nickel, J.C.
SO   *International Urogynecology Journal.* 1(4): 218–222. December 1990.

TI **Behavioral Risk Factors for Urinary Tract Infections in Women.**
AU Leibovici, L.
SO *International Urogynecology Journal.* (2)2: 105–107. June 1991.

TI **Common Urologic Problems: A Management Update.**
AU Fantl, J.A.
SO *Female Patient.* 14(1): 31, 34, 36, 38, 41–42, 47. January 1989.

TI **Differential Diagnosis of Uncomplicated Versus Complicated Urinary Tract Infection.**
AU Harrison, L.H.
SO In: Harrison, L.H. *Management of Urinary Tract Infections.* London: Royal Society of Medicine. 1990. p. 1–5.
AV Available from Royal Society of Medicine. Barbara Selves, Publications Department, 1 Wimpole Street, London. W1M 8AE. PRICE: $20.00 US plus shipping and handling. ISBN: 1853151114.

TI **Dysuria, Urgency, and Incontinence in Elderly Women with Bladder Diverticulum.**
AU Nissenkorn, I.; Gillon, G.; Servadio, C.
SO *Geriatric Medicine Today.* 9(5): 61–62, 65. May 1990.

TI **Effective Postcoital Prophylaxis of Recurrent Urinary Tract Infections in Premenopausal Women: A Review.**
AU Pfau, A.; Sacks, T.G.
SO *International Urogynecology Journal.* 2(3): 156–160. September 1991.

TI **Idiopathic Sensory Urgency and Early Interstitial Cystitis.**
AU Frazer, M.I.
SO *International Urogynecology Journal.* 4(1): 43–49. February 1993.

TI **Infection in the Elderly: Part I: Urinary Tract Infections.**
AU Barzaga, R.A., et al.
SO *Infectious Disease Practice.* 15(4): 1–7. April 1991.

TI   Interstitial Cystitis: Review of the Literature.

AU   Jensen, H.; Nielsen, K; Frimodt-Moller, C.

SO   *Urology International*. 44(4): 189–193. July-August 1989.

TI   Interstitial Cystitis: An Overlooked Cause of Pelvic Pain.

AU   Levine, D.Z.

SO   *Postgraduate Medicine*. 88(1): 101–109.

TI   Kidney and Bladder Problems Can Always Be Helped.

AU   Rob, C.; Reynolds, J.

SO   In: Rob, C. and Reynolds, J. *Caregiver's Guide: Helping Elderly Relatives Cope with Health and Safety Problems*. Boston, MA: Houghton Mifflin Company. 1991. p. 245–272.

AV   Available from Houghton Mifflin Company. 2 Park Street, Boston, MA 02108. (800)225-3362. PRICE: $12.95 (paper), $22.95 (cloth). ISBN: 0395500869.

TI   *Management of Urinary Tract Infections*.

AU   Harrison, L., ed.

SO   London: Royal Society of Medicine. 1990. 120 p.

AV   Available from Royal Society of Medicine. Barbara Selves, Publications Department, 1 Wimpole Street, London. W1M 8AE. PRICE: $20.00 US plus shipping and handling. ISBN: 1853151114.

TI   Norfloxacin Prophylaxis for Acute Recurrent Uncomplicated Urinary Tract Infection in Women.

AU   Nicolle, L.E.

SO   *International Urogynecology Journal*. 3(2): 150–154. June 1992.

TI   *Practical Urogynecology*.

AU   Wall, L.L.; Norton, P.A.; Delancey, J.O.L.

SO   Baltimore, MD: Williams and Wilkins. 1993. 399 p.

AV   Available from Williams and Wilkins. 428 East Preston Street, Baltimore, MD 21202. (800) 638-0672. PRICE: $70.00 plus $4.00 UPS shipping and handling. ISBN 0683086456.

TI   **Preventive Therapy in Urinary Tract Infection: Twenty Years' Experience.**
AU   Brumfitt, W.; Hamilton-Miller, J.M.
SO   In: Harrison, L.H. *Management of Urinary Tract Infections.* London: Royal Society of Medicine. 1990. p. 59–68.
AV   Available from Royal Society of Medicine. Barbara Selves, Publications Department, 1 Wimpole Street, London. W1M 8AE. PRICE: $20.00 US plus shipping and handling. ISBN: 1853151114.

TI   **Recognizing and Treating Acute Pyelonephritis.**
AU   Johnson, J.R.
SO   *Emergency Medicine.* 24(3): 25–27, 30–31. February 29, 1992.

TI   **Say Goodbye to Cystitis.**
AU   Nechas, E.; London, C.
SO   *Prevention.* p. 48–55, 122–123. November 1991.

TI   **Selecting Therapy for Uncomplicated UTI: Viewpoint from the USA.**
AU   Parsons, C.L.
SO   In: Harrison, L.H. *Management of Urinary Tract Infections.* London: Royal Society of Medicine. 1990. p. 7–13.
AV   Available from Royal Society of Medicine. Barbara Selves, Publications Department, 1 Wimpole Street, London. W1M 8AE. PRICE: $20.00 US plus shipping and handling. ISBN: 1853151114.

TI   **Sex and Interstitial Cystitis: Explaining the Pain and Planning Self-Care.**
AU   Webster, D.C.
SO   *Urologic Nursing.* 13(1): 4–11. March 1993.

TI   **Sexuality and IC.**
AU   Webster, D.
SO   Woodhaven, NY: Interstitial Cystitis Association. September 1991. 10 p.
AV   Available from Interstitial Cystitis Association. P.O. Box 256, Woodhaven, NY 11421. (212) 979-6058 or (800) ICA-1626. PRICE: $6.50.

TI   **Special Considerations in the Management of Acute Urinary Tract Infection.**

AU   Van Kerrebroeck, P.E.

SO   In: Harrison, L.H. *Management of Urinary Tract Infections.* London: Royal Society of Medicine. 1990. p. 69–77.

AV   Available from Royal Society of Medicine. Barbara Selves, Publications Department, 1 Wimpole Street, London. W1M 8AE. PRICE: $20.00 US plus shipping and handling. ISBN: 1853151114.

TI   **Treatment of Urinary Tract Infections in Women.**

AU   Elhilali, M.

SO   *Modern Medicine of Canada.* 45(2): 126–130. February 1990.

TI   **Urinary Incontinence in the Elderly: An Oestrogen Deficiency Disease?: A Review of the Literature.**

AU   Walter, S.; Kjaergaard, B.

SO   *Danish Medical Bulletin.* Number 8: 23–26. March 1989.

TI   **Urinary Tract Infection in Women: Current Role of Single-Dose Therapy.**

AU   Bump, R.C.

SO   *Journal of Reproductive Medicine.* 35(8): 785–791. August 1990.

TI   **Urinary Tract Infection: Selecting the Optimal Agent.**

AU   Johnson, J.R.

SO   *Drug Therapy.* 21(3): 27–32, 37. March 1991.

TI   **Urinary Tract Infections in Obstetrics and Gynecology.**

AU   Tan, J.S.; File, T. M.

SO   *Journal of Reproductive Medicine.* 35(3): 339–342. March 1990.

TI   **Urinary Tract Infections in Women: Diagnosis and Treatment.**

AU   Johnson, J.R.; Stamm, W.E.

SO   *Annals of Internal Medicine.* 111(11): 906–917. December 1, 1989.

TI   *Urinary Tract Infections.*
SO   New York, NY: National Kidney Foundation. 1990. 6 p.
CN   National Kidney Foundation.
AV   Available from National Kidney Foundation. 30 East 33rd Street, New York, NY 10016. (800) 622-9010. PRICE: Single copy free ($12.00 per 100 copies). Order Number 08–53.

TI   *Urinary Tract Infections.*
SO   Washington. DC: American College of Obstetricians and Gynecologists. March 1991. 4 p.
CN   American College of Obstetricians and Gynecologists.
AV   Available from American College of Obstetricians and Gynecologists. 409 12th Street, S.W., Washington, DC 20024-2188. (202) 638-5577. PRICE: Single copy free.

TI   **UTI: Managing the Most Common Nursing Home Infection.**
AU   Breitenbucher, R.B.
SO   *Geriatrics.* 45(5): 68–70, 75. May 1990.

TI   **Women's Attitudes and the Treatment of Urinary Tract Infections.**
AU   Elhilali, M.
SO   In: Harrison, L.H. *Management of Urinary Tract Infections.* London: Royal Society of Medicine. 1990. p. 97–104.
AV   Available from Royal Society of Medicine. Barbara Selves, Publications Department, 1 Wimpole Street, London. W1M 8AE. PRICE: $20.00 US plus shipping and handling. ISBN: 1853151114.

For More Information

CHID is available on-line through CDP Online. If you would like references to materials on other topics, you may request a special literature search of CHID from a library that subscribes to CDP Online or from the National Kidney and Urologic Diseases Information Clearinghouse, 3 Information Way, Bethesda, MD 20892-3580; (301) 654-4415.

Chapter 40

Common Genitourinary Infections

Vulvovaginal pain, itching, and burning are a triad of symptoms for which women frequently seek health care. Often accompanied by vaginal discharge, and dysuria, these symptoms account for as many as 5 million office visits a year. Proper assessment and management of these symptoms by nurses, nurse practitioners, and nurse midwives can help to substantially improve a woman's quality of life and help prevent long-term problems. Several differing syndromes or infections can be the cause of these symptoms. The most common causes are discussed, and a plan for management and prevention is presented.

Some of the most common symptoms reported by women are vulvovaginal itching, burning, pain, dysuria, and vaginal discharge. These symptoms account for a large percentage of ambulatory office visits each year. Although usually not life threatening, these symptoms and the underlying infection responsible for them can have an adverse effect on a woman's quality of life. If untreated, or improperly treated, such infections can lead to chronic vulvovaginal irritation and dyspareunia. The symptoms reported have multiple causes that are either vaginal or urinary in origin. This article addresses the most common problems responsible for the clinical presentation of vaginal discharge, itching, burning, and dysuria. A plan for assessment, treatment, and prevention is presented.

JOGNN Clinical Issues, Volume 24, Number 8, October 1995.

Vaginal Infections

Vaginitis probably is the most common infection in women during their reproductive years, resulting in 5-10 million health-care visits a year (Faro, 1994). The workup for a woman with a suspected vaginal infection should start with a complete gynecologic history. The woman's age is important in making a differential diagnosis. The most common infections seen in women of reproductive age are bacterial vaginosis (BV), candidiasis (VVC), and trichomoniasis. Although atrophic vaginitis is a common cause of vaginal discharge and burning in postmenopausal women, reproductive neoplasia also may present in this manner. For the prepubescent girl, the nurse needs to be aware that discharge may be associated with a vaginal foreign body or sexual abuse.

As with any presenting complaint, onset and associated symptoms are important in making a diagnosis Was the onset sudden or gradual? Is there pruritus? Is there odor? The nurse should ask the client to describe the quality and quantity of the discharge. The date of the last menstrual period is important for two reasons. Some infections tend to become more symptomatic with menses which helps in differentiating the etiology. Treatment may need to be modified if the client is pregnant or breastfeeding. The presence or absence of chronic disease also is important. Chronic disease may increase the likelihood of infection caused by the disease process or by the medications used for treatment. Because all clients who present with vaginal discharge, itching, and dysuria do not have an infectious process, a history of the use of feminine hygiene products and patient allergies are critical components of the history. Because some of the disorders are sexually transmitted, a complete sexual history is needed to correctly assess the client presenting with vaginal discharge. Treatment of the client and her partner is required with certain disorders.

Physical Examination

Physical examination of women with vaginal discharge should include an abdominal examination, inspection and palpation of the external genitalia, speculum and bimanual examination, and microscopic examination of the vaginal discharge. Cultures for gonorrhea and chlamydia may be done if the possibility of such diseases is indicated by history.

A complete abdominal examination can assist in ruling out upper reproductive tract infection. Percussion, palpation, and auscultation of the abdomen usually yield normal results. With cystitis, there may be suprapubic tenderness on palpation over the bladder.

The vulva, including the vestibule, should be carefully examined for evidence of edema, erythema, and fissures. Using a cotton swab can assist in localizing focal pain and help with the diagnosis of vestibulitis (Secor & Fertilla, 1992; Sobel, 1990). If the skin has been excoriated, a secondary bacterial infection may be present. The presence of vulvar lesions may indicate more than one disease process and can direct the need for additional testing. An examination of the vagina and cervix to look for erythema, petechiae, ulcerations, lesions, and discharge is necessary. Bimanual examination results in a woman with vaginitis usually are negative. Because there is no uterine or ovarian involvement, tenderness is an uncommon finding.

The vaginal discharge should be examined for amount, color, consistency, and odor. A wet mount using both normal saline and potassium hydroxide is most useful for the microscopic examination of the discharge (Kaufman & Hammill, 1990). Culture of the discharge may prove useful, especially in difficult cases. The growth of pseudo hyphae on Nicholson's or Saboraud medium is diagnostic of candidiasis (Carcio & Secor, 1992). Modified Diamond medium is used to culture for trichomoniasis. This culture should be incubated anaerobically. Growth usually is detected within 48 hours (Rein & Muller, 1989). No culture is recommended for bacterial vaginosis (Sobel, 1990).

Behavioral Suggestions to Promote Normal Vaginal Environment

- No douching
- Wear cotton fabric, especially underwear
- Maintain good perineal hygiene
- Avoid vaginal contamination
- Avoid tampons
- Use condoms
- Reduce food sources of sugar

Candida

Vulvovaginal candidiasis (VVC) is a common, irritating, and recurrent infection (Carcio & Secor, 1992). Candidiasis is the second most common vaginal infection in the United States (Sobel, 1990). It is estimated that the incidence doubled between 1981 and 1991 (Kent,

1991). As many as 75% of women will experience at least one episode of candidiasis in their lifetime; 40-45% of women will experience two or more infections. Recurrent VVC, defined as three or more episodes within a year, is present in approximately 5% of women (Carcio & Secor, 1992; "1993 Sexually transmitted disease," 1993).

Candida albicans is the most common causative organism of symptomatic infections. The incidence of nonalbicans infections also has risen dramatically. In 1970, non-albicans vaginal infections accounted for 5-10% of all infections. Today, 15-25% of VVC is non-albicans. *C. tropicalis* and *C. glabrata* are the species most frequently replacing albicans as the causative agent (Kent, 1991; Carcio & Secor, 1992).

C. albicans is found in as many as 25% of women with no symptoms (Reed & Eyler, 1993). It is unclear why some women do not experience a symptomatic infection; one theory is that the pathogenicity of *C. albicans* is low (Schaeffer, 1991). However, if the host or environment is altered, infection may result. Numerous risk factors are associated with an increased incidence of candidiasis (Eschenbach & Mead, 1992). Host alterations that can predispose to the development of a symptomatic infection include pregnancy, diabetes mellitus, obesity, and an immunosuppressed state. A woman receiving antimicrobial therapy will have an increased likelihood of infection (Sobel, 1990). Changes in the vaginal environment also can increase the number of symptomatic infections associated with candidiasis. Clothing that is too tight or made of synthetic material, douching, and a diet high in refined sugar have been implicated in vaginal candidiasis infections (Eschenbach & Mead, 1992).

The hallmark presenting symptom for candidiasis is itching. Vulvar and vaginal tissues are inflamed, so burning on urination also may be present. Because of the inflammation, dyspareunia is common. A thick, white paste-like discharge may be present, not only in the vagina, but also the labia, mons, crural folds, thighs, and buttocks. Diagnosis can be confirmed by microscopic examination or culture (Carcio & Secor, 1992; Kaufman & Hammill, 1990; Sobel, 1990).

Treatment consists of topical agents. Azole drugs, such as butoconazole, clotrimazole, terconazole, and ticonazole, are the most effective topical treatment, resulting in relief of symptoms and negative culture results ("1993 Sexually transmitted disease," 1993). Most of the products are available in cream or tablet form. The length of treatment can vary from a single dose to a 7-day therapy regimen. Although results are not conclusive, the single dose probably works better for women with uncomplicated, nonrecurrent, mild VVC. Clotrimazole and miconazole are over-the-counter medications. The nurse can advise self-medication for a woman who previously had a confirmed diagnosis of VVC. It is recommended that a woman with her first vaginal infection see her physician, nurse practitioner, or nurse midwife for a definitive diagnosis. If the infection does not respond to treatment, or recurs within 2-3 months, follow-up health care should be sought. Topical azole therapy also is recommended in pregnant and breast-feeding women (Kaufman & Hammill, 1990; "1993 Sexually transmitted disease," 1993; Sobel, 1990).

Although certainly not common, candidiasis can cause symptoms in a woman's sexual partner. The male partner may have balanitis. He will present with erythematous areas on the glans penis with pruritus. Topical azole will relieve symptoms and cure the infection. Routine treatment of partners without symptoms has not been found to be useful ("1993 Sexually transmitted disease," 1993).

For women experiencing severe burning and itching, comfort measures may be suggested. Sitz baths several times a day may help relieve the external irritation. If dysuria is a problem, pouring warm water over the vulva while voiding will dilute the urine. Sexual intercourse may need to be discontinued until tissues are no longer irritated. Tampons make the treatment less effective by absorbing the medication, so they should not be used during therapy. Prevention should be aimed at identifying any activity that might alter the vaginal environment. The client should be made aware of the predisposing factors and, if appropriate be screened for systemic disease.

Recurrent VVC

The initial approach to a client with recurrent VVC is to look for underlying causes. Diabetes mellitus, immunosuppression, and use of antibiotics and corticosteroids are conditions that can predispose women to chronic VVC; however, most cases have no apparent cause. All cases of recurrent VVC should be confirmed with a culture (Sobel, 1990).

Management of recurrent or chronic VVC can be problematic (Sobel, 1990). Oral ketoconazole 100 mg daily for 6 months has been shown to reduce the occurrence of VVC. Currently under investigation for the treatment of recurrent VVC are weekly intravaginal administration of clotrimazole and weekly oral administration of itraconazole and fluconazole ("1993 Sexually transmitted disease," 1993).

- Candidiasis is the second most common vaginal infection in the United States; as many as 75% of women will experience at least one episode of candidiasis in their lifetime.

- Diabetes mellitus, immunosuppression, and use of antibiotics and coritcosteroids are conditions that can predispose women to chronic VVC; however, most cases have no apparent cause.

Trichomoniasis

Trichomonas vaginalis is an anaerobic protozoan. It is involved in as many as 30% of all cases of vaginitis. Approximately 3 million women a year have trichomoniasis diagnosed and are treated for it. Trichomoniasis is sexually transmitted and can be recovered from as many as 80% of the sexual partners of infected women (Sparks, 1991). The infection in many partners seems to be self-limiting, and most men have no symptoms. *T. vaginalis* can live for several hours outside the body, especially in a moist environment, so transmission can be nonsexual (Sparks, 1991). Fomites such as towels and clothing have been implicated in transmission.

The presenting picture of a woman infected with *T. vaginalis* consists of profuse, yellow-green discharge, vaginal itching, dysuria, and abnormal vaginal odor. A high percentage of women with the infection also will have dypareunia. On physical examination, copious amounts of discharge and redness of the vagina that may extend to the perineum and localized hemorrhages of the cervix and vagina may be noted. Laboratory findings include an elevated pH, 10 or more leukocytes per high-power field, and the presence of the mobile protozoan (Sobel, 1990; Sparks, 1991).

T. vaginalis is a local disorder and is not thought to cause disseminated disease (Shesser, 1991). However, there is an increased incidence of postpartum endometritis in women with *T. vaginalis*. It is not clear whether *T. vaginitis* is the cause of this problem or whether it serves a vector (Thomason & Gelbert, 1989). *T. vaginalis* also has been associated with premature rupture of the membranes and premature delivery during pregnancy. Some women infected with *T. vaginalis* may experience nonspecific lower abdominal pain. Such pain probably is a result of inflammation of the paracervical nodes, but additional study is needed to clearly define this syndrome (Kent, 1991).

The treatment for *T. vaginalis* is metronidazole. Because the organism usually infects the bladder, urethra, and Bartholin's and

Skene's glands, oral therapy provides the most effective treatment. A single dose of 2 g of metronidazole can result in a 95% cure rate. The alternate regimen for treatment is metronidazole 500 mg twice a day for 7 days. The woman's sexual partner should be treated to increase the cure rate. Sexual intercourse should be avoided until both partners are free of symptoms and the course of medication is completed. Effective alternatives to metronidazole are not available ("1993 Sexually transmitted disease," 1993).

There is much controversy surrounding the management of *T. vaginalis* during pregnancy. Metronidazole readily crosses the placenta, so its use is contraindicated during the first trimester of pregnancy because of concern regarding teratogenicity (Sobel, 1990). Symptomatic relief can be obtained with the use of vaginal creams, such as clotrimazole, which may be used during the first trimester. After the first trimester, the woman can be treated with the 2-g regimen of metronidazole. Again, all partners should be treated to increase the cure rate. Breastfeeding women with *T. vaginalis* should be treated with the same regimen used for nonlactating women; however, women should avoid breastfeeding for 12 hours after treatment. The woman should be instructed to pump her breasts and discard the milk (Sparks, 1991).

If treatment failure occurs, it may be because of reinfection, noncompliance, or a resistant strain of *T. vaginalis*. Reinfection may result when the woman's partner is not treated or she has a new infected partner. It is important to explain that all partners need to be treated, and condoms should be used with a new partner. Noncompliance is more common in women receiving the 7-day course of therapy, and these women may be more effectively treated with the single-dose therapy (Sparks, 1991). Resistant strains of *T. vaginalis* have been identified; however, these strains usually respond to a higher does of metronidazole (Sparks, 1991).

Side effects commonly seen with metronidazole are nausea, vomiting, diarrhea, and a metallic taste in the mouth. Transient neutropenia and pseudomembranous colitis also have been reported (Sparks,1991). The major side effect seen with metronidazole is its disulfiram-like effect that is seen with the ingestion of alcohol. Alcohol should be avoided until 48-72 hours after ingestion of the last of the medication.

The nurse should be aware of the education needed by the client with *T. vaginalis*. Supportive care should include comfort measures that begin while the client is undergoing the examination. Once all needed specimens have been collected, the nurse practitioner can clean the discharge from the vagina with a cotton swab. This will help to provide temporary relief of symptoms. Sitz baths can help to relieve the burning and itching of the perineum.

Information concerning transmission is an important aspect of client education. The most likely mode of transmission is sexual. It has been noted that both men and women can have no symptoms and be carriers, so the exact incubation is difficult to define (Thomason & Gelbert 1989). The client may express anger at the possibility of a nonmonogamous relationship. These feelings must be explored and open communication between partners encouraged. The need for partner treatment is an important part of client education. Follow-up is not needed unless symptoms continue.

Bacterial Vaginosis

Bacterial vaginosis (BV) is perhaps one of the most frustrating of the vaginal infections to treat. It is difficult to understand this clinical condition, as can be seen by the long list of names associated with it: nonspecific vaginitis, *Hemophilus vaginalis*, corynebacterium vaginalis, and *Gardnerella vaginalis*. BV is the most common etiology of vaginal infection seen by health care professionals (Bartleson, 1992; Faro, 1994; Sparks, 1991). Several pathogens have been identified as possible causes of BV. In 1955, Garder and Dukes described a syndrome of malodorous discharge with only minimal signs of vulvovaginal inflammation and identified a gram-negative rod named *Gardnerella vaginalis* as the cause (Spiegel, Ansel, & Eschenback, 1980). Later research has found *G. vaginalis* in as many as 40% of women with no symptoms (Spiegel et al., 1980). It appears that BV may be related to the replacement of Lactobacillus in the vagina with high concentrations of anaerobic organisms such as mobilumus curtsii, bacteroides, *G. vaginalis*, and *Mycoplasma hominis* (Bartleson, 1992). The causes of the alteration in the microbial flora of the vagina are not completely understood.

BV is diagnosed by clinical findings. The woman presents with a homogeneous, white to gray discharge that adheres to the vaginal wall. The walls of the cervix and the vagina do not appear to be inflamed. The patient may report a fishy odor that usually is worse after intercourse. A wet mount examination of the discharge will reveal "clue cells." The clue cell is a vaginal epithelial cell to which coccobacillary organisms are adherent. Frequently, the margins of the cell are obscure. The smear also will show few lactobacilli and leukocytes. (If leukocytes are numerous, Trichomonas or a cervical infection caused by organisms such as *Chlamydia trachomatis* or *Neisseria gonorrhea* should be considered.) Vaginal pH usually is greater than 4.5. Three of these four signs or symptoms are required to make a positive diagnosis (Bartleson, 1992; Sobel, 1990).

The relationship of BV to sexual activity is not clear. Although BV is almost always found in sexually active women and is associated with multiple sex partners, it is not considered a sexually transmitted disease. Although the bacteria associated with BV are found in the urethras of male partners of women receiving treatment, the development appears to be related to endogenous factors (Bartleson, 1992). Treatment of partners has not been found beneficial in preventing recurrence ("1993 Sexually transmitted disease," 1993). No clinical counterpart to BV has been identified in men. Sexual abstinence should be used during the course of treatment because it may help to re-establish a normal Lactobacillus dominant flora (Sobel, 1990). The use of condoms lubricated with spermicide may predispose to BV because nonoxynol 9 has been shown to have a bactericidal effect on lactobacilli (LeVasseur, 1992; Stone, Grimes, & Madger, 1986).

The treatment for bacterial vaginosis is directed toward re-establishing the balance of flora in the vagina (Sobel, 1990). Metronidazole has been shown to relieve symptoms and to improve the vaginal flora. Metronidazole 500 mg orally twice a day for 7 days has an overall cure rate of approximately 95%. Although a single 2-g dose of metronidazole has a cure rate of only approximately 84%, it may prove to be the best option in clients with a compliance problem. Clindamycin cream and metronidazole gel can be used for 7 and 5 days, respectively. Cure rates with these products are excellent, and the client may experience fewer systemic side effects ("1993 Sexually transmitted disease," 1993).

Although BV is not invasive to the vaginal tissue, it can cause sequelae. BV in the antepartum period has been associated with adverse pregnancy outcomes (Eschenbach, 1983). Preterm labor and chorioamnionitis have been linked to the organisms associated with BV. Clindamycin cream can be used for treatment during the first trimester ("1993 Sexually transmitted disease," 1993). Oral and topical metronidazole can be used in the second trimester if clindamycin has been ineffective (Bartleson, 1992).

Recurrent or persistent cases of BV should be re-evaluated for the possibility of a coexistent infection. Clindamycin 300 mg orally twice a day for 7 days has been proven to be a successful alternative therapy in cases that seem to be resistant to metronidazole ("1993 Sexually transmitted disease," 1993). Ciprofloxacin, amoxicillin plus clavulanic acid, and cephalexin are agents being examined for use in the treatment of this syndrome (Bartleson, 1992; Reed & Eyler, 1993).

Client education includes pathogenesis of the disorder, its relationship to sexual activity, and proper use of the medication Behavioral suggestions, such as the wearing of cotton fabric and the avoidance of tampons to promote a normal vaginal environment should be stressed. Follow-up is not needed unless symptoms return.

Atrophic Vaginitis

When the woman who is estrogen deprived presents with vaginal irritation and burning, the diagnosis of atrophic vaginitis needs to be considered. Along with the itching and burning, the client may report vaginal dryness, bleeding during intercourse, and dyspareunia (Peters, 1992). It is important to remember that any condition that causes loss of ovarian function can lead to a risk of atrophic vaginitis. Atrophic vaginitis is caused by the changes associated with the loss of estrogen.

On physical examination, special attention should be given to determining whether estrogen deprivation is present. The following are signs of such deprivation:

- pubic hair is sparse;
- labia are atrophic;
- introitus may be stenotic; or
- vaginal mucosa is pale, thin, or friable.

Once it is determined that atrophic vaginitis is present, the client can be treated with estrogen replacement, or lubricants. Estrogen promotes revascularization of the vaginal tissue, thus helping to restore lubrication, and may be given orally, transdermally, and vaginally. Oral or transdermal replacement should be considered if other menopausal symptoms are present or if osteoporosis is a concern. Estrogen replacement should not be given without progestin in women with a uterus because of the increased risk of endometrial cancer (Peters, 1992). If secondary bacterial infection is present, the client will need antibiotic therapy in conjunction with these regimens (Peters, 1992).

For those women who can not or do not wish to use estrogen, vaginal lubricants or moisturizers can be used. Water-based lubricants can be used daily or just before intercourse. Daily use may relieve the sensation of dryness. Oil-based lubricants and those containing vitamin E appear to have a more sustained effect and may be used less often (Freeman, 1995). Research into the exact effect of lubricants on vaginal physiology is needed to determine the exact amount needed to correct the problem.

It is important for a woman to remain sexually active. Sexual activity slows the occurrence of pH changes and vaginal mucosa thinning (Peters, 1992). Women without a partner may need help exploring other forms of sexual activity.

Management of the different vaginitis syndromes is dependent on careful evaluation. The nurse needs to address all of the signs and symptoms during the history and physical examination. Vaginitis is a disorder that affects the client's quality of life. Accurate assessment can help avoid therapeutic failures, thus providing the client with a cure for the problem.

Vulvar Vestibulitis Syndrome

Although the most likely diagnosis of vulvar itching, burning, and pain is a vaginal infection, there may be other causes. Around the turn of the century a syndrome with no identified cause that presented with pain and burning of the vulva and severe dyspareunia on penile insertion was described (Sharp, 1993). This condition, known as vulvar vestibulitis syndrome (VVS), may affect as many as 15% of women (Secor & Fertilla, 1992).

The diagnosis of vestibulitis usually is difficult. Physical findings often are unremarkable or mimic other disorders. VVS has been defined as severe pain associated with entry to the vagina with the presence of diffuse or focal erythema and tenderness of the vestibule (Friedrich, 1987; Secor & Fertilla, 1992). A cotton-tipped applicator can be used to help ascertain vulvar tenderness. Light pressure to the introitus usually will elicit pain. Results of wet mount examination usually are negative for specific pathogens (Secor & Fertilla, 1992). Before the diagnosis can be made, careful study to rule out the common causes of vaginal infections should be done.

The etiology of VVS is unknown; however, there appear to be two forms of vestibulitis (Bazin et al., 1994). The first is associated with diffuse papilloma formation and is thought to be viral in origin. The lesions appear as micropapillomas without the presence of atypical changes. The lesions appear more vividly with the application of 5% acetic acid (Sharp, 1993). The major differential diagnosis is the human papillomavirus. The second type of vestibulitis (idiopathic) appears around the hymenal tags. The area may be smooth with patchy areas of erythema. The area is extremely tender when pressure is applied. Dyspareunia is the most common presenting symptom (Sharp, 1993).

The two types of vestibulitis have some common features. Both cause a diffuse lymphocytic infiltration of the connective tissue. The vestibular glands are not involved in the inflammatory response. The diagnosis of both usually is made by the exclusion of other pathologies. No etiologic organism has been found in most cases (Sharp, 1993).

Vestibulitis can be a chronic and recurring problem. There is no specific treatment; however, the following therapies may provide relief: moisture cream; antiviral medication; behavioral therapy; and topical anesthetic (Secor & Fertilla, 1992).

Surgery has been used in some of the more severe cases. Laser ablation of the area with the flash dye laser, has been used successfully, but additional study is needed to determine the effectiveness of the treatment. Partial vulvectomy has been done with varying success (Sharp, 1993); the reappearance of the symptoms is possible (Secor & Fertilla, 1992; Sparks, 1991). No special comfort measures have been found to be useful. Vestibulitis can be frustrating for the client and health care team.

Urinary Tract Infections

Urinary tract infections (UTI) are one of the most common problems encountered in women and may mimic vaginitis presenting with dysuria and vulvar burning. UTI should be considered part of the differential diagnosis in women presenting with these symptoms. Along with dysuria and vulvar burning, the other characteristic symptoms of cystitis are urinary frequency and suprapubic discomfort. Symptoms can cause sleep disturbances, and patients may miss time from work or have other activities of daily living interrupted by the illness.

If the client has fever, back pain, and costovertebral angle tenderness, pyelonephritis should be considered. These women are systemically unwell and may be experiencing abdominal pain, nausea, and vomiting. Leukocytosis is present with pyelonephritis.

The diagnosis of a UTI is dependent on assessment of the client's urine (Andriole, 1992). Although direct examination of the urine is readily available, it may not provide the necessary information. Bacteriuria alone may not be diagnostic of UTI. Pyuria usually is an indication of a UTI, but pus occasionally can be found in sterile urine (Andriole, 1992). Culture for the presence of the causative microorganism provides the most accurate diagnosis. Correct collection of urine specimens is critical. The use of a clean catch, midstream specimen enhances the chances of obtaining a correct diagnosis.

Urinary tract infections seem to be associated with sexual activity. A change in the frequency of sexual activity can lead to an increased incidence of UTIs. Research also has demonstrated an association between the use of a diaphragm and the occurrence of UTIs (Leiner, 1995), and UTIs have been diagnosed more frequently in women with elevated vaginal pH, absence of vaginal lactobacilli, and presence of bacterial vaginosis (Andriole, 1992).

Historic Clues to Help Determine Use of Short-Use Therapy

- Infection lasting more than 1 week
- Anatomic abnormalities
- Functional abnormalities
- Immunosuppression
- Pregnancy
- Relapse/recurrent infection

If, after a careful history is obtained, the infection is considered uncomplicated, short-course antimicrobial therapy should be considered for UTIs. There are a number of appropriate antibiotics that are effective, with treatments ranging in length from a single dose to a 3-day course. Trimethoprim or trimethoprim-sulfamethoxazole can be used as a single-dose regimen. The new quinones, such as norfloxacin and ciprofloxacin, also can be used. Failure rates for these single-dose therapy regimens are approximately 20%. If the same drugs are used for a 3-day regimen, a 95% cure rate can be expected. As many as one-third of clients with what appears to be uncomplicated cystitis may have an acute renal infection. This possibility must be considered in any failed therapy (Andriole, 1992).

Pyelonephritis can be treated with the same classes of antibiotics; however, a 10-14-day course of therapy is required. If treated on an outpatient basis, the client should be monitored carefully. If sufficient improvement is not seen within 48-72 hours, hospital admittance should be considered.

Behavioral measures to help prevent UTIs should be suggested. Voiding before and after intercourse can help to prevent infections related to sexual activity. Wiping the perineum from front to back will help prevent contamination. Intake of at least eight glasses of water a day also may reduce the chances of infection.

Conclusion

The symptomatology of vulvar-vaginal itching, burning, and pain along with vaginal discharge often are reported by women. Proper assessment, correct management, and client education can lead to the relief of these symptoms and a significant improvement in the quality of life in women experiencing these symptoms.

References

Andriole, V.T. (1992). Urinary tract infection in the 90's: Pathogenesis and management. *Infection,* 20(S4), 5251–5256.

Bartleson, N.R. (1992) Bacterial vaginosis: A subtle yet serious infection. *Nurse Practitioner Forum*, 3(3),130–134.

Bazin, S., Bauchard, C., Brison, I., Morin, C., Meisels, A. & Fortier, M. (1994). Vulva vestibulitis syndrome: An exploratory case-control study. *Obstetrics & Gynecology*, 83(1), 47–50.

Carcio, H.A., & Secor, M.C. (1992). Vulvovaginal candidiasis: A current update. *Nurse Practitioner Forum*, 3(3), 135–144.

Eschenbach, D.A. (1983). Vaginal infection. *Clinical Obstetrics and Gynecology*, 26(3), 186–202.

Eschenbach, D.A., & Mead, P.S. (1992). Managing problem vaginitis. *Patient Care*, 26(14), 137–152.

Faro, S. (1994). Bacterial vaginitis. *Clinical Obstetrics and Gynecology,* 34(3), 582–586.

Freeman, S.B. (1995). Complementary therapies for menopause. *Nurse Practitioner*, 1(1), 40–49.

Friedrich, E.G. (1987). Vulvar vestibulitis syndrome. *Journal of Reproductive Medicine*, 32(3), 110–114.

Kaufman, R.H., & Hammill, H.A. (1990). Vaginitis. *Primary Care*, 17(1), 115–125.

Kent, H.L. (1991). Epidemiology of vaginitis. *American Journal of Obstetrics and Gynecology*, 165(4), 1168–1176.

Leiner, S. (1995). Recurrent urinary tract infections in otherwise healthy adult women. *Nurse Practitioner*, 20(2), 48–55.

LeVasseur, J.J. (1992). Vulvovaginitis: Promotion of condom use to prevent sexually transmitted disease. *Nurse Practitioner Forum*, 3(3), 177–180.

1993 Sexually Transmitted Disease Treatment Guidelines. (1993). *Morbidity and Mortality Weekly Report*, 42, 1–82.

Peters, N.C. (1992). Vulvovaginitis in the postmenopausal women. *Nurse Practitioner Forum*, 3(3), 152–154.

Reed, B.D., & Eyler, A. (1993). Vaginal infections: Diagnosis and management. *American Family Physician*, 47(8), 1805–1816.

Rein, M.F., & Muller, M. (1989). Trichomonas vaginalis and trichomoniasis. In K.K. Holmes et al. (Eds.), *Sexually transmitted disease*, 2nd ed. (pp. 481–492). New York: McGraw-Hill.

Schaeffer, A.J. (1991). Vaginitis syndromes. *Seminars in Urology*, 4(1), 9–14.

Secor, M.C., & Fertilla, L. (1992). Vulvar vestibulitis syndrome. *Nurse Practitioner Forum*, 3(3), 161–168.

Sharp, H.C. (1993). Vulvovaginal conditions mimicking vaginitis. *Clinical Obstetrics and Gynecology*, 36(1), 129–136.

Shesser, R. (1991). Common vaginal infections: A concise workup guide. *The Female Patient*, 15, 53–60.

Sobel, J. D. (1990). Vaginitis in adult women. *Obstetrics and Gynecology Clinics of North America*, 17(4), 851–879.

Sparks, J.M. (1991). Vaginitis. *The Journal of Reproductive Medicine,* 36(10), 745–752.

Spiegel, C.A., Ansel, R., & Eschenback, D.A. (1980). Anaerobic bacteria in non-specific vaginitis. *New England Journal of Medicine*, 303, 409–415.

Stone, K.M., Grimes, D.A., & Madger, L.S. (1986). Personal protection against sexually disease. *American Journal of Obstetrics and Gynecology*, 150, 180–188.

Thomason, J.L., & Gelbert, S.M. (1989). Trichomonas vaginalis. *Obstetrics and Gynecology*, 74(3Pt2), 536–541.

— by Sarah B. Freeman, RN-C, PhD, FNP

Part Ten

Cancer of the Urinary Tract

Chapter 41

What You Need to Know about Bladder Cancer

The Bladder

The bladder is a hollow organ in the lower abdomen that stores urine. The kidneys filter waste from the blood and produce urine, which enters the bladder through two tubes called ureters. Urine leaves the bladder through another tube, the urethra. In women, the urethra is a short tube that opens just in front of the vagina. In men, it is longer, passing through the prostate gland and then through the penis.

What is Cancer?

Cancer is a group of diseases. More than 100 different types of cancer are known, and there are different types of bladder cancer. They all have one thing in common: abnormal cells grow and destroy body tissue.

Healthy cells that make up the body's tissues grow, divide, and replace themselves in an orderly way. This process keeps the body in good repair. Sometimes, however, some cells lose the ability to control their growth. They grow too rapidly and without any order. Too much tissue is made, and tumors begin to form. Tumors can be benign or malignant.

NIH Publication No. 93–1559.

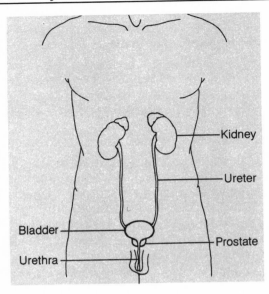

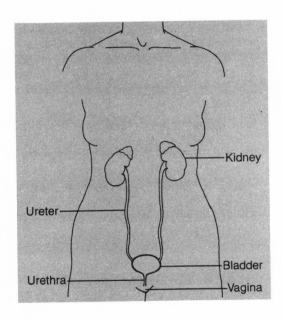

- Benign tumors are not cancer. They do not spread to other parts of the body and are seldom a threat to life. Often, benign tumors can be taken out by surgery, and they are not likely to return.

- Malignant tumors are cancer. They can invade and destroy nearby healthy tissues and organs. Cancer cells can also break away from the tumor and enter the bloodstream and lymphatic system. That is how cancer can spread to other parts of the body. This spread is called metastasis. Even if cancer is removed from the bladder, the disease sometimes returns, because cancer cells already may have spread.

Most bladder cancers develop in the inside lining of the bladder. The cancer often looks like a small mushroom attached to the bladder wall. It may also be called a papillary tumor. Often, more than one tumor is present.

Symptoms

The most common warning sign of bladder cancer is blood in the urine. Depending on the amount of blood present, the color of the urine can turn faintly rusty to deep red. Pain during urination can also be a sign of bladder cancer. A need to urinate often or urgently may be another warning sign. Often, bladder tumors cause no symptoms.

When symptoms do occur, they are not sure signs of cancer. They may also be caused by infections, benign tumors, bladder stones, or other problems. It is important to see a doctor to find out the cause of the symptoms. Any illness should be diagnosed and treated as early as possible.

Diagnosis

To diagnose bladder cancer, the doctor will take the patient's medical history and do a complete physical exam. Sometimes, the doctor can feel a large tumor during a rectal or vaginal exam. In addition, urine samples are checked under the microscope to see whether any cancer cells are present.

Often, the doctor wants the patient to have an x-ray called an intravenous pyelogram (IVP). This test lets the doctor see the kidneys, ureters, and bladder on an x-ray. An IVP normally causes little discomfort, although a few patients have nausea, dizziness, or pain from the procedure.

541

The doctor may also look directly into the bladder with an instrument called a cystoscope. In this test, a thin, lighted tube is inserted into the bladder through the urethra. If the doctor sees any abnormal areas, samples of tissue can be removed through the cystoscope. This is called a biopsy. A pathologist examines the tissue under a microscope to see whether cancer cells are present. A biopsy is needed to make a definite diagnosis of bladder cancer.

Treatment

Treatment for bladder cancer depends on a number of factors. Among these are how quickly the cancer is growing; the number, size, and location of the tumors; whether the cancer has spread to other organs; and the patient's age and general health. The doctor will develop a treatment plan to fit each patient's needs.

Staging

Before treatment begins, it is important for the doctor to know exactly where the cancer is located and whether it has spread from its original location. Staging procedures include a complete physical exam and additional blood tests and scans. The doctor may want the patient to have a CT (or CAT) scan. A CT scan is a series of x-rays put together by a computer to form a detailed picture. Ultrasound is a procedure that creates pictures of the inside of the body using high-frequency sound waves. The echoes make an image on a video screen that is much like a television. Sometimes the doctor asks for magnetic resonance imaging (MRI), in which a cross-sectional image (like a CT scan) is produced on a screen with the use of a powerful magnet instead of x-rays.

Planning Treatment

Decisions about treatment for bladder cancer are complex. Sometimes it is helpful to have more than one doctor's advice. Before starting treatment, the patient might want a second opinion about the diagnosis and treatment plan. It may take a week or two to arrange to see another doctor. This short delay will not make treatment less effective. There are a number of ways to find a doctor for a second opinion:

- The patient's doctor may be able to suggest a doctor who has a special interest in bladder cancer.

- The Cancer Information Service, at 1-800-4-CANCER, can tell callers about cancer centers and other NCI supported programs in their area.

- Patients can get the names of doctors from their local medical society, a nearby hospital, or a medical school.

Methods of Treatment

Early (superficial) bladder cancer (in which the tumors are found on the surface of the bladder wall) generally can be treated using the cystoscope in a procedure called transurethral resection (TUR). The cystoscope can remove all or part of a tumor or destroy it with an electric current.

When several tumors are present in the bladder or when there is a risk that the cancer will recur, TUR may be followed by treatment with drugs. The doctor may put a solution containing the bacillus Calmette-Guerin (BCG), a form of biological therapy, directly into the bladder. Chemotherapy (anticancer drugs) may also be put directly into the bladder.

Radiation therapy (also called radiotherapy) may be needed when the cancer cannot be removed with TUR because it involves a larger area of the bladder. X-rays destroy the ability of cancer cells to grow and divide. Internal radiation therapy, with the radioactive material placed in the bladder, may be combined with external radiation, which comes from a machine located outside the body.

For internal radiation therapy, radioactive material is inserted into the bladder through the cystoscope. This puts cancer-killing rays as close as possible to the site of the cancer while sparing most of the healthy tissues around it. The patient stays in the hospital for this treatment for 4 to 7 days.

For external radiation treatments, the patient goes to the hospital or clinic each day. Usually, treatments are given 5 days a week for 5 to 6 weeks. This schedule helps to protect normal tissue by spreading out the total dose of radiation.

When the cancer involves much of the surface of the bladder or has grown into the bladder wall, standard treatment is to remove the entire bladder. This surgery is called a radical cystectomy. In this operation, the surgeon removes the bladder as well as nearby organs. In women, this operation includes removing the uterus, fallopian tubes, ovaries, and part of the vagina. In men, the prostate and seminal vesicles are removed. Research is under way to find treatments that spare the bladder.

When cancer involves the pelvis or has spread to other parts of the body, the doctor may suggest chemotherapy, the use of anticancer drugs that travel through the bloodstream to reach cancer cells in all parts of the body. Drugs used to treat cancer may be given in different ways: some are given by mouth; others are injected into a muscle or a blood vessel. Chemotherapy is usually given in cycles—a treatment period, followed by a rest period, then another treatment period, and so on.

The patient usually receives chemotherapy as an outpatient at the hospital, at the doctor's office, or at home. Sometimes the patient may need to stay in the hospital for a short while.

Side Effects of Treatment

The methods used to treat bladder cancer are very powerful. It is hard to limit the effects of treatment so that only cancer cells are destroyed; healthy tissue may also be damaged. That's why treatment may cause unpleasant side effects. Side effects depend on the type of treatment used and on the part of the body being treated.

When the bladder is removed, the patient needs a new way to store and pass urine. Various methods are used. In one, the surgeon uses a piece of the person's small intestine to form a new pipeline. The ureters are attached to one end, and the other end is brought out through an opening in the wall of the abdomen. This new opening is called a stoma. (It is also called an ostomy or a urostomy.) A flat bag fits over the stoma to collect urine, and it is held in place with a special adhesive. A specially trained nurse or enterostomal therapist will show the patient how to care for the ostomy.

A newer method uses part of the small intestine to make a new storage pouch (called a continent reservoir) inside the body. The urine collects there and does not empty into a bag. Instead, the patient learns to use a tube (catheter) to drain the urine through a stoma. Other methods are being developed that connect a pouch made from the small intestine to a remaining part of the urethra. When this procedure is possible, a stoma and bag are not necessary because urine leaves the body through the urethra.

Radical cystectomy causes infertility in both men and women. This operation also can lead to sexual problems. In the past, nearly all men were impotent after this procedure, but improvements in surgery have made it possible to prevent this in many men. In women, the vagina may be narrower or shallower, and intercourse may be difficult.

During radiation therapy, patients may become very tired as the treatment continues. Resting as much as possible is important. Radiation treatment to the lower abdomen may cause nausea, vomiting, or diarrhea. Usually, the doctor can suggest certain foods or medications to ease these problems. Radiation therapy can also cause problems with fertility and can make sexual intercourse uncomfortable.

Chemotherapy causes side effects because it damages not only cancer cells but other rapidly growing cells as well. The side effects of chemotherapy depend on the specific drugs that are given. In addition, each patient reacts differently. Chemotherapy commonly affects blood-forming cells and cells that line the digestive tract. As a result, patients may have side effects such as lowered resistance to infection, loss of appetite, nausea and vomiting, less energy, and mouth sores. They may also lose their hair. These are short-term side effects that usually end after treatment stops. When drugs are put directly into the bladder, these side effects may be limited. However, it is common for the bladder to be irritated.

Loss of appetite can be a serious problem for patients during therapy. Patients who eat well may be better able to withstand the side effects of their treatment, so good nutrition is an important part of the treatment plan. Eating well means getting enough calories to prevent weight loss and having enough protein to build and repair muscles, organs, skin, and hair. Many patients find that eating several small meals and snacks during the day is easier than trying to eat three large meals.

The side effects that patients have during cancer treatment vary for each person. They may even be different from one treatment to the next. Doctors try to plan treatment to keep problems to a minimum. Fortunately, most side effects are temporary. Doctors, nurses, and dietitians can explain the side effects of cancer treatment and can suggest ways to deal with them. Helpful information about cancer treatment and coping with side effects is given in the NCI publications *Radiation Therapy and You, Chemotherapy and You, and Eating Hints*.

Followup Care

Regular followup exams are very important after treatment for bladder cancer. The doctor will need to check the bladder with a cystoscope and remove any superficial tumors that may have recurred. The doctor also checks for cancer cells in the urine and may suggest a chest x-ray, an IVP, or other tests.

The doctor will continue to watch the patient closely for several years, because bladder tumors can come back. If the cancer does recur, it is important for the doctor to detect it right away so additional treatment can be started.

Adjusting to the Disease

The diagnosis of bladder cancer can change the lives of cancer patients and the people who care about them. These changes in daily life can be difficult to handle. It's natural for patients and their families and friends to have many different and sometimes confusing emotions.

Patients and their loved ones may feel frightened, angry, or depressed. These are normal reactions that people have when diagnosed with a serious health problem. Others in the same situation have found that they cope with their emotions better if they can talk openly about their illness and their feelings with those who care about them.

Concerns about what the future may hold—as well as worries about tests, treatments, hospital stays, and medical bills—are common. Talking with doctors, nurses, or other members of the health care team may help to calm fears and ease confusion. Patients can take an active part in decisions about their medical care by asking questions about bladder cancer and their treatment choices. Patients, family, or friends often find it helpful to write down questions to ask the doctor as they think of them. Taking notes during visits to the doctor helps them remember what was said. Patients should ask the doctor to explain anything that is not clear.

Patients have many important questions, and the doctor is the best person to answer them. Most people ask about the extent of their cancer, how it can be treated, and how successful the treatment is likely to be. These are some other questions to ask the doctor:

- What are my treatment choices?
- What are the benefits of treatment?

- What are the risks and side effects of treatment?
- Will I need an ostomy?
- Will my sex life change?
- Will I need to change my normal activities? For how long?
- Can I keep working during treatment?
- How often will I need to have checkups ?

The doctor is the best person to give advice about treatment, working, or limiting daily activities. Patients may also wish to discuss concerns about the future, family relationships, and finances. They may find it helpful to speak with a nurse, social worker, counselor, or member of the clergy.

Sharing feelings with loved ones can help everyone feel more at ease, opening the way for others to show their concern and offer their support. Many patients feel that it helps to talk with others who are facing problems like theirs. Patients can meet other cancer patients through self-help and support groups such as those described in the next section.

Living with any serious disease can be difficult and challenging. The public library is a good source of books and articles on living with cancer. Cancer patients and their families can also find helpful suggestions in the NCI booklet called *Taking Time*.

Support for Bladder Cancer Patients

Learning to live with the changes brought about by having cancer is easier for patients and those who care about them when they have helpful information and support services. Often, the social worker at the hospital or clinic can suggest local and national groups that will help with emotional support, financial aid, transportation, home care, and rehabilitation.

If a patient has problems with a urostomy, the doctor, nurse, or enterostomal therapist can help. Also, adjusting to a stoma can be a lot easier with the advice and support of someone who has had the same problem. Many people have had bladder surgery, and several organizations offer assistance.

The Ostomy Rehabilitation Program of the American Cancer Society (ACS) and the United Ostomy Association (UOA) offer both emotional support and educational material. Information is available from local chapters (listed in the telephone book) or from the ACS and UOA national offices.

Information about other resources and services is available through the Cancer Information Service at 1-800-4-CANCER.

What the Future Holds

Each year, more than 50,000 people in the United States find out they have bladder cancer. The outlook for patients with early bladder cancer is very good. The chances of recovery from more advanced bladder cancer are improving as researchers continue to look for better ways to treat this disease.

Doctors often talk about "surviving" cancer, or they may use the word "remission" rather than "cure." Even though many bladder cancer patients recover completely, doctors use these terms because bladder cancer can recur. It is normal for patients to be concerned about their future. Sometimes they use statistics they have heard to try to figure out their chance of being cured. It is important to remember, however, that statistics are averages. They are based on the experiences of large numbers of patients, and no two cancer patients are alike. Only the doctor who takes care of the patient knows enough about his or her case to discuss the patient's chance of recovery (prognosis).

The Promise of Cancer Research

Bladder cancer is a fairly common form of cancer in the United States. Whites get bladder cancer twice as often as blacks, and men are affected two to three times as often as women. Most bladder cancers occur after the age of 55, but the disease can also develop in younger people. Scientists at hospitals and medical centers all across the country are studying bladder cancer. They are trying to learn what causes the disease and how to prevent it. They are also looking for better ways to diagnose and treat it.

Cause and Prevention

While doctors can seldom explain why one person gets bladder cancer and another doesn't, we do know that the disease is not contagious; no one can "catch" bladder cancer from another person. Scientists do not know exactly what causes this disease, but research does show that some people are more likely to develop it than others. A number of factors contribute to this higher risk.

Smoking is a major risk factor. Cigarette smokers develop bladder cancer two to three times more often than do non-smokers. Quitting smoking reduces the risk of bladder cancer, lung cancer, several other types of cancer, and a number of other diseases as well.

Workers in some occupations are at higher risk of getting bladder cancer because of exposure to carcinogens (cancer-causing substances) in the workplace. These workers include people in the rubber, chemical, and leather industries, as well as hairdressers, machinists, metal workers, printers, painters, textile workers, and truck drivers.

Treatment

The NCI is supporting many studies of new treatments for bladder cancer. When laboratory research shows that a new treatment method has promise, it is used to treat cancer patients in clinical trials. These trials are designed to answer scientific questions and to find out if a new treatment is both safe and effective. Patients who take part in clinical trials make an important contribution to medical science and may have the first chance to benefit from improved treatment methods. A person with bladder cancer who is interested in taking part in a trial should discuss this possibility with his or her doctor. (*What Are Clinical Trials All About?* is an NCI publication about treatment studies.)

One way to learn about clinical trials is through PDQ, a computerized resource of cancer treatment information. Developed by NCI, PDQ contains an up-to-date list of trials all over the country. Doctors can obtain an access code and use a personal computer to get PDQ information, or they can use the services of a medical library. Also, the Cancer Information Service, at 1-800-4-CANCER, can provide PDQ information to doctors, patients, and the public.

Medical Terms

Anesthetic (an-es-THET-ik): A drug or gas given to produce a loss of feeling.

Benign (bee-NINE): Not cancerous.

549

Biological therapy: Treatment that uses natural or laboratory-made substances that can stimulate or restore the body's immune system to fight disease more effectively. Also called immunotherapy.

Biopsy (BY-op-see): The removal of a sample of tissue to see whether cancer cells are present.

Cancer: A term for more than 100 diseases that have uncontrolled, abnormal growth of cells. Cancer cells can spread through the bloodstream and lymphatic system to other parts of the body.

CAT or CT scan: An x-ray procedure that uses a computer to produce a detailed picture of a cross-section of the body.

Catheter (KATH-a-ter): A flexible tube used to withdraw fluids from the body (or inject fluids into the body).

Chemotherapy (kee-mo-THER-a-pee): Treatment with anticancer drugs.

Clinical trial: A study of a new treatment. Each study is designed to answer scientific questions and to find better ways to treat patients.

Cystectomy (sis-TEK-to-mee): Surgery to remove the bladder.

Cystoscope (SIS-to-skope): An instrument that allows the doctor to see inside the bladder and remove tissue samples or small tumors.

Enterostomal therapist (en-ter-o-STO-mal): A health professional trained in the care of urostomies and other stomas.

Fallopian tube (fa-LOW-pee-an): A tube through which the egg from the ovary reaches the uterus.

Infertility: The inability to have children.

Impotent: Unable to have an erection.

Intravenous pyelogram (in-tra-VEE-nus PIE-uh-lo-gram): An x-ray study of the urinary system. Also called IVP.

Lymph (limf): The almost colorless fluid that bathes body tissues and contains cells that help fight infection.

Lymph nodes: Small, bean-shaped organs located along the lymphatic system. Nodes filter bacteria or cancer cells that may travel through the lymphatic system. Also called lymph glands.

Lymphatic system (lim-FAT-ik): The tissues and organs (including the bone marrow, spleen, thymus, and lymph nodes) that produce and store cells that fight infection, and the channels that carry lymph.

Magnetic resonance imaging (mag-NET-ik REZ-o-nans IM-a-jing): A procedure in which a magnet linked to a computer is used to create detailed pictures of areas inside the body. Also called MRI.

Malignant (ma-LIG-nant): Cancerous (see Cancer).

Metastasis (me-TAS-ta-sis): The spread of cancer from one part of the body to another. Cells in the metastatic tumor (the second tumor) are like those in the original tumor.

Oncologist (on-KOL-o-jist): A doctor who specializes in treating cancer.

Ovaries (O-var-eez): Two small, round organs on each side of the uterus that produce eggs and female sex hormones.

Papillary tumor (PAP-I-lar-ee): A tumor shaped like a small mushroom with its stem attached to the inner lining of the bladder.

Pathologist (path-OL-o-jist): A doctor who identifies diseases by studying cells and tissues removed from the body.

Pelvis: The area between the hips.

Prognosis (prog-NO-sis): The probable outcome of a disease; the prospect of recovery.

Prostate gland (PROS-tate): A gland in the male reproductive system just below the bladder. It surrounds part of the urethra, the canal that empties the bladder.

Radiation therapy (ray-dee-AY-shun THER-a-pee): Treatment with high energy rays from x-rays or other sources of radiation.

Radical cystectomy (RAD-I-kal sis-TEN-to-mee): Surgery to remove the bladder as well as nearby tissues and organs.

Seminal vesicles (SEM-in-al VES-ikulz): Glands that help produce semen.

Small intestine: The part of the digestive tract that extends from the stomach to the large intestine.

Staging: The process of learning whether cancer has spread from its original site to another part of the body.

Stoma: An opening in the abdominal wall; also called an ostomy or urostomy.

Surgery: An operation.

Transurethral resection (TRANZ-yuREE-thral ree-SEK-shun): Surgery performed with a special instrument inserted through the urethra. Also called TUR.

Tumor: An abnormal mass of tissue.

Ultrasound: A test that bounces sound waves off tissues and internal organs and changes the echoes into pictures (sonograms). Tissues of different densities reflect sound waves differently.

Ureter (yur-EE-ter): The tube that carries urine from each kidney to the bladder.

Urethra (yur-EE-thra): The tube that empties urine from the bladder.

Urine: (YUR-in): Liquid waste.

Urologist (yur-OL-o-jist): A doctor who specializes in diseases of the urinary organs in females and the urinary and sex organs in males.

Uterus (YOO-ter-us): The organ that holds a baby before birth. Also called the womb.

Resources

Information about cancer is available from many sources, including the ones listed below. You may wish to check for additional information at your local library or book store or from support groups in your community.

Cancer Information Services (CIS)

The Cancer Information Service, a program of the National Cancer Institute, provides a nationwide telephone service for cancer patients and their families and friends, the public, and health professionals. The staff can answer questions and can send booklets about cancer. They also know about local resources and services. One toll-free number, 1-800-4-CANCER (1-800-422-6237), connects callers all over the country to the office that serves their area. Spanish-speaking staff members are available.

American Cancer Society (ACS)

The American Cancer Society is a voluntary organization with a national office (1599 Clifton Road, NE, Atlanta, GA 30329) and local units all over the country. It supports research, conducts educational programs, and offers many services to patients and their families. It provides free booklets on cancer and on sexuality. To obtain booklets or to learn about services and activities in local areas, call the Society' s toll-free number, 1-800-ACS-2345 (1-800-227-2345), or the number listed under American Cancer Society in the white pages of the telephone book.

United Ostomy Association (UOA)

The United Ostomy Association is another organization with chapters in many cities. It offers a number of booklets for people with ostomies. In addition, volunteers will visit a patient to offer support and encouragement. The national office at 36 Executive Park, Irvine, CA 92714, phone 1-714-660-8624, can provide the address of the nearest chapter.

For Further Information

Cancer patients, their families and friends, and others may find the following booklets useful. They are available free of charge by calling 1-800-4-CANCER or writing:

Office of Cancer Communications
National Cancer Institute
Building 31, Room 10A24
Bethesda, MD 20892

Booklets About Cancer Treatment

- *Radiation Therapy and You: A Guide to Self-Help During Treatment*
- *Chemotherapy and You: A Guide to Self-Help During Treatment*
- *Eating Hints: Recipes and Tips for Better Nutrition During Cancer Treatment*
- *Questions and Answers About Pain Control (also available from the American Cancer Society)*
- *What Are Clinical Trials All About?*

Booklets About Living With Cancer

- *Taking Time: Support for People With Cancer and the People Who Care About Them*
- *Facing Forward: A Guide for Cancer Survivors*
- *When Cancer Recurs: Meeting the Challenge Again*
- *Advanced Cancer: Living Each Day*

Chapter 42

Urethral Cancer

What Is Cancer of the Urethra?

Cancer of the urethra, a rare type of cancer, is a disease in which cancer (malignant) cells are found in the urethra. The urethra is the tube that empties urine from your bladder, the hollow organ in the lower abdomen that stores urine. In women, the urethra is about 1 ½ inches long and opens to the outside of the body above the vagina. In men, the urethra is about 8 inches long and goes through the prostate gland and then through the penis to the outside of the body. Cancer of the urethra affects women more often then men.

Like most cancers, cancer of the urethra is best treated when it is found (diagnosed) early. There may be no symptoms of early cancer of the urethra. You should see your doctor if you have a lump or growth on your urethra, pain or bleeding when you urinate, or difficulty urinating.

If you have symptoms, your doctor will examine you and feel for lumps in the urethra. In men, a thin lighted tube called a cystoscope may be inserted into the penis so your doctor can see inside the urethra. If your doctor finds cells or other signs that are not normal, a small piece of tissue (called a biopsy) may be cut out and looked at under a microscope for cancer cells.

Your chance of recovery (prognosis) and choice of treatment depend on the stage of your cancer (whether it is just in one area or has spread to other places) and your general state of health.

National Cancer Institute, CancerNet online information service.

Stages of Cancer of the Urethra

Once cancer of the urethra is found, more tests will be done to find out if cancer cells have spread to other parts of the body (staging). Your doctor needs to know the stage of your disease to plan treatment. For cancer of the urethra, patients are grouped into stages depending on where the tumor is and whether it has spread to other places. The following stage groupings are used for cancer of the urethra:

Anterior Urethral Cancer

The part of the urethra that is closest to the outside of your body is called the anterior urethra, and cancers that start here are called anterior urethral cancers.

Posterior Urethral Cancer

The part of the urethra that connects to your bladder is called the posterior urethra, and cancers that start here are called posterior urethral cancers.

Because the posterior urethra is closer to the bladder and other tissues, cancers that start here are more likely to grow through the inner lining of the urethra and affect nearby tissues.

Urethral Cancer Associated with Invasive Bladder Cancer

Occasionally, patients who have bladder cancer also have cancer of the urethra. This is called urethral cancer associated with invasive bladder cancer.

Recurrent Urethral Cancer

Recurrent cancer means that the cancer has come back (recurred) after it has been treated. It may come back in the same place, or in another part of the body.

How Cancer of the Urethra Is Treated

There are treatments for all patients with cancer of the urethra. Three kinds of treatment are used:

- surgery (taking out the cancer in an operation)
- radiation therapy (using high-dose x-rays or other high-energy rays to kill cancer cells)
- chemotherapy (using drugs to kill cancer cells).

Surgery is the most common treatment for cancer of the urethra. Your doctor may take out the cancer using one of the following operations:

- Electrofulguration uses an electric current to remove the cancer. The tumor and the area around it are burned away and then removed with a sharp tool.
- Laser therapy uses a narrow beam of intense light to kill cancer cells.
- Cystourethrectomy removes the bladder and the urethra.

In men, the part of the penis containing the urethra that has cancer may be removed in an operation called a partial penectomy. Sometimes the entire penis is removed (penectomy). You may need plastic surgery to make a new penis if all or part of the penis is removed. The bladder and prostate may also be removed in an operation called cystoprostatectomy. Lymph nodes in the pelvis may also be removed (lymph node dissection). Lymph nodes are small bean-shaped structures that are found throughout the body. They produce and store infection-fighting cells.

In women, surgery to remove the urethra, the bladder, and the vagina (anterior exenteration) may also be done. Lymph nodes in the pelvis may be removed (lymph node dissection). Plastic surgery may be needed to make a new vagina after this operation.

If the urethra is removed, your doctor will need to make a new way for the urine to pass from your body. This is called urinary diversion.

If your bladder is removed, your doctor will need to make a new way for you to store and pass urine. There are several ways to do this. Sometimes your doctor will use part of the small intestine to make a tube through which urine can pass out of the body through an opening (stoma) on the outside of the body. This is sometimes called an ostomy or urostomy. If you have an ostomy, you will need to wear a special bag to collect urine. This special bag, which sticks to the skin around the stoma with a special glue, can be thrown away after it is used. This bag does not show under clothing, and most people take care of these bags themselves. Your doctor may also use part of your small intestine to make a new storage pouch (a continent reservoir) inside the body where the urine can collect. You would then need to use a tube (catheter) to drain the urine through a stoma.

Radiation therapy uses x-rays or other high-energy rays to kill cancer cells and shrink tumors. Radiation may come from a machine outside the body (external radiation therapy) or from putting materials that produce radiation (radioisotopes) through thin plastic tubes (internal radiation therapy) in the area where cancer cells are found. Radiation may be used alone or with surgery and/or chemotherapy.

Chemotherapy uses drugs to kill cancer cells. Chemotherapy may be taken by mouth, or it may be put in the body through a needle in a vein or muscle. Chemotherapy is called a systemic treatment because the drug enters the bloodstream, travels through the body and can kill cancer cells outside the urethra.

Treatment by Stage

Your treatment depends on where the cancer is found, whether it has spread to other areas in the body, your sex, your age and your overall health.

You may receive treatment that is considered standard based on its effectiveness in a number of patients in past studies, or you may choose to go into a clinical trial. Not all patients are cured with standard therapy and some standard treatments may have more side effects than are desired. For these reasons, clinical trials are designed to find better ways to treat cancer patients and are based on the most up-to-date information. Clinical trials are going on in many parts of the country for patients with cancer of the urethra.

If you want more information, call the Cancer Information Service at 1-800-4-CANCER (1-800-422-6237).

Anterior Urethral Cancer

Treatment is different for men and women. If you are a woman, your treatment may be one of the following:

1. Electrofulguration.
2. Laser therapy.
3. External and/or internal radiation therapy.
4. Radiation therapy followed by surgery or surgery alone to remove the urethra and the organs in the lower pelvis (anterior

exenteration), or the tumor only, if it is small. A new way is made for urine to pass out of the body (urinary diversion).

If you are a man, your treatment may be one of the following:

1. Electrofulguration.
2. Laser therapy.
3. Surgery to remove a part of the penis (partial penectomy).
4. Radiation therapy.

Posterior Urethral Cancer

Treatment is different for men and women. If you are a woman, your treatment will probably be radiation therapy followed by surgery or surgery alone to remove the urethra, the organs in the lower pelvis (anterior exenteration), or the tumor only, if it is small. Lymph nodes in the pelvis are usually removed (lymph node dissection), and lymph nodes in the upper thigh may or may not be removed. A new way is made for urine to pass out of the body (urinary diversion).

If you are a man, you will probably have radiation therapy followed by surgery or surgery alone to remove the bladder and prostate (cystoprostatectomy) and the penis and urethra (penectomy). Lymph nodes in the pelvis are usually removed (lymph node dissection), and lymph nodes in the upper thigh may or may not be removed. A new way is made for urine to pass out of the body (urinary diversion).

Urethral Cancer Associated with Invasive Bladder Cancer

Because people with bladder cancer sometimes also have cancer of the urethra, the urethra may be removed at the same time the bladder is taken out (cystourethrectomy). If the urethra is not removed when you have surgery for bladder cancer, your doctor may follow you closely so you can be treated if you develop cancer of the urethra.

Recurrent Urethral Cancer

Your treatment depends on what treatment you received before. If you had surgery, you may have radiation therapy and surgery to remove the cancer. If you had radiation therapy, you may have surgery to remove the cancer. Clinical trials are testing chemotherapy for cancer of the urethra that has spread to other parts of the body.

To Learn More

To learn more about cancer of the urethra, call the National Cancer Institute's Cancer Information Service at 1-800-4-CANCER (1-800-422-6237). By dialing this toll-free number, you can speak with someone who can answer your questions.

The Cancer Information Service can also send you free booklets. The following general booklets on questions related to cancer may be helpful:

— What You Need to Know About Cancer
— Taking Time: Support for People with Cancer and the People Who Care About Them
— What Are Clinical Trials All About?
— Chemotherapy and You: A Guide to Self-Help During Treatment
— Radiation Therapy and You: A Guide to Self-Help During Treatment
— Eating Hints for Cancer Patients
— Advanced Cancer: Living Each Day
— When Cancer Recurs: Meeting the Challenge Again

There are many other places you can get information about cancer treatment and services to help you. You can check the social service office at your hospital for local and national agencies that help with your finances, getting to and from treatment, care at home, and dealing with your problems. The American Cancer Society and the United Ostomy Association, for example, have many free services. Their local offices are listed in the white pages of the telephone book.

You can also write to the National Cancer Institute at this address:

National Cancer Institute
Building 31, Room 10A24
9000 Rockville Pike
Bethesda, MD 20892

What is PDQ?

PDQ is a computer system that gives up-to-date information on cancer treatment. It is a service of the National Cancer Institute (NCI) for people with cancer and their families, and for doctors, nurses, and other health care professionals.

PDQ tells about the current treatments for most cancers. The information in PDQ is reviewed each month by cancer experts. It is updated when there is new information. The patient information in PDQ also tells about warning signs and how the cancer is found. PDQ also lists information about research on new treatments (clinical trials), doctors who treat cancer, and hospitals with cancer programs. The treatment information in this summary is based on information in the PDQ treatment summary for health professionals on this cancer.

How to Use PDQ

You can use PDQ to learn more about current treatment for your kind of cancer. Bring this material from PDQ with you when you see your doctor. You can talk with your doctor, who knows you and has the facts about your disease, about which treatment would be best for you. Before you start your treatment, you might also want to seek a second opinion from a doctor who treats cancer.

Before you start treatment, you also may want to think about taking part in a clinical trial. A clinical trial is a study that uses new treatments to care for patients. Each study is based on past studies and what has been learned in the laboratory. Each trial answers certain scientific questions in order to find new and better ways to help cancer patients. During clinical trials, more and more information is collected about new treatments, their risks, and how well they do or do not work. If clinical trials show that the new treatment is better than the treatment currently being used, the new treatment may become the "standard" treatment. Listings of clinical trials are a part of PDQ. Many cancer doctors who take part in clinical trials are listed in PDQ.

If you want to know more about cancer and how it is treated, or if you wish to learn about clinical trials for your kind of cancer, you can call the National Cancer Institute's Cancer Information Service. The number is 1-800-4-CANCER (1-800-422-6237). The call is free and a trained information specialist will talk with you and answer your questions.

PDQ may change when there is new information. Check with the Cancer Information Service to be sure that you have the most up-to-date information.

561

Chapter 43

Resources on Urothelial Tract Cancer

Legend

TI   Title
AU   Authors
SO   Source
AD   Address

Citations

TI   *Survival of Patients with Upper Urothelial Tumor*
AU   Salinas Sanchez AS; Hernandez Millan IR; Segura Marti M;
      Martinez Martin M; Ruiz Mondejar R; Pastor Guzman JM;
      Virseda Rodriguez
SO   Arch Esp Urol 1995;48(7):688–700
AD   Servicio de Urologia, Hospital General de Albacete, Espana.

TI   *Metachronous Metastasis in Ureteral Stump Secondary to Ipsilateral Renal Adenocarcinoma*
AU   Pereira Arias JG; Aurtenetxe Goiriena JJ; Prieto Ugidos N;
      Zabalza Estevez I; Marana Fernandez M; Bernuy Malfaz C
SO   Arch Esp Urol 1995;48(7):746–8
AD   Servicio de Urologia, Hospital de Galdacano, Vizcaya, Espana.

NCI/PDQ, CancerLit Search, January 1996.

TI *Transitional Cell Carcinoma of the Ureter and Cyclophosphamide: Apropos of a Case*
AU Ponsot Y; Guerin JG; Carmel M
SO Prog Urol 1995;5(4):578–9
AD Service d'Urologie, Centre Hospitalier Universitaire de Sherbrooke, Quebec, Canada.

TI *P53 and Human Papillomavirus DNA in Renal Pelvic and Ureteral Carcinoma Including Dysplastic Lesions*
AU Furihata M; Yamasaki I; Ohtsuki Y; Sonobe H; Morioka M; Yamamoto A; Terao N; Kuwahara M; Fujisaki N
SO Int J Cancer 1995;64(5):298–303
AD Department of Pathology II, Kochi Medical School, Japan.

TI *Benign Neoplasms of the Urethra in Women*
AU Uzunova I
SO Khirurgiia (Sofiia) 1994;47(5):29–30

TI *Clinical Investigation of Renal Pelvic and Ureteral Cancer with Special Reference to Adjuvant Chemotherapy*
AU Shinohara M; Okazawa A; Suzuki M; Itakura H; Munakata A; Kinoshita K
SO Nippon Hinyokika Gakkai Zasshi 1995;86(8):1375–82
AD Department of Urology, Tokyo Metropolitane Komagome General Hospital.

TI *A Clinical Study of Associated Bladder Tumor in Patients with Renal Pelvic and Ureteral Tumor*
AU Sugano O; Shouji N; Horigome T; Uchi K; Katou H
SO Nippon Hinyokika Gakkai Zasshi 1995;86(8):1383–7
AD Department of Urology, Yamagata Prefectural Central Hospital.

TI *Squamous Cell Carcinoma of the Ureter as a Late Complication of Ureterocutaneostomy—a Case Report*
AU Sekine S; Sakurai S; Ito M
SO Nippon Hinyokika Gakkai Zasshi 1995;86(8):1402–5
AD Department of Urology, Niigata Prefectural Yoshida Hospital.

Index

Index

567